Decoding Polycystic Ovarian Syndrome (PCOS)

Decoding Polycystic Ovarian Syndrome (PCOS)

Editors

Kanthi Bansal MD DGO FICOG
Director
Safal Fertility Foundation and Bansal Hospital
Ahmedabad, Gujarat, India
E-mail: kanthibansal@gmail.com
Website: www.safalivf.com

Pooja Sharma Dimri MD DNB FMIS
Consultant Gynecologist
Obstetrician and Gynec–Laparoscopic Surgeon
Bellevue, Cloudnine, and Mahavir Hospitals
Mumbai, Maharashtra, India

Apoorva Pallam Reddy MS DNB (OBG)
Consultant
Department of Endoscopy and Fertility
Mathrutva Fertility Center
Bengaluru, Karnataka, India

Foreword
Sadhana K Desai

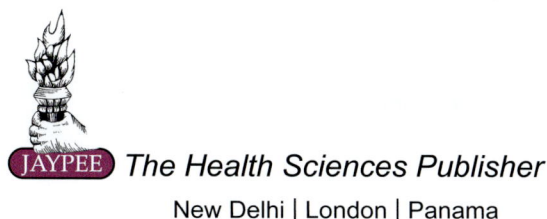

JAYPEE The Health Sciences Publisher
New Delhi | London | Panama

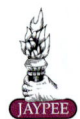 **Jaypee Brothers Medical Publishers (P) Ltd.**

Headquarters
Jaypee Brothers Medical Publishers (P) Ltd.
4838/24, Ansari Road, Daryaganj
New Delhi 110 002, India
Phone: +91-11-43574357
Fax: +91-11-43574314
E-mail: jaypee@jaypeebrothers.com

Overseas Offices

J.P. Medical Ltd.
83, Victoria Street, London
SW1H 0HW (UK)
Phone: +44 20 3170 8910
Fax: +44(0) 20 3008 6180
E-mail: info@jpmedpub.com

Jaypee Highlights Medical Publishers Inc.
City of Knowledge, Building 235, 2nd Floor
Clayton, Panama City, Panama
Phone: +1 507-301-0496
Fax: +1 507-301-0499
E-mail: cservice@jphmedical.com

Jaypee Brothers Medical Publishers (P) Ltd.
17/1-B, Babar Road, Block-B, Shaymali
Mohammadpur, Dhaka-1207
Bangladesh
Mobile: +08801912003485
E-mail: jaypeedhaka@gmail.com

Jaypee Brothers Medical Publishers (P) Ltd.
Bhotahity, Kathmandu, Nepal
Phone: +977-9741283608
E-mail: kathmandu@jaypeebrothers.com

Website: www.jaypeebrothers.com
Website: www.jaypeedigital.com

© 2017, Jaypee Brothers Medical Publishers

The views and opinions expressed in this book are solely those of the original contributor(s)/author(s) and do not necessarily represent those of editor(s) of the book.

All rights reserved. No part of this publication may be reproduced, stored or transmitted in any form or by any means, electronic, mechanical, photocopying, recording or otherwise, without the prior permission in writing of the publishers.

All brand names and product names used in this book are trade names, service marks, trademarks or registered trademarks of their respective owners. The publisher is not associated with any product or vendor mentioned in this book.

Medical knowledge and practice change constantly. This book is designed to provide accurate, authoritative information about the subject matter in question. However, readers are advised to check the most current information available on procedures included and check information from the manufacturer of each product to be administered, to verify the recommended dose, formula, method and duration of administration, adverse effects and contraindications. It is the responsibility of the practitioner to take all appropriate safety precautions. Neither the publisher nor the author(s)/editor(s) assume any liability for any injury and/or damage to persons or property arising from or related to use of material in this book.

This book is sold on the understanding that the publisher is not engaged in providing professional medical services. If such advice or services are required, the services of a competent medical professional should be sought.

Every effort has been made where necessary to contact holders of copyright to obtain permission to reproduce copyright material. If any have been inadvertently overlooked, the publisher will be pleased to make the necessary arrangements at the first opportunity.

Inquiries for bulk sales may be solicited at: jaypee@jaypeebrothers.com

Decoding Polycystic Ovarian Syndrome (PCOS)

First Edition: **2017**

ISBN: 978-93-86322-85-2

Printed at: Samrat Offset Pvt. Ltd.

Dedicated to

*Polycystic Ovarian Syndrome (PCOS)
Patients*

Contributors

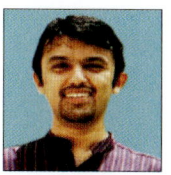

Aditya Khurd
Director
Dr Khurd's Infertility, ICSI and IVF Centre
Pune, Maharashtra, India

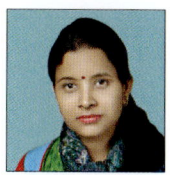

Anu Agarwal
Director
Vansh Fertility and Test Tube Baby Center
Varanasi, Uttar Pradesh, India

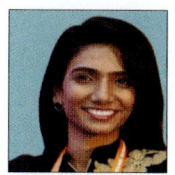

Apoorva Pallam Reddy
Consultant
Department of Endoscopy and Fertility
Mathrutva Fertility Center
Bengaluru, Karnataka, India

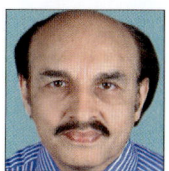

AK Pancholia
Head
Department of Medicine
Arihant Hospital and Research Centre
Indore, Madhya Pradesh, India

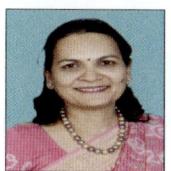

Asha Baxi
Director
Disha Fertility and Surgical Center
Indore, Madhya Pradesh, India

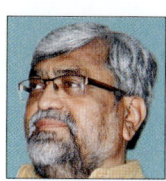

CB Nagori
Director
Dr Nagori's Institute for Infertility and IVF
Ahmedabad, Gujarat, India

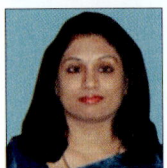

Chandana A
Consultant Gynec–Endoscopic Surgeon
Chandana Health Care Clinic
Bengaluru, Karnataka, India

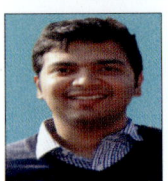

Dhaval Baxi
Associate Gynecologist
Disha Fertility and Surgical Center
Indore, Madhya Pradesh, India

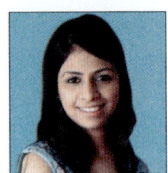

Dolly Sandhu Gill
Embryologist
Canada

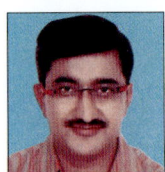

Hitesh J Bhatt
Medicolegal Consultant
Mumbai, Maharashtra, India

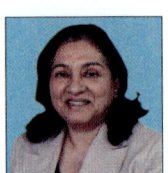

Jaideep Malhotra
Managing Director
Rainbow IVF
Agra, Uttar Pradesh, India

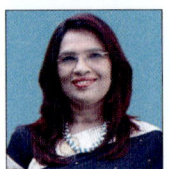

Kanthi Bansal
Director
Safal Fertility Foundation and Bansal Hospital
Ahmedabad, Gujarat, India

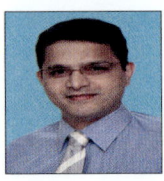

Kedar Ganla
Consultant Fertility Physician
Ankoor Fertility Clinic
Mumbai, Maharashtra, India

Contributors

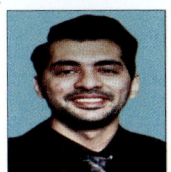

Keshav Malhotra
Director, Rainbow IVF
Malhotra Nursing Home
Agra, Uttar Pradesh, India

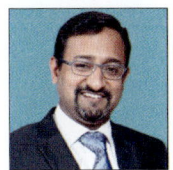

Kundan Vasant Ingale
Consultant and Director
Nirmiti Clinic
Centre for Assisted Reproduction and Endoscopy
Pune, Maharashtra, India

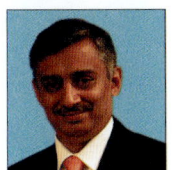

Manish Banker
Director
Nova IVI Fertility
Ahmedabad, Gujarat, India

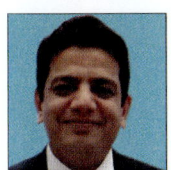

Milind R Shah
Professor and Head
Department of Obstetrics and Gynecology
Gandhi Natha H Medical College
Mumbai, Maharashtra, India

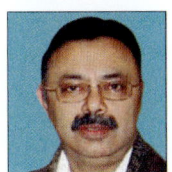

Narendra Malhotra
Managing Director
Global Rainbow Healthcare
Agra, Uttar Pradesh, India

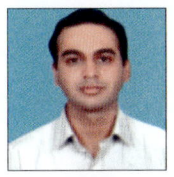

Nirmal N Gujarathi
Clinical Associate and Coordinator
Nanavati Super Speciality Hospital
Mumbai, Maharashtra, India

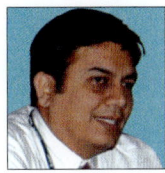

Parul Kotdawala
Endoscopy Surgeon
Department of Obstetrics and Gynecology
VS Hospital and NHL Municipal Medical College
Ahmedabad, Gujarat, India

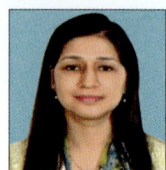

Pooja Sharma Dimri
Consultant Gynecologist,
Obstetrician and Gynec–Laparoscopic Surgeon
Bellevue, Cloudnine, and Mahavir Hospitals
Mumbai, Maharashtra, India

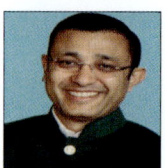

Rajeev Agarwal
Director
Care IVF
Kolkata, West Bengal, India

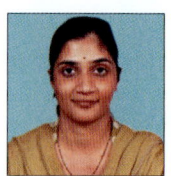

Reena Gupta
Nova IVI
Ahmedabad, Gujarat, India

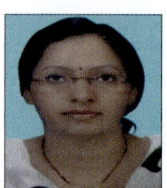

Ritu Bijarnia
Consultant
Radhakrishna Multispeciality Hospital
IVF Centre
Bengaluru, Karnataka, India

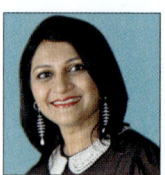

Rupal N Shah
Medical Director
Rupal Hospital for Women
Women's Health Centre of Excellence
Surat, Gujarat, India

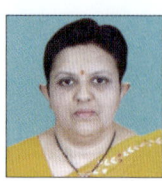

Sadhana Khurd
Director
Dr Khurd's Infertility, ICSI and IVF Centre
Pune, Maharashtra, India

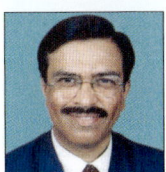
Sanjeev Khurd
Director
Dr Khurd's Infertility, ICSI and IVF Centre
Pune, Maharashtra, India

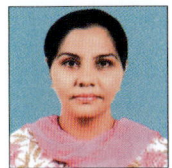
Shalini Gainder
Associate Professor
Department of Obstetrics and Gynecology
Postgraduate Institute of Medical Education and Research
Chandigarh, India

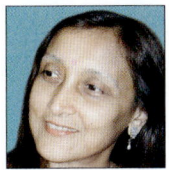
Sonal Panchal
Director
Dr Nagori's Institute for Infertility and IVF
Ahmedabad, Gujarat, India

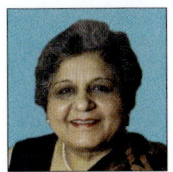
Sonia Malik
Director and Head
Southend Fertility and IVF
New Delhi, India

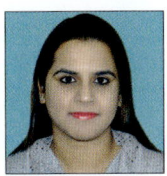
Suyesha Khanijao
Jr Consultant
Southend Fertility and IVF
New Delhi, India

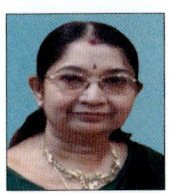
T Ramani Devi
Consultant
Obstetrics, Gynecology and Infertility
Tiruchirappalli, Tamil Nadu, India

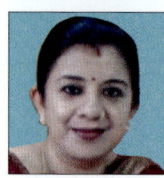

Vidhya V Bhat
Director
Radhakrishna Multispeciality Hospital
IVF Centre
Bengaluru, Karnataka, India

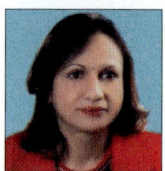

Vidya Pancholia
Head
Department of Obstetrics and Gynecology
Arihant Hospital and Research Centre
Indore, Madhya Pradesh, India

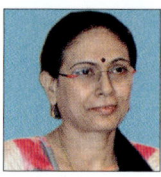

Yasodhara Pallam Reddy
Consultant
Sri Durga Hospital
Nellore, Andhra Pradesh, India

Foreword

It is an honor to pen a Foreword for the book of great clinical utility, titled *Decoding Polycystic Ovarian Syndrome,* edited by an eminent assisted reproductive technology and infertility specialist Dr Kanthi Bansal, and co-edited by Dr Pooja Sharma Dimri and Dr Apoorva Pallam Reddy.

In an age, when conventional diagnostic aids and therapeutic treatments are being challenged and replaced by newer innovations, the gynecologists, particularly infertility specialists must know all the recent advances with their advantages and pitfalls in managing women with polycystic ovarian syndrome (PCOS).

The PCOS is a condition where gynecologists have debated on its definition, diagnosis and management every few years. In-depth knowledge of pathophysiology of the PCOS and update in management of it is necessary for postgraduates as well as practicing gynecologists.

The chapters in this book cover, in detail, various problems and their management that PCOS women come across. I am sure that this book will find its place as a ready reckoner in the library of medical colleges, gynec-endocrinologists and infertility specialists. The experts have worked hard to address various issues related to PCOS.

I congratulate Dr Kanthi Bansal and her team for bringing out this book!

Sadhana K Desai MD FRCOG (Eng) FICOG
Emeritus Professor
Department of Obstetrics and Gynecology
Bombay Hospital Institute of Medical Sciences
Founder Director
Fertility Clinic and IVF Centre
Mumbai, Maharashtra, India

Message

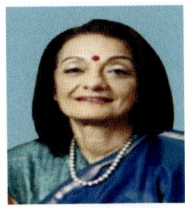

Polycystic ovarian syndrome (PCOS) is a silent disorder that creates havoc on young bodies, and is one of the most critical, underserved, underdiagnosed and underfunded conditions affecting the women's health. There is a huge health disparity when it comes to PCOS diagnosis, funding and support, as 50% of women and girls with PCOS are undiagnosed. Additionally, it often takes the women several years and, on an average, they see almost seven doctors before they can find someone who can help them with the condition.

Despite being one of the most common women's disorders with serious long-term health consequences, the PCOS awareness and support organizations receive less amount from the government, corporate, or community funding than any other health condition receives.

Our vision is that the PCOS be treated as a public health priority and hence we created the PCOS Society of India, which is a multidisciplinary organization of gynecologists, endocrinologists, dermatologists and other associated specialists, who attend to PCOS women. I am delighted that Dr Kanthi Bansal, who is one of the patrons of the PCOS Society, is editing this book. This book will help to update the knowledge on PCOS amongst the medical community.

I wish her and her team all the best and congratulate her on this stupendous creation!

Duru Shah
MD FRCOG FCPS FICS FICOG DGO FICMCH DFP
Director
Gynaecworld
Center for Assisted Reproduction and Women's Health
Panel Consultant
Breach Candy Hospital, Jaslok Hospital and Global Hospital
Mumbai, Maharashtra, India
Founder President
PCOS Society of India

Message

As we are all aware, polycystic ovarian syndrome (PCOS) was first reported in modern medical literature by Stein and Leventhal in 1935. We have come a long way since then, and it is now recognized as a common, heterogeneous and heritable disorder affecting women throughout their reproductive period and beyond.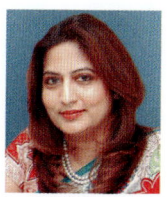

The PCOS is characterized by hyperandrogenism, ovulatory dysfunction, and polycystic ovaries, but there is considerable inter-individual variation in presentation. Although not required for diagnosis, the presence of insulin resistance and hyperinsulinemia is common and places those affected at increased risk of diabetes and cardiovascular disease. Thus, the PCOS adversely affects endocrine, metabolic, and cardiovascular health in the long term.

In addition, the prevalence of PCOS varies depending on which criteria are used to make the diagnosis, but may be as high as 15–20% when the European Society for Human Reproduction and Embryology/American Society for Reproductive Medicine (Rotterdam) criteria are used. An alarming fact is that the rise of PCOS is inexorable and stretches across the continents, affecting more women irrespective of caste, creed, religion and social background.

Hence, it is of paramount importance that we have greater depth of understanding of this multisystemic disease and keep ourselves updated regarding the latest advances on diagnosis, treatment and long-term implications. Implementing these in our daily practice will significantly improve our therapeutic approaches to the patients' complaints, including subfertility, obesity, menstrual problems, and pregnancy complications.

This excellently put together book is a step in this direction. I have no doubt that this book will go a long way toward improving our knowledge and understanding of the PCOS.

I congratulate Dr Kanthi Bansal, Dr Pooja Sharma Dimri, and Dr Apoorva Pallam Reddy, for this endeavor!

Nandita Palshetkar MD FCPS FICOG
Professor
Obstetrics and Gynecology
Dr DY Patil Medical College, Hospital and Research Center
Navi Mumbai, Maharashtra, India
President, MOGS

Preface

"Books are the quietest and most constant of friends; they are the most accessible and wisest of counselors, and the most patient of teachers."
—**Charles William Eliot**

Polycystic ovarian syndrome (PCOS) is a heterogeneous condition with a range of clinical, endocrine and metabolic manifestations. The increasing prevalence of the condition and plethora of presentation along with the consequences on fertility make it a complex disorder. It puts up a mighty challenge to gynecologists, dermatologists and endocrinologists alike. Though there are numerous publications and books on the PCOS, this subject provokes a lot of discussion and controversy about pathophysiology, diagnosis and therapy. We thought there was a need to evaluate comprehensively the latest trends in the management of this disorder, hence this book was conceived.

This book *Decoding Polycystic Ovarian Syndrome* is divided into 5 sections comprising 20 chapters. The sections deal with the basics, diagnosis, areas of concern, and management of the PCOS. The chapters have been written by expert gynecologists, sonologists, laparoscopic surgeons, and fertility experts, who have contributed to various aspects of the spectrum. In addition, a section is dedicated to the important issue of PCOS and fertility. The text is accompanied by tables, boxes, and key points, that make the content reader-friendly. This book combines the latest research and knowledge with the experiences of the authors.

We believe that this book will be useful for the postgraduates and practicing gynecologists to deal with the management of PCOS patients. Hopefully, it will add to our knowledge and information about this enigmatic syndrome.

Kanthi Bansal
Pooja Sharma Dimri
Apoorva Pallam Reddy

Acknowledgments

"Feeling gratitude and not expressing it is like wrapping a present and not giving it."
—**William Arthur Ward**

A book in the hands of a reader is a combined effort of so many people, most of them behind the scenes. This book also is a culmination of the hard work of many individuals, who contributed in various capacities to convert an idea into reality. The following lines are our sincere effort to acknowledge and thank all those who helped us in our endeavor.

First and foremost, we want to thank all the contributing authors, who shared their clinical acumen and experience in the form of chapters, and added gems of knowledge to the book in spite of their busy schedules. This book would not have been possible without their cooperation. A special mention is for Ms Shilpa Damodar, who worked tirelessly for the compilation and editing work and did a wonderful job of 'smoothing out the hard edges'. Also, no words can thank enough all the staff we work with, who make our life easier and help us to carry out our academic pursuits. Special thanks go to Dr Sadhana K Desai for the Foreword.

We want to sincerely thank M/s Jaypee Brothers Medical Publishers (P) Ltd. New Delhi, India, and the entire team, for all the support.

We offer our heartfelt gratitude to all the patients who keep faith in our abilities and allow us to enhance our knowledge and learning. Last but not least, we express our gratitude to our family members for their continuous and unconditional support.

Contents

Section 1
BASICS

1. Polycystic Ovarian Syndrome (PCOS)—The Mounting Syndrome   3
Sonia Malik, Suyesha Khanijao
History   *3*
Studies on PCOS Prevalence in India   *4*
Reasons for Rising Numbers   *6*

2. Etiology of Polycystic Ovarian Syndrome   9
Rupal N Shah
Environmental Factors Causing Polycystic Ovarian Syndrome   *9*
Genetic Association of Polycystic Ovarian Syndrome   *10*

Section 2
DIAGNOSES

3. Diagnosis of Polycystic Ovarian Syndrome   17
Rajeev Agarwal, Apoorva Pallam Reddy
Characteristic Features of Polycystic Ovarian Syndrome   *17*
Diagnostic Criteria of PCOS in Reproductive Age Group   *21*
Diagnosis of PCOS in Adolescents   *26*
Diagnostic Criteria of PCOS in Peri- and Postmenopausal Women   *27*
Diagnosis of Exclusion   *28*

4. Ultrasound in Polycystic Ovarian Syndrome   34
Sonal Panchal, CB Nagori
Techniques for Baseline Scan of Ovaries   *34*
Ultrasound Criteria of Polycystic Ovary   *37*
Ovarian Volume   *38*
Pathophysiology and Ultrasound Findings   *40*
Assessment of Stromal Abundance   *41*
Stromal Abundance and Hormonal Implications   *43*
Arrangement of Follicles   *44*

Section 3: POLYCYSTIC OVARIAN SYNDROME AND FERTILITY

5. Infertility in Polycystic Ovarian Syndrome — 53
Asha Baxi, Dhaval Baxi
- Epidemiology and Diagnosis 53
- Pathophysiology of PCOS-associated Infertility 54
- Etiology of Excessive Follicular Growth 54
- Etiology of Follicular Arrest 54
- Insulin Resistance and Hyperinsulinemia 55
- Disruption of Hypothalamic-Pituitary-Gonadal Axis in PCOS 57
- Deregulation of Ovarian Steroidogenesis 57
- Genetic Factors in PCOS 58

6. Ovulation Inductions in Polycystic Ovarian Syndrome — 61
Kanthi Bansal
- History of Ovarian Stimulation 61
- Pathophysiology of Ovulation 62
- Management of Ovulation Induction 62
- Principles of Ovulation Induction 65
- Ovulation Induction by Oral Ovulogens 65
- Surgical Management of Ovulation Induction by Laparoscopic Ovarian Drilling 73
- Complications 74

7. Assisted Reproductive Technology in Polycystic Ovarian Syndrome — 78
Manish Banker, Reena Gupta
- Indications for ART in PCOS 78
- Challenges in Ovulation Induction in PCOS for ART 79
- Protocols for Stimulation 80
- PCOS and OHSS 82
- ART Outcomes in PCOS 83
- In Vitro Maturation 86

8. Complications in Assisted Reproductive Technique — 92
Kedar Ganla
- Anesthesia-related Complications 92
- Procedure-related Complications 93
- Long-term Effects on Fertility 102

9. Embryology in Polycystic Ovarian Syndrome — 107
*Keshav Malhotra, Dolly Sandhu Gill
Jaideep Malhotra, Narendra Malhotra*

Extraovarian Factors   *107*
Intraovarian Factors   *109*
Oocyte in Polycystic Ovary   *110*
Spindle Assessment and Reactive Oxygen Species   *112*
Mitochondrial Assessment and Metabolism   *115*
Embryo in Polycystic Ovary   *116*
Strategies for Managing PCOS in the Lab   *117*
In Vitro Maturation   *118*

Section 4
AREAS OF CONCERN

10. Polycystic Ovarian Syndrome in Lean and Obese Women — 129
Kundan Vasant Ingale

Changes in Body Weight and Menstruation   *129*
Neuroendocrine Abnormalities in Polycystic Ovarian Syndrome   *130*
Impact of Obesity on Polycystic Ovarian Syndrome   *131*

11. Polycystic Ovarian Syndrome in Adolescents — 138
Sanjeev Khurd, Sadhana Khurd, Aditya Khurd

History and Pathogenesis   *139*
Pathogenesis of Polycystic Ovarian Syndrome   *140*
Polycystic Ovarian Syndrome Diagnosis in Adults   *141*
Adolescence   *141*
Adolescents and Polycystic Ovarian Syndrome   *141*
Principles of Management   *144*
Actual Management Protocols   *144*

12. Implications of Polycystic Ovarian Syndrome on Pregnancy — 155
Milind R Shah, Nirmal N Gujarathi

Pathophysiology of Polycystic Ovarian Syndrome   *157*
Polycystic Ovarian Syndrome and Pregnancy   *158*
Maternal Complications   *159*
Fetal Complications   *160*
Diet and Medication Concerns in PCOS Pregnancy   *163*

13. Psychological and Cognitive Problems in Polycystic Ovarian Syndrome — 168
Vidya Pancholia, AK Pancholia
Reduced Quality of Life Indicators *169*
Depression *170*
Bipolar Disorders *171*
Eating Disorders *172*
Anxiety and Fears *172*
Self-esteem and Body Satisfaction *173*
Potential Mechanisms *173*
Management *174*

14. Long-term Sequel of Polycystic Ovarian Syndrome — 180
Anu Agarwal
Metabolic Dysfunction in Polycystic Ovarian Syndrome *180*
Psychological Features of Polycystic Ovarian Syndrome *186*
Management of Long-term Complications *186*

15. Medicolegal Aspects of Polycystic Ovarian Disease — 191
Hitesh J Bhatt
Legal Implications *191*

Section 5: MANAGEMENT

16. Lifestyle Modifications in Polycystic Ovarian Syndrome — 197
T Ramani Devi
Diagnosis of Polycystic Ovarian Syndrome *197*
Diet in Polycystic Ovarian Syndrome *198*
Exercise Recommendations *201*

17. Drilling the Ovaries: What is the Latest Evidence? — 204
Vidhya V Bhat, Ritu Bijarnia
Management *204*
Techniques of Laparoscopic Ovarian Surgery *206*
Safety and Complications *211*
Advantages *212*

18. Hirsutism — 217
Pooja Sharma Dimri, Chandana A
Pathophysiology *217*
Causes of Hirsutism *219*

Evaluation and Diagnosis *219*
Management of Hirsutism *221*
Pharmacologic Intervention *222*

19. Adjuvants in Polycystic Ovarian Syndrome — 227
Apoorva Pallam Reddy, Yasodhara Pallam Reddy
Rationale for Use of Adjuvants *227*
Adjuvants Used *228*

20. Recent Advances in Polycystic Ovarian Syndrome — 247
Parul Kotdawala, Shalini Gainder
Classification of PCOS: Is there a Need for a New Consensus? *247*
Treatment of PCOS *250*
Impact on Quality of Life *252*
Obesity and Its Impact: Role of Bariatric Surgery in PCOS *253*
Cardiovascular Health Factors *253*
Genetics and PCOS *253*
Animal Models of PCOS *255*
Pregnancy in PCOS Women *256*
PCOS and Cancer *256*
Perimenopause and Menopause *257*

Index — 261

SECTION 1

BASICS

1. Polycystic Ovarian Syndrome—The Mounting Syndrome
2. Etiology of Polycystic Ovarian Syndrome

CHAPTER 1

Polycystic Ovarian Syndrome —The Mounting Syndrome

Sonia Malik, Suyesha Khanijao

INTRODUCTION

Polycystic ovarian syndrome (PCOS) is an endocrine disorder without any permanent cure. It is a lifestyle disease affecting a growing number of urban Indian women. Medical practitioners have noted a recent rise in PCOS cases in urban India and attribute it to 'Westernization,' modernization, stress, and lifestyle changes. We are in the middle of an alarming trend. More and more women are being diagnosed with polycystic ovarian syndrome (PCOS). The disorder is not new, but it is increasing at a dazzling rate. The prevalence of PCOS is increasing throughout the world in parallel with the rising prevalence of type 2 diabetes mellitus (T2DM). Use of different diagnostic criteria may partly account for it, as has recently been shown in a study from Mumbai.[1] PCOS has also been noted to affect 28% of unselected obese and 5% of lean women. In 2006, based on the US data and traditionally lower prevalence estimates, the anticipated economic burden of PCOS in Australia was AU $400 million (menstrual dysfunction 31%, infertility 12% and PCOS-associated diabetes 40% of total costs), representing a major health and economic burden.[2] Although there are no such studies from India, but most gynecologists and endocrinologists are perceiving an increase in the number of PCOS adding to the economic health burden of the country.[3]

HISTORY

Hippocrates (460–377 BC) noted, "But those women whose menstruation is less than three days or is meager, are robust, with a healthy complexion and a masculine appearance; yet they are not concerned about bearing children nor do they become pregnant" (Diseases of Women 1.6).[4] In Ayurveda, Acharya Sushruta[5,6] has mentioned *Bandhya* a type of, 'yonivyapada', whose symptom is amenorrhea or oligomenorrhea. Similarly, Acharya Charaka has described *Arajasaka*, a yonivyapada indicating amenorrhea.

But it was about 80 years back, a seminal publication in a journal transformed the perception of this disorder. The report by Irving Freiler Stein and Michael Leventhal titled, 'Amenorrhea Associated with Polycystic Ovaries', has proven to be a remarkably lasting and influential publication. Popularly known as the

'Stein-Leventhal syndrome', this condition was little understood and females were treated for their immediate gynecologic problems. The long-term sequelae were not well known. The growth in the related literature has been increasing exponentially ever since: the 50 years between 1950 and 2000 saw a little more than 8,000 publications on the topic, whereas the 15-year period between 2001 and 2015 has seen more than 20,000 related publications, a greater than 8-fold increase in the publication rate after 2000,[2] thus focusing on not only the growing interest in this disorder but also leading to a better understanding of the disorder.

Polycystic ovarian syndrome is becoming very common affecting women of all ages from adolescence to menopause. The presentation varies across communities and ages, making this a syndromic disorder. Though the most common features usually include excessive weight gain, oligomenorrhea/amenorrhea, increased triglyceride and insulin levels in the blood, acne, hirsutism and hypermenorrhea, it is also associated with menstrual disorders and infertility, usually occurring due to chronic anovulation. PCOS is a heterogeneous disorder of uncertain cause. There is some evidence that it is a genetic disease. This includes the familial clustering of cases, greater concordance in monozygotic compared with dizygotic twins and heritability of endocrine and metabolic features of PCOS. Environment and nutrition, however, seem to be playing a major role in the evolution of this disorder. Ayurveda[5] suggests that this is a *vata* type disorder (*Apanvata*), though the involvement of other can be there but in some measure. *Vata* predominance manifests with painful menses, severe menstrual irregularity, low weight, coldness *Pitta* predominance manifests as hair loss, acne, painful menses, clots and heart problems. *Kapha* predominance manifests as increased weight, infertility, hirsutism and diabetic tendencies. This varied interpretation of symptoms in the other streams on medicines also suggests that this syndrome is truly heterogeneous in nature. A study by Kar et al.[7] from Odisha defines the prevalence of different phenotypes of the disorder and its implications. Various studies from different parts of India suggest that not only is the disorder gaining prominence, but it is also suggesting a relationship with diabetes and metabolic syndrome in the later years. The presence of hypertension in adolescents who are obese, is a risk factor for developing metabolic syndrome in later years in life (Indian good practice guidelines) and studies also indicate that presence of PCOS indicates both diabetes and metabolic syndrome in their families.[8]

The worldwide prevalence of polycystic ovarian syndrome ranges from 2.2 to 26%. The World Health Organization estimates that it affects 116 million women worldwide as of 2010 (3.4% of women).[9] The rates of polycystic ovarian syndrome have been reportedly high among Indian women compared to their Caucasian counterparts, with an estimated prevalence of 9.13% in Indian adolescents.[10] Statistics reveal that, in India, 1 out of every 5 women in the reproductive age, and as high as 2 out of every 5 adolescents, are diagnosed with PCOS. PCOS prevalence in India is as high as 22%, which is much higher as compared to that in developed countries.

STUDIES ON PCOS PREVALENCE IN INDIA (TABLE 1.1)

The PCOS is believed to be a disease of upper class or rich people. Shweta et al. conducted a study in Tamil Nadu and concluded that the proportion of

TABLE 1.1 Prevalence of PCOS—various studies

Region	Place	No. of subjects	Study type	Age	Year	Criteria used	Prevalence	Study
North	Lucknow	1520	Community based	18–25	2013	MI or H or both	3.7%	Gill et al.
North	New Delhi	175	Case control	13–18	2010	Rotterdam	46.18%	Ganie et al.
South	Andhra Pradesh	460	Cross-sectional	15–18	2011	Rotterdam	9.13%	Nidhi et al.
South	Kerela and Kottayam	200	Cross-sectional survey	18–31	2013	Rotterdam	15%	Vijan and Sonia et al.
South	Nellore (Andhra Pradesh)	80	Cross-sectional	19–35	2012–14	Rotterdam	15.4%	Akumar et al.
West	Mumbai	778	Cross-sectional	15–24	2014	Rotterdam AES	22.5% 10.7%	Beenajoshi et al.

participants diagnosed with PCOS was higher among urban participants in comparison to rural participants.[10] The prevalence of obesity, overweight, and insulin resistance, associated with PCOS pathogenesis, appear to be higher among members of higher socioeconomic strata living in urban areas; medical researchers have attributed this to more sedentary lifestyles and access to more calorie-dense foods and labor-saving devices in urban and higher socioeconomic populations.[11] Gill et al. calculated that prevalence of PCOS in women between the ages of 18 years and 25 years from Lucknow, north India, is 3.7%. Majority of these girls were lean but have abdominal obesity.[12] Nidhi et al. prospectively studied 460 girls aged 15–18 years from a residential college in Andhra Pradesh, South India. The authors have reported a prevalence of PCOS in 9.13% of the adolescents.[13] Williamson et al. reported that PCOS women of different ethnicity presented with different clinical manifestation of PCOS.[14] Studies conducted on Indian PCOS women suggested that abnormalities of the insulin receptor are more common in Indian women with PCOS compared to white women with PCOS.[15] The prevalence of PCOS in Nellore district is 15.4%. Several factors influencing the occurrence of this syndrome have been investigated earlier.[16] Beena Joshi et al. tried to look at the prevalence using both the Rotterdam and Androgen Excess Society (AES) criteria and concluded the prevalence of PCOS in Mumbai was 22.5% by Rotterdam and 10.7% by criteria. This indicates that the disorder is better picked up if the ASRM/ESHRE criteria are used. Non-obese comprised 71.8% of PCOS diagnosed by Rotterdam criteria. Mild PCOS (oligomenorrhea and polycystic ovaries on USG) was the most common phenotype (52.6%). The prevalence of PCOS depends on the choice of diagnostic criteria. They demonstrated that PCOS is an emerging disorder during adolescence and screening could provide opportunity to target the group for promoting healthy lifestyle and, early interventions, to prevent future morbidities.[1]

Metropolitan Cities

In 2000, a multicentric study involving six urban cities (Chennai, Bengaluru, Hyderabad, Mumbai, Kolkata, and New Delhi) in India among the age group of 20–40 years indicated that the prevalence rate of obesity was 31%. Our study showed a 37.5% prevalence rate of obesity in women with PCOS.[16] A national survey of diabetes and IGT conducted in 2000 AD in six major cities of India showed a 13.1% prevalence of IGT and 5% prevalence of diabetes in the younger age group (20–40 years) of the general population.[17]

REASONS FOR RISING NUMBERS

A recent editorial by Aziz et al.[2] challenges the view that the incidence of the disorder is rising but, at the same time, recognizing this enigmatic disorder has a genetic predisposition and is, therefore, being passed on down the generations. An error in the insulin metabolism leading to hyperinsulinemia and hyperandrogenemia has been attributed to it. There are, however, no reports to compare the incidence of the disease in the past centuries with the present and it is probably because of better recognition and definition of diagnostic criteria that the syndrome is better recognized and diagnosed. The reasons have been attributed to this sudden explosion of PCOS are obesity, changing lifestyle and environmental toxins. However, an mentioned above,[2] published prevalence studies from many countries do not find a higher incidence of PCOS in the obese population thus giving credence to the fact that the disorder affects only those who have a genetic predisposition to the disorder.[18]

India has been labeled as the 'diabetic capital of the world' due to an alarming increase in the number of cases of both diabetes and metabolic syndrome. Since PCOS is a disorder of insulin metabolism, it is possible that there may be an increasing number of cases of PCOS as well. Further studies are warranted, especially from India, to know whether the incidence is rising or not, and what are the contributing factors.

KEY POINTS

- PCOS is a syndrome showing an alarming rise worldwide.
- Prevalence is high in India, adding to the economic health burden of the country.
- One out of every five women in the reproductive age and as high as two out of every five adolescents in India, are diagnosed with PCOS.
- The disorder has a heterogeneous origin with both genetic factors, and lifestyle and environmental influences.
- Rise in incidence and prevalence is parallel to increase in cases of diabetes mellitus.
- More studies are warranted from India to understand the contributory factors and possible prevention.

REFERENCES

1. Joshi B, Mukherjee S, Patil A, Purandare A, Chauhan S, Vaidya R. A cross-sectional study of polycystic ovarian syndrome among adolescent and young girls in Mumbai, India. Indian J Endocrinol Metab. 2014;18(3):317-24.
2. Aziz R, Marin C, Hoq L, Badamgarav E, Song P. Healthcare-related economic burden of the polycystic ovarian syndrome during the reproductive lifespan. J Clin Endocrinol Metab. 2005;90:4650-8.
3. Ganie MA, Kalra S. Polycystic ovarian syndrome – A metabolic malady, the mother of all lifestyle disorders in women – Can Indian health budget tackle it in future? Indian Journal of Endocrinology and Metabolism. 2011;15(4):239-41. doi:10.4103/2230-8210.85571.
4. Hanson AE. Hippocrates: diseases of women. Signs (Chic). 1975;1:567-84.
5. Sharma PV. *Charaka Samhita* (English Translation) Chaukambha Orientalia. Varanasi: 1981.
6. Srikantha Mruthi KR. *Sushruta Samhita* (English Translation) Chaukambha Orientale. Varanasi: 2001. pp. 170-3.
7. Kar S, et al. Anthropometric, clinical, and metabolic comparisons of the four Rotterdam PCOS phenotypes: A prospective study of PCOS women. Journal of Human Reproductive Sciences. 2013;6(3):194-200.

8. Shabir I, Ganie MA, Zargar MA, Bhat D, Mir MM, Jan A, Shah ZA, Jan V, Rasool R, Naqati A. Prevalence of metabolic syndrome in the family members of women with polycystic ovarian syndrome from North India. Indian J Endocr Metab. 2014;18:364-9.
9. Malik S, Jain K, Talwar P, Prasad S, Dhorepatil B, Devi G, et al. Management of Polycystic ovarian syndrome in India. Fertil Sci Res. 2014;1:23-43.
10. Balaji S, Amadi C, Prasad S, BalaKasav J, Upadhyay V, Singh AK, Surapaneni KM, Joshi A. Urban Rural Comparisons of Polycystic ovarian syndrome Burden among Adolescent Girls in a Hospital Setting in India. BioMed Research International. Volume 2015. Article ID 158951,.
11. Pathak G, Nichter M. Polycystic ovarian syndrome in globalizing India: An ecosocial perspective on an emerging lifestyle disease. Social Science and Medicine 2015; 146:21-8.
13. Nidhi R, Padmalata V, N Gagarathna R, Amritanshu R. Prevalence of polycystic ovarian syndrome in Indian adolescents. J Pediatr Adolesc Gynecol. 2011;24:223-7.
14. Williamson K, Gunn AJ, Johnson N, Milsom SR. The impact of ethnicity on the presentation of polycystic ovarian syndrome. Aust NZJ Obstet Gynaecol. 2001;41: 202-6.
15. Norman RJ, Mahabeer S, Masters S. Ethnic differences in insulin and glucose response to glucose between white and Indian women with polycystic ovarian syndrome. Fertil Steril. 1995;63:58-62.
16. Nagaraja Bhuvanashree, Sandhya Gupta, Medabalmi Anitha. Epari Venkatarao. Annals of tropical health and medicine. 2013;6(6):632-6.
17. Snehalatha C, Ramchandran A, Kapur A, Vijay V. Age-specific prevalence and risk associations for impaired glucose tolerance in urban southern Indian population. J Assoc Physicians India. 2003;51:766-9.
18. Holte J, Gennarelli G, Berne C, Bergh T, Lithell H. Elevated ambulatory daytime blood pressure in women with polycystic ovarian syndrome: A sign of a prehypertensive state? Hum Reprod. 1996;11:23-8.

CHAPTER 2

Etiology of Polycystic Ovarian Syndrome

Rupal N Shah

INTRODUCTION

Polycystic ovarian syndrome (PCOS) is a common disorder of premenopausal women, characterized by hyperandrogenism and chronic anovulation.[1,2] Genetic and environmental contributors combine with obesity, ovarian dysfunction and hormonal changes to contribute to the etiology of PCOS.[3,4] Many genetic studies in PCOS have been underpowered, and the results of published candidate gene studies have been disappointing. The underlying hormonal imbalance encompass a combination of increased androgens and/or hyperinsulinemia secondary to insulin resistance. Lack of ideal methods to assess either hyperandrogenism or insulin resistance hampers the understanding of pathophysiology. Hyperandrogenism is detected in around 60–80% of women with PCOS, and insulin resistance is a pathophysiological contributor in around 50–80% cases.[5] Obesity increases the hormonal dysfunction and consequences—hyperandrogenism, hirsutism, infertility and pregnancy complications—both independently and by exacerbating PCOS.[6,7] Obesity also increases risk of impaired glucose tolerance, diabetes and coronary artery disease.[8]

ENVIRONMENTAL FACTORS CAUSING POLYCYSTIC OVARIAN SYNDROME

Although the pathogenesis of PCOS remains unclear, the syndrome appears to have environmental and genetic components. Starting from early life and extending throughout lifecycle, environmental insults may affect susceptible women, who finally demonstrate the clinical phenotype of PCOS. Excessive dietary intake emerges as the major environmental determinant of PCOS. Over nutrition leading to obesity is widely recognized to have an aggravating impact, while another detrimental dietary factor may be the high content of advanced glycated end products (AGEs) in food. Environmental exposure to industrial products, particularly bisphenol A (BPA), may also exacerbate the clinical course of PCOS. AGEs and BPA may act as endocrine disruptors in the pathogenesis of the syndrome. PCOS appears to portray the harmful influence of the modern environment and lifestyle on the reproductive and metabolic balance of inherently predisposed individuals.[9]

Ibanez hypothesized that insult during pregnancy may cause intrauterine growth retardation (IUGR), which probably induces a "thrifty phenotype" in small for gestational age babies. These have a high-risk of suffering from insulin resistance, which may result in hypertension, glucose intolerance, adrenal axis hyperactivity with relative cortisol excess, functional hyperandrogenism and PCOS later in life, especially if they are exposed to environmental factors such a sedentary lifestyle and a diet rich in saturated fat.[10] This environmental factors may cluster in certain families because exercise and diet control are greatly influenced by parental lifestyle. The metabolic abnormalities can impart additional insult to the pregnancies of these small for gestational age (SGA) and PCOS patients, and these defects might be transmitted to another generation without the participation of any genetic abnormality.[11]

Women with epilepsy are found to have a higher prevalence of reproductive disorders including PCOS. Bilo et al. identified PCOS in 13 of 50 women (26%) with epilepsy. Among the 16 patients, not on treatment, 5 (31%) were diagnosed with PCOS, suggesting that epilepsy, independent of antiepileptic drugs, increases the risk of PCOS. Valproic acid, an anti-epileptic drug widely used to treat epilepsy, bipolar disorder, and migraine, is associated with features of polycystic ovarian syndrome.[12]

GENETIC ASSOCIATION OF POLYCYSTIC OVARIAN SYNDROME

The PCOS is a genetically heterogeneous syndrome in which the genetic contribution remains incompletely analyzed. PCOS is an inherently difficult condition to study genetically because of its heterogeneity, difficult retrospective diagnosis in postmenopausal women, associated subfertility, incompletely understood etiology, and gene effect size.[13]

Familial aggregation of PCOS suggesting a genetic etiology has been clearly established.[14,15] Studies of family members with PCOS indicate that an autosomal dominant mode of inheritance occurs for many families with this disease. Cooper et al.[16] reported that a history of oligomenorrhea was more common in the mothers and sisters of PCOS women than in controls. The proposed mechanism of inheritance was autosomal dominant with decreased penetrance. Givens et al. have reported multiple cases showing affected women in several generations.[17] Diagnostic criteria for PCOS were hirsutism and enlarged ovaries. High prevalence of metabolic disorders such as diabetes mellitus and abnormal lipid profile was found in both male and female members in families. In one family, there were several males with oligospermia and one with Klinefelter's syndrome (47,XXY). Elevated luteinizing hormone (LH)/follicle-stimulating hormone (FSH) ratios were present in some males and 89% of their daughters had PCOS. Another study observed that fathers of women with PCOS can be abnormally hairy; female siblings and mother may show oligomenorrhea.[18] Research has suggested that in a large cohort of women with PCOS, a family history of type 2 diabetes in a first-degree family member is associated with an increased risk of metabolic abnormality, impaired glucose tolerance, and type II diabetes.[18] In addition, a Dutch twin-family study showed a PCOS heritability of 0.71 in monozygotic twin sisters, versus 0.38 in dizygotic twins and other sisters.[19]

Genes related to PCOS can be grossly classified as follows:
- *Genes related to androgen biosynthesis and action and their regulation:* CYP17, CYP11A, CYP19, LH gene, sex hormone-binding globulin (SHBG) genes, etc.
- *Genes involved in insulin resistance and metabolic disorders:* INSR (insulin receptor gene), insulin growth factor system genes, peroxisome proliferator-activated receptor-γ (PPAR-γ), Calpain-10
- *Genes encoding inflammatory cytokines:* Paraoxanase (PON1), TNF-alfa, TNFR2 gene, IL-6.

Wickenheisser et al. reported that *CYP17* promoter activity was 4-fold greater in cells of patients with PCOS. This research suggests that the pathogenesis of PCOS may be in part related to the gene regulation of *CYP17*.[20] However, in a study that assessed candidate genes for PCOS using microsatellite markers to look for association in 4 genes—*CYP19*, *CYP17*, *FST*, and *INSR*—only 1 marker near the *INSR* gene was found to be significantly associated with PCOS.[21] The authors concluded that a susceptibility locus for PCOS (designated PCOS 1) exists in 19p13.3 in the *INSR* region, but it cannot be concluded that the *INSR* gene itself is responsible.[21]

Subsequent studies have found additional associations, such as those of 15 regions in 11 genes previously described to influence insulin resistance, obesity, or type 2 diabetes.[22] Individuals with PCOS were found more likely to be homozygous for a variant upstream of the *PON1* gene and homozygous for an allele of interest in *IGF2*. Interestingly, the *PON1* gene variant resulted in decreased gene expression, which could increase oxidative stress. The exact result of the *IGF2* variant is unclear, but *IGF2* stimulates androgen secretion in the ovaries and adrenal glands.[22]

In study by Goodarzi et al. the leucine allele was found to be associated with protection against PCOS, as compared to the valine allele at position 89 in *SRD5A2*.[23] The leucine allele is associated with a lower enzyme activity.[23] When the results of this study are combined with those of an observational study by Vassiliadi et al. based on urinary steroid profiles in women with PCOS, further support can be found for an important role for 5-alpha reductase in the pathogenesis of this syndrome.[24] In a genome-wide association study for PCOS in a Han Chinese population, 3 strong regions of association were identified, at 2p16.3, 2p21, and 9q33.3.[25] The polymorphism most strongly associated with PCOS at the 2p16 locus was near several genes involved in proper formation of the testis, as well as a gene that encodes a receptor for luteinizing hormone (LH) and human chorionic gonadotropin (hCG). This polymorphism was also located 211kb upstream from the follicle-stimulating hormone receptor *(FSHR) gene*, which encodes the follicle-stimulating hormone (FSH) receptor.[25]

The polymorphisms most strongly associated with PCOS at the 2q21 locus encode a number of genes, including the *THADA* gene, which has previously been associated with type 2 diabetes. In addition, 6 significant polymorphisms were identified as being associated with PCOS at the 9q33.3 locus near the *DENND1A* gene, which interacts with the *ERAP1 gene*. Elevation in serum ERAP1 has been previously associated with PCOS and obesity.[25]

Other genetic variations that regulate gene and phenotype expression, such as telomere length also play an important role in the etiology of PCOS. In a Chinese study, significant reduction of telomere length was observed in PCOS patients compared with healthy controls. There is correlation between oxidative stress and PCOS and between oxidative stress and telomere length. One possible mechanism is that the all factors associated withPCOS, such as androgen excess, abdominal adiposity, insulin resistance, and obesity, could contribute to raised oxidative stress that leads to telomere shortening.[26]

SUMMARY

The PCOS arises from an interaction of genetic and environmental factors. It is more likely to be polygenic or oligogenic in origin.[27] Genes involved in steroidogenesis, carbohydrate metabolism and major histocompatibility region, Insulin metabolism are likely to be involved.[28] Environmental factors like dietary intake and lack of physical activity are important contributors to the development of PCOS.

KEY POINTS

- A combination of genetic and environmental factors predisposes to PCOS
- Complex interplay of genetic tendency, hyperandrogenism, insulin resistance, dietary intake and obesity
- Genes related to sex steroid synthesis, insulin receptor metabolism and inflammatory cytokines are likely to be involved
- Inheritance of PCOS shows autosomal dominant inheritance
- Environmental factors such as prenatal insult and IUGR and medical conditions like epilepsy have a role
- Lifestyle modifications like optimum dietary intake and exercise important part of management.

REFERENCES

1. Dunaif A, Givens JR, Haseltine F, Merriam GR (Eds). The polycystic ovarian syndrome. Blackwell Scientific, Cambridge, MA. 1992.
2. Franks S. Polycystic ovarian syndrome. N Engl J Med. 1995;333:853-61.
3. Legro R, Strauss J. Molecular progress in infertility: polycystic ovarian syndrome. Fertil Steril. 2002;78:569-76.
4. Doi S, Al-Zaid M, Towers P, et al. Ovarian steroids modulate neuroendocrine dysfunction in polycystic ovarian syndrome. J Endocrinol Invest. 2005;28:882-92.
5. Legro R, Castracane V, Kauffman R. Detecting insulin resistance in polycystic ovarian syndrome: purposes and pitfalls. Obstet Gynecol Surv. 2004;59:141-54.
6. Balen A, Conway G, Kaltsas G, et al. Polycystic ovarian syndrome: the spectrum of the disorder in 1741 patients. Hum Reprod. 1995;10:2107-11.
7. Kiddy D, Sharp P, White D, et al. Differences in clinical and endocrine features between obese and non-obese subjects with polycystic ovarian syndrome: an analysis of 263 consecutive cases. Clin Endocrinol (Oxf). 1990;32:213-20.
8. Shaw L, Bairey Merz C, Azziz R, et al. Postmenopausal women with a history of irregular menses and elevated androgen measurements at high risk for worsening

cardiovascular event-free survival: results from the National Institutes of Health—National Heart, Lung, and Blood Institute sponsored Women's Ischemia Syndrome Evaluation. J Clin Endocrinol Metab. 2008;93:1276-12.
9. Diamanti-Kandarakis E, Christakou C, Marinakis E. Phenotypes and enviromental factors: their influence in PCOS. Curr Pharm Des. 2012;18(3):270-82.
10. Ibanez L, Vellas C, Potau N, et al. PCOS after precocious puberty: ontogeny of the low birthweight effects. Clinical endocrinology (Oxf). 2001;55:667-72.
11. Escobar-Morreale HF, Luque-Ramirez M, San Millan JL. The molecular-genetic basis of functioanl hyperandrogenism and the PCOS: Endocer Rev. 2005;26(2):251-82.
12. Bilo L, Meo R, Valentino R, Di Carlo C, Striano S, Nappi C. Characterization of reproductive endocrine disorders in women with epilepsy. J Clin Endocrinol Metab. 2001;86:2950-6.
13. Barber TM, Franks S. Genetic basis of polycystic ovarian syndrome. Expert review of endocrinology and metabolism. 2010;5(4):549-61.
14. Givens JR. Familial ovarian hyperthecosis: a study of two families. Am J Obstet Gynecol. 1971;11:959-72.
15. Wilroy RS, Givens JR, Weser WL, Coleman SA, Andersen RN, Fish SA. Hyperthecosis—an inheritable form of polycystic ovarian disease. Birth Defects. 1975;11:81-5.
16. Cooper HE, Spellacy WN, Prem KA, Cohen WD. Hereditary factors in Stein-Leventhal syndrome. Am J Obstet Gynecol. 1968;100:371-87.
17. Givens JR. Familial polycystic ovarian disease. Endocrinol Metab Clin North Am. 1988;17:1-17.
18. Ehrmann DA, Kasza K, Azziz R, Legro RS, Ghazzi MN. Effects of race and family history of type 2 diabetes on metabolic status of women with polycystic ovarian syndrome. J Clin Endocrinol Metab. 2005;90(1):66-71.
19. Vink JM, Sadrzadeh S, Lambalk CB, Boomsma DI. Heritability of polycystic ovarian syndrome in a Dutch twin-family study. J Clin Endocrinol Metab. 2006;91(6):2100-4.
20. Wickenheisser JK, Quinn PG, Nelson VL, Legro RS, Strauss JF 3rd, McAllister JM. Differential activity of the cytochrome P450 17alpha-hydroxylase and steroidogenic acute regulatory protein gene promoters in normal and polycystic ovarian syndrome theca cells. J Clin Endocrinol Metab. 2000;85(6):2304-11.
21. Tucci S, Futterweit W, Concepcion ES, et al. Evidence for association of polycystic ovarian syndrome in caucasian women with a marker at the insulin receptor gene locus. J Clin Endocrinol Metab. 2001;86(1):446-9.
22. San Millan JL, Corton M, Villuendas G, Sancho J, Peral B, Escobar-Morreale HF. Association of the polycystic ovarian syndrome with genomic variants related to insulin resistance, type 2 diabetes mellitus, and obesity. J Clin Endocrinol Metab. 2004;89(6):2640-6.
23. Goodarzi MO, Shah NA, Antoine HJ, Pall M, Guo X, Azziz R. Variants in the 5 alpha-reductase type 1 and type 2 genes are associated with polycystic ovarian syndrome and the severity of hirsutism in affected women. J Clin Endocrinol Metab. 2006;91(10):4085-91
24. Vassiliadi DA, Barber TM, Hughes BA, et al. Increased 5 alpha-reductase activity and adrenocortical drive in women with polycystic ovarian syndrome. J Clin Endocrinol Metab. 2009;94(9):3558-66.
25. Chen ZJ, Zhao H, He L, et al. Genome-wide association study identifies susceptibility loci for polycystic ovarian syndrome on chromosome 2p16.3, 2p21 and 9q33.3. Nat Genet. 2011;43(1):55-9.
26. Li Q, et al. A possible new mechanism in the pathophysiology of PCOS: the discovery that leukocyte telomere length is strongly associated with PCOS. J Clin Endo Crinol Metab. 2014;99(2):E234-E40.
27. Urbanek M. The genetics of the polycystic ovarian syndrome. Nat Clin Pract Endocrinol Metab. 2007;3:103-11.
28. Carey AH, Chan KL, Short F, White D, Williamson R, et al. Evidence for a single gene effect causing polycystic ovaries and male pattern baldness. Clin Endocrinol (Oxf). 1993;38:653-8.

SECTION 2

DIAGNOSES

3. Diagnosis of Polycystic Ovarian Syndrome
4. Ultrasound in Polycystic Ovarian Syndrome

CHAPTER 3

Diagnosis of Polycystic Ovarian Syndrome

Rajeev Agarwal, Apoorva Pallam Reddy

INTRODUCTION

The polycystic ovarian syndrome (PCOS) is one of the most common endocrine-reproductive–metabolic disorders, affecting women across all age groups. Despite the progress in understanding the pathophysiology, little is known regarding the onset and etiology. It has a wide spectrum of phenotypic manifestations like oligo-ovulation or anovulation, hyperandrogenism (either clinical or biochemical), and the presence of polycystic ovaries.

Since its first description by **Irving F Stein, Sr and Michael L Leventhal** in 1935, the criteria of diagnosis, symptoms, and causative factors are subject to debate. Over the last several decades, significant efforts have been made to classify PCOS; however, global consensus regarding a PCOS criterion remains controversial. Owing to the vast spectrum of the condition and its varied manifestations based on age, the existing epidemiologic and/or basic research data have not been sufficient in providing the foundation needed to derive an evidence-based definition of the syndrome. The current proposed criteria are predominantly based on expert opinion and this only adds to the ambiguity.

Till date 3 ESHRE/ASRM-sponsored PCOS consensus workshops have been organized to establish consensus in dealing with PCOS. The first one in Rotterdam, Netherlands 2003, focused on diagnostic criteria for PCOS Rotterdam ESHRE/ASRM-Sponsored PCOS Consensus Workshop Group.[1] The second in Thessaloniki, Greece 2007, dealt with infertility management in PCOS.[2] The third PCOS consensus workshop—took place in Amsterdam, the Netherlands, in October 2010 and attempted to summarize current knowledge and to identify gaps in knowledge regarding various women's health aspects of PCOS.

This chapter aims to summarize the best available evidence for diagnosing PCOS.

CHARACTERISTIC FEATURES OF POLYCYSTIC OVARIAN SYNDROME

The current available definitions for PCOS essentially rely on three characteristics namely-androgen excess, chronic anovulation, and ovarian morphology on USG to make the diagnosis.

Androgen Excess

Clinical hyperandrogenism: Clinical hyperandrogenism may include seborrhea, hirsutism (defined as excessive terminal hair that appears in a male pattern), acne, or androgenic alopecia. Hirsutism is defined as a modified Ferriman Gallway score >7.

Biochemical hyperandrogenism: Refers to an elevated serum androgen level and typically includes an elevated total, bioavailable, or free serum testosterone (T) level.

Given variability in T levels and the poor standardization of assays, it is difficult to define an absolute level that is diagnostic of PCOS or other causes of hyperandrogenism. It is recommended to be familiar with local assays. Samples for laboratory studies should be drawn early in the morning, with the patient in a fasting state; in women with regular menses, samples should be preferably taken between days 5 and 9 of the menstrual cycle.[3]

The limitations of defining androgen excess by the measurement of circulating androgen levels were:
- There are multiple androgens that may not be considered (Rittmaster, 1993).
- There is wide variability in the normal population.
- Normal ranges have not been well established using well-characterized control populations.
- Age and body mass index (BMI) have not been considered when establishing normative values for androgen levels (Moran et al., 1999; Bili et al., 2001).
- Few normative data are present in adolescent and older women.
- Androgens are suppressed more rapidly by hormonal suppression than other clinical features and may remain suppressed even after discontinuation of hormonal treatment.

In order to overcome these limitations, the Royal College of Obstetricians and Gynaecologists (RCOG) recommends using free androgen index (defined as total testosterone divided by sex hormone binding globulin [SHBG] × 100, to give a calculated free testosterone level) as a measurement for hyperandrogenism.

Other androgens, such as androstenedione, dehydroepiandrosterone sulfate (DHEA-S), may be normal or slightly above the normal range in patients with PCOS. Levels of SHBG are usually low in patients with PCOS. Hence, they are not including in making a diagnosis.

Chronic Ovulatory Dysfunction

Ovulatory dysfunction is undoubtedly the most common presenting feature in PCOS women. Women with oligomenorrhea or amenorrhea have about a 90% chance of being diagnosed with PCOS, and up to 95% of PCOS affected adults have oligomenorrhea or amenorrhea.[4] Although cycle abnormalities are common during the reproductive years, as many as one-third of women with PCOS may ovulate spontaneously. Anovulation may manifest as frequent bleeding at intervals <21 d or infrequent bleeding at intervals >35 d. Occasionally, bleeding may be anovulatory despite falling at a normal interval (25–35 days). A midluteal progesterone documenting anovulation (P4 <3 ng/mL) or a follicular monitoring may help with the diagnosis, if bleeding intervals appear to suggest regular ovulation. It may be noted that with advancement of age there is increased probability of having regular cycles.

Menstrual disturbance carries both short term and long term implications as the extent of irregularity is directly proportional to the severity of PCOS and risk of metabolic syndrome.

PCOM on Ultrasound

Ultrasound characteristics for polycystic ovarian morphology (PCOM) were, for the first time, described at the Rotterdam consensus in 2003. The PCO morphology has been defined by—the presence of 12 or more follicles 2–9 mm in diameter and/or an increased ovarian volume >10 mL (without a cyst or dominant follicle) in either ovary.[1,5]

The subjective appearance of PCO, the follicular distribution and stromal echogenicity should not be substituted for this definition. Although increased stromal volume is a feature of PCO (Bucket et al., 2003), it has been shown that the measurement of the ovarian volume is a good surrogate for the quantification of stromal volume in clinical practice.

The following technical recommendations have been highlighted by the Rotterdam consensus while performing ultrasound for PCOS:
- State-of-the-art equipment is required and should be operated by appropriately trained personnel.
- Whenever possible, the transvaginal approach should be utilized, particularly in obese patients.
- Regularly menstruating women should be scanned in the early follicular phase (cycle days 3±5). Oligo-/amenorrheic women should be scanned either at random or between days 3 and 5 after a progestin-induced withdrawal bleeding.
- Calculation of ovarian volume is performed using the simplified formula for a prolate ellipsoid (0.5 × length × width × thickness) (Swanson et al., 1981).
- Follicle number should be estimated in both longitudinal and anteroposterior cross-sections of the ovaries. The size of follicles <10 mm should be expressed as the mean of the diameters measured on the two sections.

In PCOS patients, ultrasound not only provides an opportunity to screen for endometrial hyperplasia but also predicts the risk of hyperstimulation, OHSS and metabolic dysfunction.

Revised USG Criteria

Since initial proposal of use of USG in 2003, a heightened prevalence of polycystic ovaries has been described in healthy women with regular menstrual cycles, which has questioned the accuracy of these criteria and marginalized the specificity of polycystic ovaries as a diagnostic criterion for PCOS.

Owing to the advancement in technology and improved imaging, there is surfacing of evidence to increase the threshold of number of follicles per ovary. In a diagnostic test study done in women of age group 18–35 years, diagnostic potential for PCOS was highest for follicle number per ovary (FNPO) (0.969), followed by follicle number per cross section (FNPS) (0.880) and ovarian volume OV (0.873). An FNPO threshold of 26 follicles had the best compromise between sensitivity (85%) and specificity (94%) when discriminating between controls and PCOS. Similarly, an FNPS threshold of nine follicles had 69% sensitivity and 90% specificity, and an OV of 10 cm^3 had 81% sensitivity and 84% specificity.[6]

In a study by Michael et al, diagnostic thresholds by **3D ultrasound** for PCO with 100% specificity as determined by receiver operator characteristic (ROC) curves were ≥20 for mean FNPO, ≥10 for maximum FNPS, and ≥13 cm^3 for ovarian volume. Both 2D and 3D transvaginal ultrasound were highly accurate in the diagnosis of PCO, but different thresholds should be utilized for each modality **(Table 3.1)**.[7]

TABLE 3.1 Diagnostic strengths and weaknesses of the main features of PCOS as adapted from the NIH evidence-based methodology workshop on PCOS

Criterion	Strengths	Limitations
Androgen excess	• Included as a component in all major classifications • A major clinical concern for patients • Animal models employing androgen excess resemble but do not fully mimic human disease	• Measurement is performed only in blood. • Concentrations differ during time of day. • Concentrations differ with age. • Normative data are not clearly defined. • Assays are not standardized across laboratories. • Clinical hyperandrogenism is difficult to quantify and may vary by ethnic group. • Tissue sensitivity is not assessed.
Ovulatory dysfunction	• Included as a component in all major classifications • A major clinical concern for patients Infertility a common clinical complaint	• Normal ovulation is incompletely understood. • Normal ovulation varies over a woman's lifetime. Ovulatory dysfunction is difficult to measure objectively.
Polycystic ovarian morphology	• Historically associated with syndrome • May be associated with hypersensitivity to ovarian stimulation	• Technique dependent • Difficult to obtain standardized measurement • Lack of normative standards across the menstrual cycle and lifespan (notably in adolescence) as ovarian morphology varies with age • Technology required to accurately image not universally available • Imaging possibly inappropriate in certain circumstances (e.g. adolescence)

DIAGNOSTIC CRITERIA OF PCOS IN REPRODUCTIVE AGE GROUP

The following sets of diagnostic criterion have been proposed over the past three decades to achieve some uniformity in diagnosing PCOS.

National Institute of Health Criterion, 1990

For most of the 20th century, PCOS was a poorly understood condition. In 1990, the National Institutes of Health (NIH) held a conference on PCOS to create both a working definition of the disorder and diagnostic criteria. The outcome of this conference, the NIH criteria, served as a standard for researchers and clinicians for more than a decade.
- Oligomenorrhea and/or anovulation
- Signs of androgen excess (clinical or biochemical)
- Exclusion of other disorders that can result in menstrual irregularity and hyperandrogenism.

All the three criteria should be fulfilled.

Rotterdam Criteria, 2003

The second definition was based on the consensus opinion of 27 PCOS experts, who met in Rotterdam, the Netherlands, May 2003.

This consensus, which was partly sponsored by ESHRE and partly by ASRM, introduced as ultrasound features suggesting PCOM. Adding PCOM to the existing NIH criterion to make it more complex. A diagnosis of PCOS is made if any two out of three criteria are met, after exclusion of secondary conditions that might cause these findings. The 3 criteria were:
1. Signs of clinical or biochemical hyperandrogenism (HA)
2. Chronic ovulatory dysfunction (OD)
3. PCOM.

This essentially expanded the diagnosis of PCOS to include women who either had PCOM in combination with HA, or PCOM in combination with OD (OD is a slightly broader term than oligo/amenorrhea, and includes other forms of OD beyond just oligoanovulation, possibly reflected in, e.g. polymenorrhea). This led to a substantial increase in the number of patients diagnosed with PCOS, as well as broadened the heterogeneity of PCOS phenotypes as compared with the NIH definition.[8]

Androgen Excess and PCOS Society, 2006

In 2006 a task forceassembled by the Androgen Excess and PCOS Society (AEPCOS), composed of five investigators from the United States and six from Europe and Australia conducted a systematic review of published literature to identify the link between PCOS phenotypes and independent morbidity.

The literature cleared distinguished two categories of PCOS women; PCOS with hyperandrogenism and nonhyperandrogenic PCOS. There was substantial body of evidence suggesting that hyperandrogenism seemed to be the strongest determinant of the PCOS pathophysiology and a key predictor of the associated metabolic dysfunction. The nonhyperandrogenic PCOS women exhibited similar metabolic and long term sequelae as that of the non PCOS controls. This led to the establishment of AEPCOS society guidelines.

AE-PCOS Diagnostic Criteria

Need to fulfill both the criteria:
- Clinical or biochemical hyperandrogenism
- Ovulatory dysfunction or/and PCOM

However, all criteria are consistent in that, PCOS is considered a diagnosis of exclusion.

NIH Evidence-based Methodology Workshop 2012

The PCOS in itself is considered an enigma at various levels. The controversies in the diagnostic criteria has only added to confusion and has made it difficult to develop evidence from literature as the criterion used for diagnosis were widely varied in the studies. This has resulted in "delay in progress in understanding the syndrome".

In order to establish some clarity, the NIH in 2012 undertook an evidence-based methodology PCOS workshop which, among other topics, addressed the "benefits and drawbacks" of existing diagnostic criteria.[9]

After scrutinizing all the available criteria, the panel recommended the use of the broader ESHRE/ASRM (Rotterdam) 2003 criteria, but added that this must be accompanied with a detailed description of the PCOS phenotype **(Table 3.2)**.

TABLE 3.2 Evolution of the diagnostic criteria for polycystic ovarian syndrome

Parameter	NIH 1990	ESHRE/ASRM 2003	AE-PCOS 2006	NIH 2012 extension of ESHRE/ASRM 2003
Criterion	HA OA	HA OD PCOM	HA Ovarian dysfunction (OD and/or PCOM)	HA OD PCOM
Limitations	Two of two criteria required	Two of three criteria required	Two of two criteria required	Two of three criteria required and identification of specific phenotypes included: A: HA + OD + PCOM B: HA + OD C: HA + PCOM D: OD + PCOM

Abbreviations: AE-PCOS, Androgen Excess & PCOS Society; ASRM, American Society for Reproductive Medicine; ESHRE, European Society for Human Reproduction and Embryology; HA, hyperandrogenism; NIH, National Institutes of Health; OA, oligoanovulation; OD, ovulatory dysfunction; PCOM, polycystic ovarian morphology
Source: Adapted from Lizneva. Criteria, prevalence, and phenotypes of PCOS. Fertil Steril 2016.

Phenotypic Approach for PCOS Impact on Metabolic Risks and Reproductive Risks

Azziz et al. were the first to introduce the concept of adding a phenotype to every case of PCOS. Considering the four essential features of PCOS, ovulatory dysfunction, hirsutism, hyperandrogenemia, and polycystic ovaries, the task force identified nine different phenotypes that could be considered as being PCOS **(Table 3.3)**.

The task force noted that there were ample data to support an increased risk of metabolic dysfunction in women with the following phenotypes:
- Hirsutism and/or hyperandrogenemia, and oligo-ovulation with and without polycystic ovaries (phenotypes A–F)
- Hyperandrogenemia and/or hirsutism, and normo-ovulation with polycystic ovaries (phenotype G–I)[10]

Current evidence generally did not support an increased metabolic dysfunction among women with polycystic ovaries only, with or without oligo-ovulation (phenotype J).[11]

Characteristic Features of Classic PCOS (Phenotypes A and B)

Features more specific to classic PCOS:
- More pronounced menstrual dysfunction
- Increased insulin levels
- Higher rates of insulin resistance and risk for metabolic syndrome
- Higher body mass index and prevalence of obesity
- More severe forms of atherogenic dyslipidemia
- Increased risk of hepatic steatosis
- The highest AMH levels.

Characteristic Features of Ovulatory PCOS (Phenotype C)

- Intermediate levels of serum androgens, insulin, atherogenic lipids, hirsutism scores and prevalence of metabolic syndrome
- More seen in higher socioeconomic status
- Higher incidence of ovulatory cycles due to more favorable insulin levels and fat tissue distribution.

Characteristic Features of Nonhyperandrogenic PCOS (Phenotype D)

- Mildest degree of endocrine and metabolic dysfunction
- Lowest prevalence of metabolic syndrome
- Lower LH to FSH ratios, lower total and free T levels, and higher sex hormone-binding globulin levels
- Higher incidence of regular cycles.

It should be stressed that the incidence of metabolic dysfunction in PCOS is significantly increased by the concomitant presence of obesity. The practical application of this phenotypic approach in routine clinical practice would be helpful to identify those women with PCOS who are at the highest risk for metabolic dysfunction.

TABLE 3.3 Potential phenotypes of PCOS by NIH, 1990; Rotterdam 2003; and AE-PCOS, 2006

Panel terminology	Diagnostic criteria	Potential PCOS phenotypes									
		NIH						AE-PCOS/Rotterdam 1			Rotterdam 2
		A	B	C	D	E	F	G	H	I	J
Androgen excess	Hyperandrogenemia	+	−	+	+	−	+	+	−	+	−
	Hyperandrogenism*	+	+	−	+	+	−	+	+	−	−
Ovulatory dysfunction	Oligoanovulation	+	+	+	+	+	+	−	−	−	+
Polycystic ovarian morphology	Polycystic ovaries	+	+	+	−	−	−	+	+	+	+
	NIH 1990 criteria	×	×	×	×	×	×				
	Rotterdam 2003 criteria	×	×	×	×	×	×	×	×	×	×
	AE PCOS 2006 criteria	×	×	×	×	×	×	×	×	×	

*Clinical signs or symptoms of excess androgen

This classification also allows researchers to categorize their outcomes on a finite number of PCOS phenotypes, permitting comparisons with other well-defined PCOS populations.

Pitfalls of Phenotype Classification

Despite there being sufficient evidence supporting the notion that different phenotypes have different metabolic risk, there is another school of thought that there is not much difference between the subtypes. In a study done on German patients, Cupisti et al. did not observe any significant difference in insulin resistance, BMI, and dyslipidemia between the various PCOS phenotypes.[12] Likewise, Wijeyaratne et al.[13] and Melo et al.[14] did not observe any difference in the prevalence of metabolic syndrome between the various PCOS phenotypes in women from Sri Lanka and Brazil, respectively. It is noteworthy, however, that the use of poor-quality androgen assays in the majority of these studies could have resulted in the misclassification of patients who actually have hyperandrogenemia (i.e. with classic PCOS) as nonhyperandrogenic.

The assessment of the PCOS phenotype is indeed a complex multistep process, which requires multiple clinical and laboratory assessments, pelvic ultrasound, which might require several visits for some subjects. This might also cause delay and decrease in the actual number of cases. Even with the various intricacies posed, NIH's 2012 phenotypic extension of the Rotterdam definition has been shown to be the most convenient approach when conducting research and clinical practice.

Ultrasound Features Predictive of Degree of Reproductive and Metabolic Disturbance in PCOS

The phenotypic approach imparts maximum causal effect on hyperandrogenism for most of the metabolic risks. Although PCOM is included as one the diagnostic criteria in the most widely accepted Rotterdam criterion, the relevance of ultrasound features in predicting degree of symptomatology, response to treatment, and/or health risks in PCOS is uncertain.

Of the studies that have reported associations among sonographic markers and clinical indices, most—but not all—have noted positive relationships among androgens, gonadotropins and menstrual cycle length with follicle counts, stromal area (SA), stromal echogenicity, and/or ovarian volume (OV).[15] There are reports of positive associations among follicle number, OV, and stromal features with markers of insulin resistance.[16] A cross sectional observational study done by Christ et al. over 49 women diagnosed with PCOS based on NIH criterion to evaluate the predictability of sonographic markers on reproductive and metabolic outcome, concluded that AFC, but not OV, was positively associated with total testosterone (p=0.610), androstenedione (p=0.490), and LH:FSH (p=0.402). Follicles <4 mm were negatively associated with various metabolic markers, whereas larger follicles (5–8 mm) showed positive associations. Stromal markers were not associated with cardiometabolic measures. The probability of dominant follicles >10 mm were best predicted by age.[17]

DIAGNOSIS OF PCOS IN ADOLESCENTS

Adolescence is a period of hormonal and reproductive transition. It is possible that PCOS may begin to manifest itself in adolescence but may not be readily diagnosed until adulthood due to the lack of consensus on how PCOS should be defined in adolescents. All PCOS diagnostic criteria were derived for adults, not adolescents. Although essentially the definition of PCOS in adolescents follows the general principles outlined for adult women, there are several caveats that need to be considered when evaluatingthis age group, particularly in girls whose presentationdoes not meet the full presentation seen in adults **(Table 3.4)**.

Furthermore, most of the PCOS features may overlap or mimic the normal physiological puberty transitions:

Oligomenorrhea: It is common after menarche during normal puberty and is therefore not specific to adolescents with PCOS. Anovulatory cycles is noted in 85%, 59% and 25% of menstrual cycles in the first, third and fifth year after menarche respectively. On the other hand approximately two-thirds of adolescents with PCOS will have menstrual symptoms, and for one-third it will be the presenting symptom, with the spectrum from primary amenorrhea to frequent dysfunctional bleeding.[18]

Hyperandrogenism: Anovulatory cycles are associated with higher serum androgen and LH levels. Mild hirsutism and more commonly acne are noted as frequently as 50% in adolescents. However, severe forms of hirsutism and androgenic alopecia should be viewed more cautiously during diagnosis. There are no well-defined cut-off points for androgen levels during normal pubertal maturation and this can be further exacerbated by obesity.[19]

PCOM: The Rotterdam criteria were not validated for adolescents and the lack of feasibility to do a transvaginal ultrasound adds to the trouble in diagnosis. Multifollicular ovaries can be found in approximately 26% of adolescents.Moreover, during puberty ovarian volume is typically greater compared with adults.[20]

However, two years from menarche most of the transitions from adolescence to adulthood are achieved and by the age of 18 years, thevast majority of girls who have PCOS will have developed thephenotype clearly.[21] After two years after menarche the threshold for ovarian size, the total and free T levels in adolescents are generally comparable to those in adults. Although menstrual dysfunction is a commonly encountered during normal reproductive maturation, prolonged adolescent oligomenorrhea at age 14–19 years has been found to be predictive of persistent ovarian dysfunction later in life.[22] Based on the above observations 2 sets of PCOS criteria were suggested for adolescents two years after menarche. One by an ESHRE/ASRM working group[23] and the other by a clinical practice guidelines committee of the Endocrine Society.

As per these recommendations, when PCOS is not evident by adult standards, the disorder could be considered in adolescents based on the presence of
- increased serum androgens levels and/or progressive hirsutism, in association with
- persistent oligo/amenorrhea for at least two years after menarche and/or primary amenorrhea by age 16 years
- and/or an ovarian volume >10 cm^3, after exclusion of secondary causes.

TABLE 3.4 Diagnostic criteria for polycystic ovarian syndrome in adolescents

Parameter	ESHRE/ASRM, 2012	ESHRE Society, 2013
Criteria	• Clinical or biochemical hyperandrogenism[a] • Oligo-/anovulation[b] • Polycystic ovarian morphology[c]	• Clinical or biochemical hyperandrogenism[a] • Persistent oligo-/anovulation[b]
Limitation	Three of three criteria required with exclusion of other etiologies	Two of three criteria required with exclusion of other etiologies

Note: ASRM, American Society of Reproductive Medicine; ESHRE, European Society for Human Reproductive and Embryology
[a] Increased serum androgens and/or progressive hirsutism
[b] Oligo-/amenorrhea for at least 2 years, or primary amenorrhea by age 16 years
[c] Ovarian volume > 10cm^3
Source: Lizneva. Criteria, prevalence, and phenotypes of PCOS. Fertil Steril 2016

The follicle number per ovary was not considered as a part of the diagnostic criterion in either of the two groups.

It should be noted, however, that neither of the proposed criteria have yet to be validated.

One of the studies by Kenigsberg et al. proposed that USG cannot accurately detect follicle number, and is a poor imaging modality for characterizing PCOs in adolescents. They recommended the use of MRI as a diagnostic imaging modality for adolescents in whom diagnosis of PCOS remains uncertain after clinical and laboratory evaluation.[24]

DIAGNOSTIC CRITERIA OF PCOS IN PERI- AND POSTMENOPAUSAL WOMEN

Diagnosing PCOS in the peri- and postmenopause is more challenging than that in adolescents. The menopausal transition of women with PCOS is poorly understood, but many aspects of the syndrome appear to improve. In a cross-sectional study by Johnstone et al. in 161 PCOS women, odds of meeting Rotterdam criteria for PCOS and of biochemical hyperandrogenism decrease with age. Even the phenotypes of PCOS ameliorate with age. Women gain menstrual cyclicity,[25] experience a decrease in the ovarian volume, AMH and number of ovarian follicles,[26] all of which can ameliorate the clinical presentation of PCOS. Androgen levels decline with age in all women irrespective of their PCOS status. Serum testosterone declines by 50% between the ages of 20 and 40 years. As the basal level of androgens is elevated in PCOS women, the androgens levels, despite being normal, are higher than their non PCOS counterparts. The assessment of androgen levels is complicated further due to lack of age related cut offs for testosterone levels and imprecise assays for measurement **(Table 3.5)**.[27]

In 2013, an endocrine society appointed committee of experts, based on limited evidence, formulated the presumptive PCOS definition for postmenopause. The committee stressed on the fact that it is unlikely that new onset PCOS can occur in the perimenopausal age and therefore recommended to make the diagnosis of PCOS in postmenopausal women based on a previous medical history of

TABLE 3.5 Suggested diagnostic criteria for polycystic syndrome in postmenopausal women

Parameter	Endocrine Society, 2013
Criteria	Clinical or biochemical hyperandrogenism[a] Prolonged oligoamenorrhea[a]
Limitation	Two of two criteria required with exclusion of other etiologies

[a] Based on well-documented long term previous medical history
Source: Lizneva. Criteria, prevalence, and phenotypes of PCOS. Fertil Steril 2016

TABLE 3.6 Other diagnoses to be excluded in all women before making a diagnosis of PCOS

Disorder	Test	Abnormal values	Study for further evaluation and treatment of abnormal findings; First Author; Year
Thyroid disease	Serum TSH	TSH > the upper limit of normal suggests hypothyroidism TSH < the lower limit, usually <0.1 mIU/L, suggests hyperthyroidism	Ladenson, 2000
Prolactin excess	Serum prolactin	> Upper limit of normal for the assay (27 ng/mL)	Melmed, 2011
Nonclassical congenital adrenal hyperplasia	Early morning (before 8 am) serum 17-OHP	200–400 ng/dL depending on the assay (applicable to the early follicular phase of a normal menstrual cycle as levels rises with ovulation), but a cosyntropin stimulation test (250 µg) is needed if levels fall near the lower limit and should stimulate 17-OHP > 1000 ng/dL	Speiser, 2010

menstrual dysfunction and the presence of hyperandrogenemia during the reproductive period.[28] The presence of PCOM was considered a supportive sign; however, it was unlikely to be found owing to age-related changes in ovarian morphology.

DIAGNOSIS OF EXCLUSION

The single most important criterion that was unanimously agreed by all the groups across decades was to make the diagnosis of PCOS only after excluding other causes of hyperandrogenism and anovulation. The conditions to be excluded were further divided into two categories.[28]
1. To be excluded in all women **(Table 3.6)**.
2. To be excluded in select women with severe phenotypes **(Table 3.7)**.

TABLE 3.7 Diagnoses to be excluded in select women, depending on presentation

Other diagnosis*	Suggestive features in the presentation	Tests to assist in the diagnosis	Study for further evaluation and treatment of abnormal findings; First Author; Year
Pregnancy	Amenorrhea (as opposed to oligomenorrhea), other signs and symptoms of pregnancy, including breast fullness, uterine cramping, etc.	Serum or urine hCG (positive)	Morse, 2011
HA including functional HA	Amenorrhea, clinical history of low body weight/BMI, excessive exercise, and a physical exam in which signs of androgen excess are lacking; multifollicular ovaries are sometimes present	Serum LH and FSH (both to low normal), serum estradiol (low)	Wang, 2008
Primary ovarian insufficiency	Amenorrhea combined with symptoms of estrogen deficiency, including hot flashes and urogenital symptoms	Serum FSH (elevated), serum estradiol (low)	Nelon, 2009
Androgen-secreting tumor	Virilization, including change in voice, male pattern androgenic alopecia, and clitoromegaly; rapid onset of symptoms	Serum T and DHEAS levels (markedly elevated), ultrasound imaging of ovaries, MRI of adrenal glands (mass or tumor present)	Carmina, 2006
Cushing's syndrome	Many of the signs and symptoms of PCOS can overlap with Cushing's (i.e striae, obesity, dorsocervical fat (i.e buffalo hump, glucose intolerance); however, Cushing's more likely to be present when a large number of signs and symptoms, especially those with high discriminatory index (e.g myopathy, plethora, violaceous striae, easy brusing) are present, and this presentation should lead to screening	24-hour urinary collection of urinary free cortisol (elevated), late night salivary cortisol (elevated), overnight dexamethasone suppression test (failure to suppress morning serum cortisol level)	Nieman, 2008

Contd...

Contd...

Other diagnosis*	Suggestive features in the presentation	Tests to assist in the diagnosis	Study for further evaluation and treatment of abnormal findings; First Author; Year
Acromegaly	Oligomenorrhea and skin changes (thickening, tags, hirsutism, hyperhidrosis) may overlap with PCOS. However, headaches, peripheral vision loss, enlarged jaw (macrognathia), frontal bossing, macroglossia, increased shoe and glove size, etc. are indications for screening	Serum free IGF-1 level (elevated), MRI of pituitary (mass or tumor present)	Melmed, 2009

*Additionally there are very rare causes of hyperandrogenic chronic anovulation that are not included in this table because they are so rare, but they must be considered in patients with an appropriate history. These include other forms of congenital adrenal hyperplasia (e.g. 11 β-hydroxylase deficiency, 3 β-hydroxysteroid dehydrogenase), related congenital disorders of adrenal steroid metabolism or action (e.g. apparent/cortisone reductase deficiency, apparent DHEA sulfotransferase deficiency, glucocorticoid resistance), virilizing congenital adrenal hyperplasia (adrenal rests, poor control, fetal programming), syndromes of extreme IR, drugs, portohepatic shunting, and disorders of sex development.

Role of AMH in Diagnosing PCOS

Serum anti-Müllerian hormone (AMH) levels are 2-4 fold higher in women with PCOS than in healthy women and is found in all PCOS populations.[29] This increase in serum AMH was first thought to be due to the higher number of preantral and small antral follicles. However, production of AMH by granulosa cells was found *in vitro* to be 75-fold higher in anovulatory PCOS and 20-fold higher in normo ovulatory PCOS than in normal ovaries.[30]

Given the strong correlation of AMH in the pathophysiology of PCOS and the fact that AMH would be theoretically more accurate than AFC, as it reflects also the excess of small follicles nonvisible on ultrasound, various authors have proposed using AMH as the standard in diagnosis of PCOS. Owing to the constant change in the cut off for follicles with the evolution of ultrasound and poor AMH assays, it is not possible, so far, to propose a consensual and universal diagnostic threshold for serum AMH in the prediction of PCOS. Some authors have proposed a cut off at 35 pmol/L (4.9 ng/mL) with the enzyme immunoassayAMH-EIA (EIA AMH/MIS kit) ("Immunotech", ref A16507) provided by Beckman Coulter (France) had a good specificity (97%) and a better sensitivity than the AFC (92%) to distinguish women with PCOS from normal women.[31] However, till robust evidence develops in this area, AMH should be used only as a prognostic tool and is still considered premature to make the diagnostic transition.

CONCLUSION

PCOS, a heterogeneous complex genetic trait of unclear etiology, has a prevalence ranging from 6% to 10% in unselected women. It affects not only current lifestyle with ovulatory and menstrual irregularity, subfertility and infertility, clinically evident hyperandrogenism, but also has significant long term sequelae like increased cardiovascular and diabetic complications, sleep apnea, anxiety, depression and malignancy risk due to metabolic dysfunction. Hence, the need is for early and accurate diagnosis. The current available evidence recommends maintaining the broad, inclusionary diagnostic criteria of Rotterdam (which includes the "classic NIH" and AE-PCOS criteria) while specifically identifying the phenotype:
- Androgen excess + ovulatory dysfunction
- Androgen excess + polycystic ovarian morphology
- Ovulatory dysfunction + polycystic ovarian morphology
- Androgen excess + ovulatory dysfunction + polycystic ovarian morphology.

These criterion need to be modified when trying to make the diagnosis in adolescent and perimenopausal age groups.

KEY POINTS

- Androgen excess, chronic ovulatory dysfunction and polycystic ovarian morphology are the key characteristic features for PCOS.
- Women of different age groups require different criterion for making a diagnosis of PCOS.
- Of the various existing criteria, Rotterdam criterion is widely accepted.
- Subdividing PCOS based on their phenotype and its practical application in routine clinical practice would be helpful to identify PCOS women, who are at the highest risk for metabolic dysfunction.
- Diagnosis of PCOS is always a diagnosis of exclusion.

REFERENCES

1. Revised 2003 consensus on diagnostic criteria and long-term health risks related to polycystic ovarian syndrome (PCOS). Hum Reprod. 2004;19:41-7.
2. Thessaloniki ESHRE/ASRM-Sponsored PCOS Consensus Workshop Group. Consensus on infertility treatment related to polycystic ovarian syndrome. Fertil Steril. 2008;89:505-22.
3. American Association of Clinical Endocrinologists. American Association of Clinical Endocrinologists position statement on metabolic and cardiovascular consequences of polycystic ovarian syndrome. National Guideline Clearinghouse. Available at http://guideline.gov/summary/summary.aspx?doc_id=7108. Accessed: August 28, 2009.

4. Consensus on women's health aspects of polycystic ovarian syndrome (PCOS): the Amsterdam ESHRE/ASRM-Sponsored 3rd PCOS Consensus Workshop Group Fertility and Sterility®. 2012;97(1):0015-0282.
5. Jonard S, Robert Y, Cortet C, Decanter C, Dewailly D. Ultrasound examination of polycystic ovaries: is it worth counting the follicles? Hum Reprod. 2003;18:598-603.
6. Lujan ME. Updated ultrasound criteria for polycystic ovarian syndrome: reliable thresholds for elevated follicle population and ovarian volume. Human Reproduction. 2013;28(5):1361-8.
7. Michael C. Diagnosis of polycystic ovaries by three-dimensional transvaginal ultrasound Michael C. Allemand Fertil Steril. 2006;85:214-9.
8. Lizneva D. Criteria, prevalence, and phenotypes of polycystic ovarian syndrome. Fertil Steril. 2016;106:6-15. 2016 by American Society for Reproductive Medicine.
9. Adapted from National Institutes of Health Evidence-based Methodology Workshop on Polycystic ovarian syndrome, December 3-5, 2012.
10. Glueck CJ, Papanna R, Wang P, Goldenberg N, Sieve-Smith L. Incidence and treatment of metabolic syndrome in newly referred women with confirmed polycystic ovarian syndrome. Metabolism. 2003;52:908-15.
11. Michelmore K, Ong K, Mason S, Bennett S, Perry L, Vessey M, Balen A, Dunger D. Clinical features in women with polycystic ovaries: relationships to insulin sensitivity, insulin gene VNTR and birth weight. ClinEndocrinol (Oxf). 2001;55:439-46.
12. Cupisti S, Haeberle L, Schell C, Richter H, Schulze C, Hildebrandt T, et al. The different phenotypes of polycystic ovarian syndrome: no advantages for identifying women with aggravated insulin resistance or impaired lipids. Exp Clin Endocrinol Diabetes. 2011;119:502-8.
13. Wijeyaratne CN, SeneviratneRde A, Dahanayake S, Kumarapeli V, Palipane E, Kuruppu N, et al. Phenotype and metabolic profile of South Asian women with polycystic ovarian syndrome (PCOS): results of a large database from a specialist endocrine clinic. Hum Reprod. 2011;26:202-13.
14. Melo AS, Vieira CS, Romano LG, Ferriani RA, Navarro PA. The frequency of metabolic syndrome is higher among PCOS Brazilian women with menstrual irregularity plus hyperandrogenism. Reprod Sci. 2011;18:1230-6.
15. Takahashi K, Eda Y, Abu-Musa A, Okada S, Yoshino K, Kitao M. Transvaginal ultrasound imaging, histopathology and endocrinopathy in patients with polycystic ovarian syndrome. Hum Reprod. 1994;9:1231-6.
16. Sikka P, Gainder S, Dhaliwal LK, Bagga R, Sialy R, Sahdev S. Ultrasonography of the ovaries and its correlation with clinical and endocrine parameters in infertile women with PCOS. Int J FertilWomens Med. 2007;52:41-7.
17. Christ JP. Ultrasound features of polycystic ovaries relate to degree of reproductive and metabolic disturbance in polycystic ovarian syndrome. Fertil Steril. 2015 by American Society for Reproductive Medicine. 2015;103:787-94.
18. Apter D. Endocrine and metabolic abnormalities in adolescents with a PCOS-like condition: consequences for adult reproduction. Trends Endocrinol Metab. 1998;9:58-61.
19. Rosenfield RL, Ghai K, Ehrmann DA. Diagnosis of the polycystic ovarian syndrome in adolescence: comparison of adolescent and adult hyperandrogenism. J Pediatr Endocrinol Metab. 2000;13(Suppl 5):1285-9.
20. Fruzzetti F, Campagna AM, Perini D, Carmina E. Ovarian volume in normal and hyperandrogenic adolescent women. Fertil Steril. 2015;104:196-9.
21. Legro RS, Arslanian SA, Ehrmann DA, Hoeger KM, Murad MH, Pasquali R, et al. Diagnosis and treatment of polycystic ovarian syndrome: an Endocrine Society clinical practice guideline. J Clin Endocrinol Metab. 2013;98:4565-92.

22. Glueck CJ, Woo JG, Khoury PR, Morrison JA, Daniels SR, Wang P. Adolescent oligomenorrhea (age 14-19) tracks into the third decade of life (age 20-28) and predicts increased cardiovascular risk factors and metabolic syndrome. Metabolism. 2015;64:539-53.
23. Fauser BC, Tarlatzis BC, Rebar RW, Legro RS, Balen AH, Lobo R, et al. Consensus on women's health aspects of polycystic ovarian syndrome (PCOS): the Amsterdam ESHRE/ASRM-Sponsored 3rd PCOS Consensus Workshop Group. Fertil Steril. 2012;97:28-38.e25.
24. Kenigsberg LE. Clinical utility of magnetic resonance imaging and ultrasonography for diagnosis of polycystic ovarian syndrome in adolescent girls. Fertil Steril. 2015;104:1302-9.
25. Elting MW, Korsen TJ, Rekers-Mombarg LT, Schoemaker J. Women with polycystic ovarian syndrome gain regular menstrual cycles when ageing. Hum Reprod. 2000;15: 24-8.
26. Alsamarai S, Adams JM, Murphy MK, Post MD, Hayden DL, Hall JE, et al. Criteria for polycystic ovarian morphology in polycystic ovarian syndrome as a function of age. J Clin Endocrinol Metab. 2009;94:4961-70.
27. Pinola P, Piltonen TT, Puurunen J, Vanky E, Sundstrom-Poromaa I, Stener-Victorin E, et al. Androgen profile through life in women with polycystic ovarian syndrome: a Nordic multicenter collaboration study. J Clin Endocrinol Metab. 2015;100:3400-7.
28. Legro RS, et al. Diagnosis and treatment of polycystic ovarian syndrome: an endocrine society clinical practice guideline. J Clin Endocrinol Metab. 2013;98:4565-92.
29. Laven JS, Mulders AG, Visser JA, Themmen AP, De Jong FH, Fauser BC. Anti-Müllerian hormone serum concentrations in normoovulatory and anovulatory women of reproductive age. J ClinEndocrinol Metab. 2004;89(1):318-23. doi:10.1210/jc.2003-030932
30. Pellatt L, Hanna L, Brincat M, Galea R, Brain H, Whitehead S, et al. Granulosa cell production of anti-Müllerian hormone is increased in polycystic ovaries. J Clin Endocrinol Metab. 2007;92(1):240-5. doi:10.1210/jc.2006-1582
31. Dumont A, et al. Role of anti-Müllerian hormone in pathophysiology, diagnosis and treatment of polycystic ovarian syndrome: a review. Reproductive Biology and Endocrinology. 2015;13:137.

CHAPTER 4

Ultrasound in Polycystic Ovarian Syndrome

Sonal Panchal, CB Nagori

INTRODUCTION

Polycystic ovarian syndrome (PCOS) is a complex endocrine condition in which ovulatory dysfunction and androgen excess are cardinal features.[1] It affects about 10% of women in reproductive age.[2] Approximately 20–30% of women with infertility have polycystic ovaries and about half of these have signs and symptoms of PCOS. The earliest description of polycystic ovaries appears to date from 1845 as 'sclerocystic ovaries'.[3] Other names suggested are polyfollicular syndrome or ovarian dysmetabolic syndrome. Diagnosis of polycystic ovarian syndrome (PCOS) has always been a controversial and debatable issue. It has been defined in different ways by different college of thoughts European Society for Human Reproduction and Embryology (ESHRE)-American Society for Reproductive Medicine (ASRM), Androgen Society, etc. But as for the fertility group, most people still accept the ESHRE-ASRM consensus 2003 as a guideline. According to ESHRE/ASRM consensus 2003[4] the diagnosis of polycystic ovarian syndrome consists of at least two of the three following criteria:
1. Oligo and/or anovulation
2. *Hyperandrogenism:* Biochemical or clinical
3. Polycystic ovaries on ultrasound.

Therefore, the diagnosis of PCOS depends on clinical findings, laboratory testing and ultrasound.

TECHNIQUES FOR BASELINE SCAN OF OVARIES

B mode ultrasound assessment of the ovaries consists of assessment of ovarian diameters and volume and counting of antral follicles as quantitative and qualitative assessment of stromal density. Once the ovary is located, the probe is rotated to find out the longest diameter of ovary and is stored as one frame on a dual screen. Then probe is rotated 90° to get a true transverse axis of ovary. The largest longitudinal, transverse and AP diameter of the ovary is measured in centimetres (cm), and ovarian volume can be calculated by the formula (x x y x z x 0.523) **(Fig. 4.1)**.

Numbers of antral follicles are counted in ovary by performing a 2-dimensional sweep across the whole ovary. This method is very feasible and reliable when

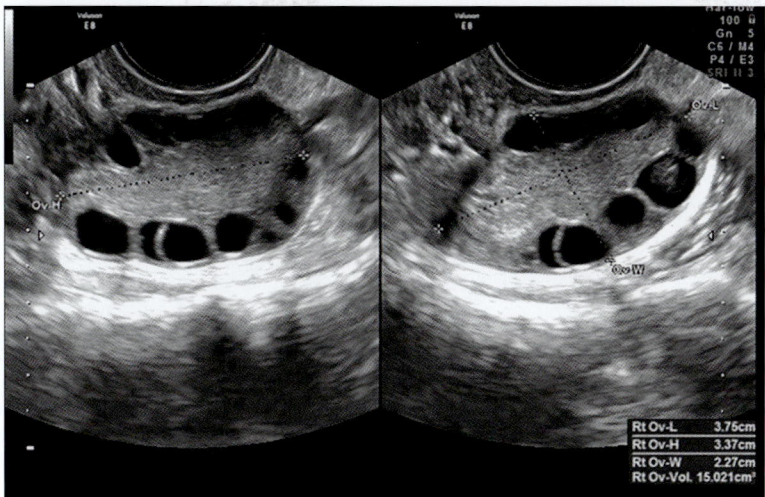

Fig. 4.1 Longitudinal and transverse sections of ovary

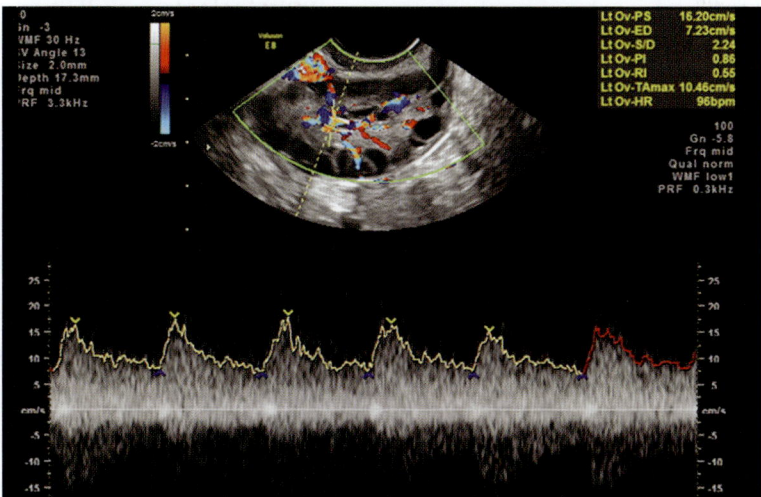

Fig. 4.2 Measuring ovarian stromal flows

number of antral follicles is approximately 10–15. But, when number of follicles is much more as in polycystic ovaries, the calculation using B mode scroll may be inaccurate.

Stromal echogenecity is compared with the echogenecity of myometrium, especially if ovary and uterus are at almost same depth from probe. Normally ovarian stroma is hypoechoic or isoechoic to myometrium, but in PCO it is hyperechoic as compared to the myometrium.

Color or power Doppler box is then placed on the ovary, so that whole ovary in included in colour box. Doppler is used to observe presence of vessels in ovarian stroma **(Fig. 4.2)**. The vessel that is close to any of the follicles is not a stromal vessel. If blood vessels are seen, pulse Doppler is used for quantitative assessment of the flows—intraovarian resistance index (RI) and peak systolic velocity (PSV).

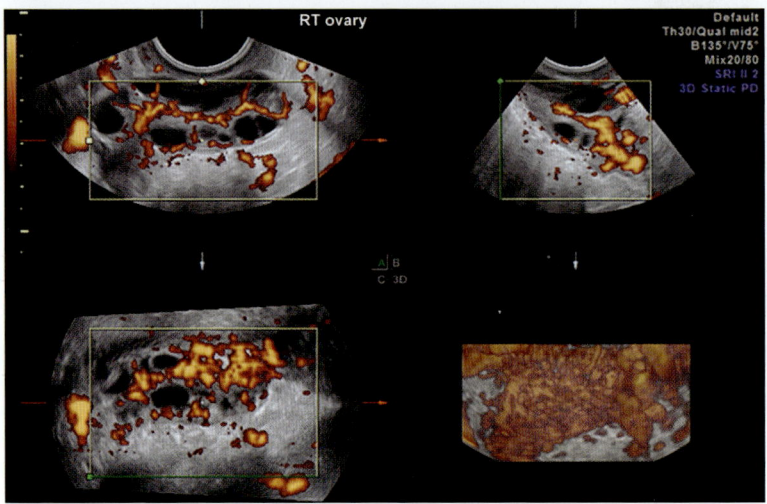

Fig. 4.3 3D power Doppler volume of ovary

For color Doppler pulse repetition frequency (PRF) is set at 0.3, wall filters lowest with optimum gains and balance settings. For pulse Doppler PRF is set at 1.3 usually but may be lowered of required and wall filters are set at 30 Hz, as stromal flows on baseline scan are low velocity flows. The vessel selected for interrogation is that which shows brightest color on color Doppler, though one may opt to take the readings for three different vessels that appear the brightest on color and take a mean of these values as stromal flows.

After having completed the Doppler study, volume studies are initiated. Three dimensional ultrasound provides a new method for objective quantitative assessment of follicle count, ovarian volume, stromal volume and blood flow in the ovary.[5] Power Doppler box is set to include whole ovary and then 3D volume of ovary is acquired **(Fig. 4.3)**. This volume of ovary is used to calculate ovarian volume, stromal volume, and to count number of antral follicles. Global vascular indices vascularity index (VI), flow index (FI) and vascularity flow index (VFI) may be calculated from the same ovarian volume.

Antral follicles can be counted by using inversion mode rendering **(Fig. 4.4)** or using a software called Sono automated volume calculation (AVC) **(Fig. 4.5)**. Sono AVC is based on inversion mode rendering, but further color codes each follicle and also shows x, y and z diameters, mean diameter and volume of each follicle on result sheet **(Fig. 4.6)**. Region of interest (ROI) is selected to include the whole ovary in all three orthogonal planes on acquired ovarian volume and selecting the right/left ovary on the screen and initiating the software will calculate the number of antral follicles. Postprocessing also may be done if the operator is not convinced with the calculations made by the scanner automatically.

A software called VOCAL (Volume calculation by computer) is used to define ovarian volume **(Fig. 4.7)**. VOCAL calculates volume of any structure by rotating it 180°. A rotating angle of 6°–30° can be selected. A circumference is drawn around the structure of interest at every step of rotation and at the end of 180°, total volume is calculated by the scanner computer. On this calculated ovarian volume with power Doppler, applying volume histogram assesses the global vascularity

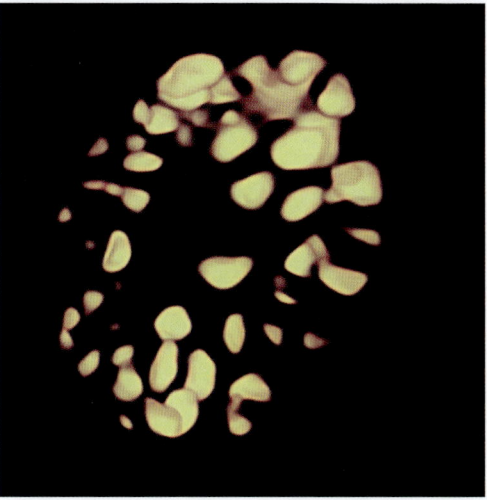

Fig. 4.4 Follicles as seen on inversion mode rendering

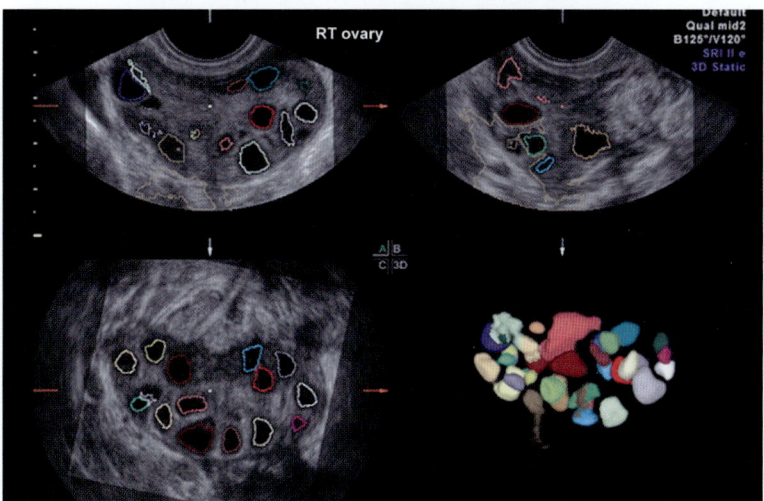

Fig. 4.5 Antral follicles as seen on Sono AVC

in the selected volume and presents it as vascularity index (VI), flow index (FI) and vascularity flow index (VFI) **(Fig. 4.8)**. VI is an index for abundance of flow in the selected volume, FI is an index for average intensity of flow in a selected volume and VFI is a perfusion index. Applying threshold volume on the same VOCAL calculated volume will define stromal volume when threshold is set to differentiate follicles from rest of the ovarian tissue **(Fig. 4.9)**.

ULTRASOUND CRITERIA OF POLYCYSTIC OVARY

As per ESHRE-ASRM 2003 consensus (Rotterdam criteria) polycystic ovary is defined as above 10 cc in volume and/or has more than 12 antral follicles. These seem to appear very clear and objective criteria for the diagnosis of polycystic

DR.NAGORI INSTITUTE

Date of Exam: 22.04.2010 Page 3/4
Exam Type:

Name NAYANA G 730 Pat. ID D10878-10-03-04-5

Ovary: Left
Total#: 12

Nr.	d(V) mm	dx mm	dy mm	dz mm	mn. d mm	V cm³
1	9.3	17.0	9.6	5.8	10.8	0.42
2	7.6	10.7	8.2	5.2	8.0	0.23
3	7.4	11.0	7.5	5.7	8.1	0.21
4	5.8	6.9	6.4	4.7	6.0	0.10
5	5.7	13.5	7.7	4.2	8.5	0.10
6	5.7	6.6	6.2	4.7	5.8	0.10
7	5.4	6.8	6.6	3.9	5.8	0.08
8	5.0	7.6	5.4	3.7	5.6	0.07
9	4.6	5.6	4.5	4.1	4.7	0.05
10	3.0	5.4	3.0	1.8	3.4	0.01
11	2.2	3.3	2.1	1.6	2.4	<0.01
12	2.1	3.2	2.3	1.7	2.4	<0.01

Ovary: Right
Total#: 10

Nr.	d(V) mm	dx mm	dy mm	dz mm	mn. d mm	V cm³
1	13.1	20.7	15.6	7.9	14.7	1.18
2	9.7	13.6	11.7	6.5	10.6	0.48
3	8.6	10.7	9.0	7.0	8.9	0.33
4	7.2	10.1	7.2	5.5	7.6	0.20
5	7.0	9.6	6.6	5.8	7.3	0.18
6	5.1	7.2	5.7	3.4	5.4	0.07
7	4.7	6.2	5.2	3.4	4.9	0.05
8	4.2	5.7	4.6	3.1	4.4	0.04
9	3.2	3.6	3.4	2.8	3.3	0.02
10	3.1	3.7	3.0	2.7	3.1	0.02

Endo Thickness 4.89 mm

Pelvic Floor

funneling yes no
urethral kinking yes no

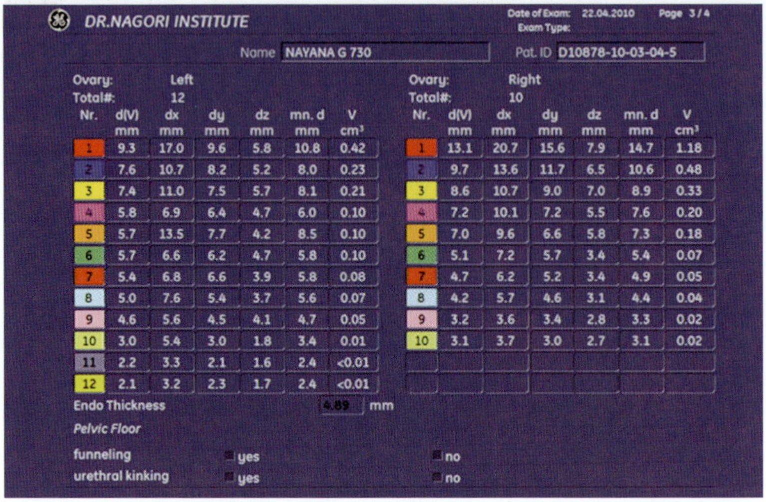

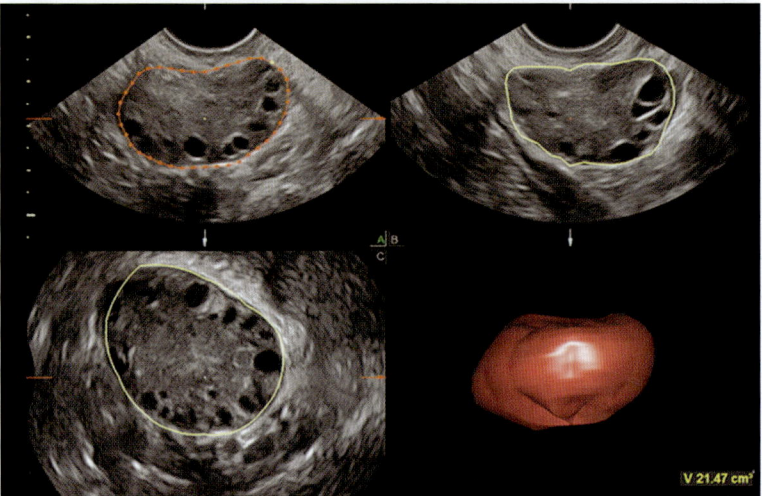

Fig. 4.6 Result sheet of Sono AVC

Fig. 4.7 Ovarian volume calculated by VOCAL

ovaries evidently. But then the problem is that ovaries of significant percentage of the patients diagnosed as polycystic ovarian syndrome do not fulfil these criteria on one hand and on the other hand several patients whose ovaries show these characters otherwise do not show any clinical signs and symptoms of polycystic ovarian syndrome. These mean both these ultrasound features need to be evaluated for their relevance to polycystic ovaries and polycystic ovarian syndrome.

OVARIAN VOLUME

'Enlarged spherical ovaries >10 cc on ultrasound, has shown good correlation between diagnosis of polycystic morphology and histopathological criteria for

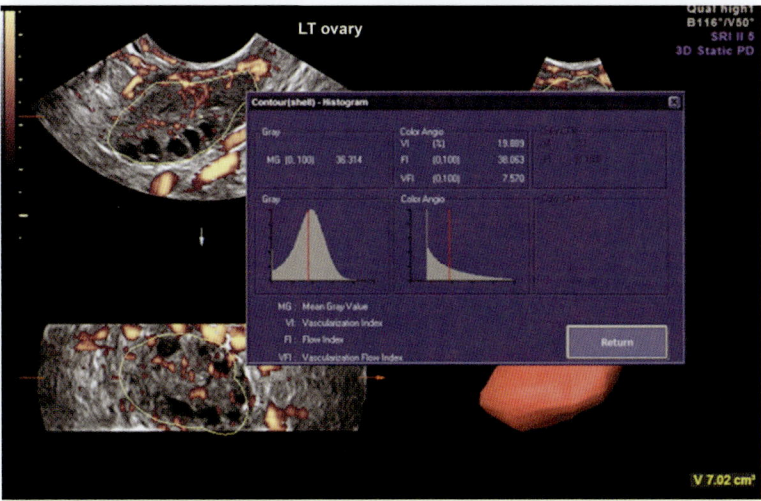

Fig. 4.8 3D power Doppler volume histogram of ovary

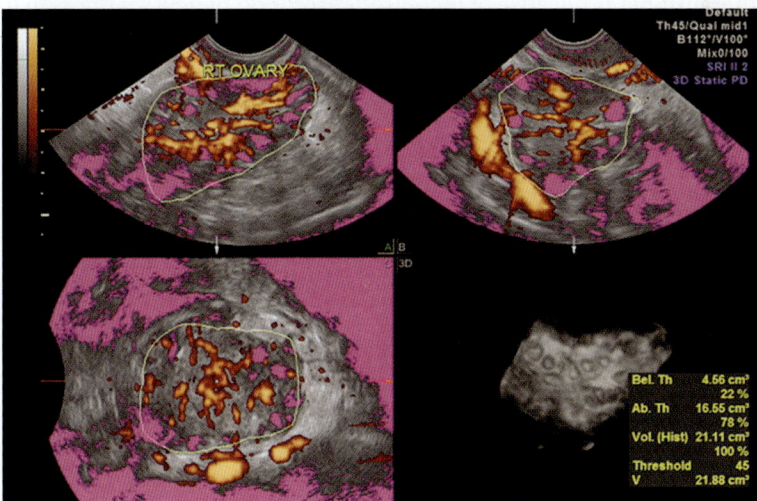

Fig. 4.9 Stromal volume calculated using threshold volme after VOCAL of ovary

polycystic ovaries.'[6] But the ovarian volume setting the threshold at 7 cc offered the best compromise between specificity (91.2%) and sensitivity (67.5%). In comparison, specificity and sensitivity were 98.2% and 45% respectively with threshold at 10 cc.[7] Ovarian volume 6.6 cc has shown 91% sensitivity and 91% specificity for polycystic ovarian syndrome.[8] Moreover, according to S. Kupesic, ovaries that are normal in volume can be polycystic as demonstrated by histological and biochemical studies (in 20%). Polycystic ovarian morphology has therefore been found to be a better discriminator than ovarian volume between polycystic ovarian syndrome and control women.[9] This discussion indicates that ovarian volume alone cannot be used as a parameter for diagnosis of polycystic ovaries. Therefore, morphological features of polycystic ovaries like number and arrangement of the follicles and stromal characteristics need consideration.

Antral Follicle Count

Antral follicle count (AFC) of 12/more (2-9 mm) has been used as a characteristic for polycystic ovaries according to Rotterdam criteria. Setting the threshold at 12 for 2-9 mm FNPO offered the best compromise between specificity (99%) and sensitivity (75%).[10]

The mean follicular number per ovary (FNPO) of follicles 2-5 mm in size was significantly higher in polycystic ovaries than in controls, while it was similar within 6-9 mm range. Within 2-5 mm range, significant relationship was found between FNPO and androgens but FNPO in the range of 6-9 mm was significantly and negatively related to body mass index and fasting serum insulin level.[11] Obesity and IR may enhance follicular excess by dysregulation of AMH through pathway of hyperandrogenemia.[12]

Though a study by Dewailly et al. in 2011 shows that FNPO > 19 had a sensitivity of 81% and specificity of 92% for PCO. And adding AMH >35 pmol/L as an additional parameter will increase the sensitivity to 92% and specificity to 97%.[13] The higher number is because of increased resolution of new scanners to identify follicles smaller than 2 mm. According to a study in 2013, an average value of 26 or more follicles per ovary is a reliable threshold for detecting polycystic ovaries in women with frank manifestation of PCOS. Sensitivity and specificity for diagnosis of PCOS for FNPO (26) was 85% and 94% and for OV (10 cc) was 81% and 84%. But the same study has also quoted that the lower follicle threshold may be required to detect milder variants of the syndrome.[14]

Moreover, polycystic ovaries with advancing age may show lesser number of follicles. AFC also thus cannot be used as the characteristic of polycystic ovaries. This indicates even antral follicle count cannot be diagnostic of PCO. Moreover, PCOM (size and follicle number) though is consistently found in PCOS patients, it may be seen in 25% of normal controls also.[15]

Stromal Abundance

Though not included in the Rotterdam criteria, stromal abundance is an important feature of PCO. Hyperdense stroma and stromal abundance have been described with polycystic ovaries since the first definition of the syndrome by Stein-Leventhal. Patients having long standing PCOS and long standing anovulation have denser stroma. Most severe form of stromal abundance, hyperthecosis, presents large ovaries with almost absence of cystic lesions: solid looking ovaries **(Figs 4.10A and B)**.

PATHOPHYSIOLOGY AND ULTRASOUND FINDINGS

Polycystic ovaries are a result of chronic anovulation. Mildly raised androgen levels, in early follicular phase in PCOS patients, leads to recruitment of several follicles. It is believed that androgen leads to early follicular development, but further progression is not normal due to hyperinsulinemia and/or other metabolic influence linked to obesity.[16] All these follicles do not become dominant.

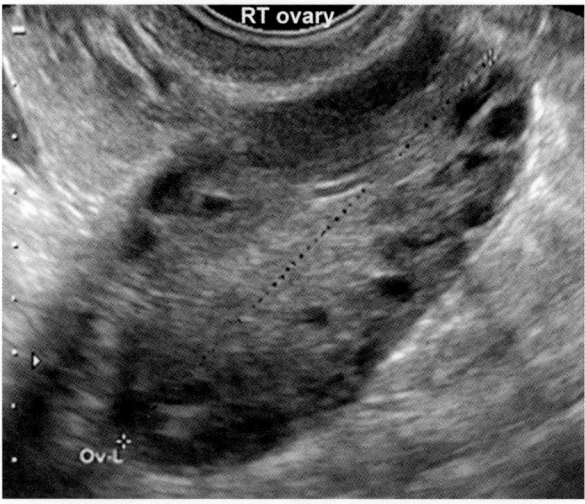

Fig. 4.10A Solid looking polycystic ovary

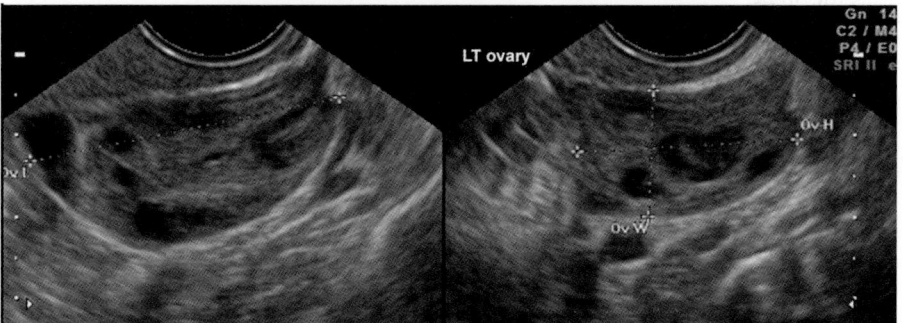

Fig. 4.10B Normal ovaries

This is because there is partial conversion of androgen to estrogen and there is also cumulative effect of minimal estradiol production by multiple follicles leading to negative feedback for FSH and positive feedback for LH. All these factors lead to maturation arrest of these follicles and premature luteinization leading to atresia. These luteinized atretic follicles ultimately contribute to the stroma leading to stromal abundance. Even when the cycle is ovulatory, in PCO patients the recruited antral follicles are more resulting in increase in atretic follicles which contribute to higher stromal density.

Stromal abundance can present as increased echogenecity because stroma is densely packed.

ASSESSMENT OF STROMAL ABUNDANCE

Polycystic ovaries show a hyperechoic stroma but assessment of this hyperechogenecity is subjective not only to the operator but also to equipment settings.[17,18] Though ovarian stroma can be stamped as hyperecoic when it is more echogenic than myometrium. This hyperechogenecity is especially useful for its

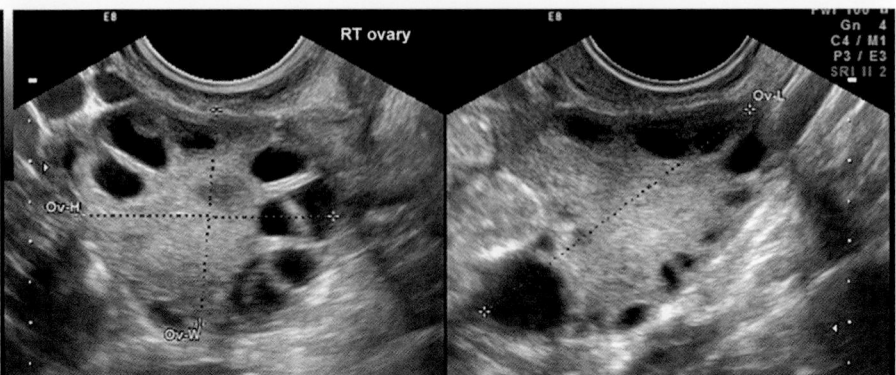

Fig. 4.11A Dense hyperechoic stroma of polycystic ovary

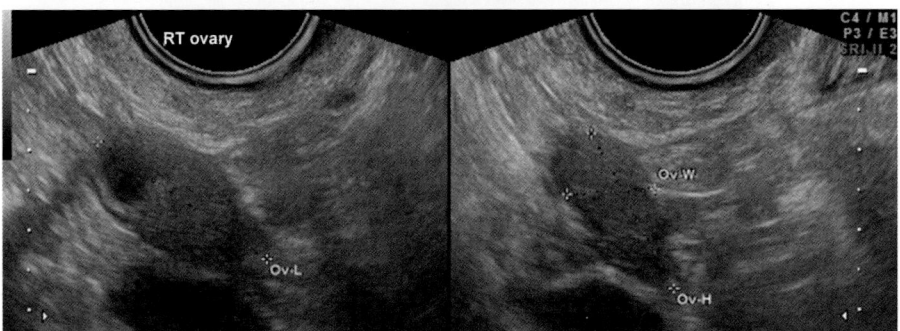

Fig. 4.11B Low reserve ovaries: small size and <3 antral follicles

differentiation from multicystic ovaries that are normally seen in adolescence and have multiple follicles, of variable sizes and nonhyperechogenic stroma. Increased stromal echogenecity for diagnosis of PCO has a sensitivity of 94% and specificity of 90%[19] **(Figs 4.11A and B)**.

But recent studies have shown that mean stromal echogenecity or total ovarian echogenecity as measured by histogram are not different in controls and PCOS. But Stromal index (stromal echogenecity/total ovarian echogenecity was significantly higher in PCOS than controls.[20]

Not only the echogenecity but also total stromal volume is also increased in polycystic ovaries. This can be measured on ultrasound as stromal area in the most longitudinal section of ovary on 2D US. As for echogenecity, this also has been found to be sensitive for diagnosis of polycystic ovarian disease. Stromal area : 4.6 cm^2 has 91% sensitivity and 86% specificity for diagnosis of PCOS. The ovarian area can also be measured in this same section. Ovarian area of 5.3 cm^2 has 93% sensitivity and 91% specificity for diagnosis of PCOS.[21]

But the ratio of stromal area to ovarian area has been found to be more reliable. **(Box 4.1)** stromal area/ovarian area (S/A) ratio also has a strongest correlation with S. androgens especially testosterone and androstenedione and insulin.[22] Stromal area/ovarian area ratio of > 0.34 is diagnostic of PCOS and can be correlated with S. androstenedione. Mean stromal area/mean ovarian area ratio of 0.34 and above also has a specificity of 100% in the same study.[23]

BOX 4.1 Sensitivity for diagnosis of polycystic ovarian syndrome

• Ovarian volume	13.21 cc	21%
• Ovarian area	7 cm²	4%
• Stromal area	1.95 cm²	62%
Stromal/total area	0.34	100%

TABLE 4.1 Ovarian volume on sonography

Ovarian volume	Right	Left
Normal	5.3 ± 2.0 cc	5.7 ± 1.6 cc
PCOD	12.2 ± 4.7cc	10.5 ± 3.6 cc[20]

STROMAL ABUNDANCE AND HORMONAL IMPLICATIONS

The proportion revealed between the stroma and the ovary surface in the median section (S/A ratio) had been indicated as a reliable marker for hyperandrogenism. Hyperandrogenic subjects showed higher values of stromal area and S/A ratio, with no difference in ovarian volume and ovarian area.[24] S/A has also been found to be the best significant predictor of elevated androgen and testosterone levels. This parameter may be used in routine clinical practice for improving US diagnosis of PCOS.[23] Stromal to ovarian ratio is lower in normal females. Stromal abundance may be better assessed by stromal volume than with stromal area. Stromal volume can be assessed by using threshold volume on vocal calculated ovarian volume.

3D ultrasound provides a new method for objective quantitative assessment of follicle count, ovarian volume, stromal volume and blood flow in the ovary.[25] Ovarian volume calculation by 3D US has been found to be useful over 2D evaluation of ovarian long diameter or volume by 2D US.

Right ovary is larger in PCOS patients, whereas left ovary is larger in normal patients **(Table 4.1)**.

Theca cells of PCOS women hyper respond to gonadotrophins (LH) and produce excess androgens. This is due to an escape of their normal down regulation to gonadotrophins. This dysregulation is linked to excess of insulin and IGF-1. Hyperinsulinemia is a key factor to the pathogenesis of PCOS. Insulin augments LH stimulated androgen production by stromal cells. Androgen in turn causes proliferation of stromal and theca cells. This leads to increased stroma in the PCO. Stromal volume was positively correlated with serum androstenedione concentrations in patients with polycystic ovarian syndrome.[26] Increased androstenedione secretion as shown earlier is due to hyperinsulinemia.[27]

A prospective study of 50 polycystic ovarian syndrome patients with 50 non PCOS patients was done over a period six months with clinical examination, baseline ultrasound scan with 2D and 3D ultrasound and fasting and postprandial insulin levels. Group A: 50 patients with normal ovulation, no hirsutism, normal menstrual cycle and normal ovarian size and group B: 50 patients with PCOS, according to Rotterdam criteria. Age range of patients for both groups was between 25 and 35 with mean age for group A was 30.4 years, mean age for group B was 29.7 years. Mean BMI in both the groups was 28, range from 25–32 kg/m². Patients with BMI < 25 kg/m², proven diabetes mellitus, other endocrinological derangement thyroid, adrenal, etc.), follicles larger than 9 mm or residual corpus luteum on day 3 and ovarian mass lesions (cystic/solid) were excluded from the study cohort. Ovarian volume and stromal volume were calculated by applying threshold volume to the VOCAL calculated volume. The threshold was set to differentiate follicles from stroma. Fasting and postprandial insulin levels were checked for all on the same day. Insulin estimation was done by chemiluminescence method. For postprandial insulin measurement patient was given 75 g of glucose after fasting blood sample and then blood sample for PP insulin was taken after 2 hours. The average values of ovarian and stromal volumes and AFC was checked for both ovaries in each patient. Two-tailed Pearson correlation was checked for ovarian volume, stromal volume and stromal volume to ovarian volume ratio with fasting insulin and postprandial insulin level each. Ovarian and stromal volumes were compared and correlated with both fasting and postprandial insulin levels. Positive correlation was seen between ovarian and stromal volumes and fasting and postprandial insulin levels. With Pearson correlation significance level of 0.01 (2-tailed) the correlation for:

- Ovarian volume to fasting insulin is 0.651
- Ovarian volume to PP insulin is 0.409
- Stromal volume to fasting insulin is 0.736
- Stromal volume to PP insulin is 0.428

Stromal and ovarian volumes and AFC correlated significantly well with the fasting insulin levels, more than with postprandial insulin levels in obese PCOS patients. It is the stromal volume that can be best correlated with fasting insulin levels followed by ovarian volumes and AFC.[28]

A similar study has also been done earlier. Study by Pache et al. has shown that the degree of insulin resistance can be correlated with ovarian volume and stromal echogenecity.[29] A retrospective observational study done with 50 PCOS patients showing correlation between ovarian and stromal volumes with fasting and postprandial insulin levels. But in this study neither BMI, nor age group were defined. In PCOS patients a strong and similar correlation was seen between ovarian and stromal volumes to fasting and postprandial insulin levels.

ARRANGEMENT OF FOLLICLES

The antral and atretic follicles get arranged peripherally or are dispersed in the stroma and thus may categorize polycystic ovary as peripheral and general cystic pattern. In peripheral cystic pattern there is typical garland like arrangement of follicles and in generalized cystic pattern, the follicles can be seen throughout the ovary[30] **(Figs 4.12A and B)**. Though one school of thought believes that peripheral cystic pattern polycystic ovaries and generalized cystic pattern polycystic ovaries have different histopathological and endocrine bases.[31] According to another theory, the ovary is multifollicular in adolescence. Follicles that are < 9 mm are exposed to LH and undergo atresia and make stroma denser giving rise to generalized cystic polycystic ovary. As the disease progresses, gradually the follicles in the central part of the ovary, in the effort and process of recruitment

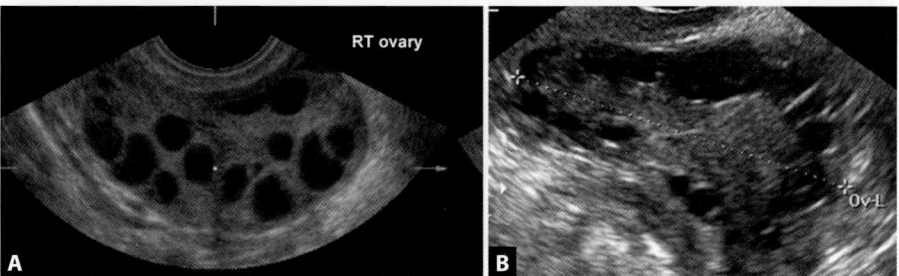

Figs 4.12A and B (A) Generalized polycystic pattern; (B) Peripheral polycystic pattern: polycystic ovary

reach the periphery or are pushed out to periphery by expanding stroma. These undergo atresia ultimately leading to peripheral cystic polycystic ovary.[25,32] So multicystic ovary to generalized cystic PCO, and then to peripheral cystic PCO is a process of evolution of the disease.

Stromal Vascularity

Based on 3D US, women with PCOS have an increased stromal volume and vascularity. Even with same echogenecity, PCOS has more stromal flow. In polycystic ovaries even on 3rd day of the cycle intraovarian stromal flow is seen and they have moderate to low resistance flow with RI of 0.50–0.58.[33]

Elevated LH levels may be responsible for increased stromal vascularization due to neoangiogenesis, catecholaminergic stimulation and leukocyte and cytokine activation. This vascularity is inversely related to LH/FSH ratio. Tonic secretion of LH in early follicular phase in PCOS is also associated with theca and stromal cell hyperplasia and consequent androgen production. This androgen hypersecretion is responsible for not only increased follicular recruitment but also for vasoconstrictive effect on the uterine arteries. This effect is thought to be due to activation of specific receptors in arterial walls and collagen and elastin deposition in smooth muscle cells. Uterine artery PI is > 3 and sometimes the diastolic flow is absolutely absent. Even in later phases of the cycle this effect continues. This leads to inadequate perfusion of the endometrium and is thought to be responsible for blastocyst implantation failure and high abortion rate in PCOS.

Stromal Vascularity and Hormonal Implications

Looking to the hormonal correlation with the Doppler findings, it is evident that in patients in whom the hormonal milieu is worse the Doppler findings are more prominent. As discussed earlier the peripheral cystic pattern of PCO is an advanced stage then generalized cystic pattern and so the intraovarian vascularity and uterine artery resistance are more in peripheral polycystic ovaries than in generalized polycystic ovaries. In 22% of GCP PCO intraovarian vessels are not recognized.[34] Stromal vascularity is significantly higher in women with PCOS who are hyperandrogenic and lean rather than normoandrogenic and obese.[35] Fertile controls and PCOS women had similar total ovarian 3D power Doppler flow indices. Normal weight PCOS women had significantly higher total ovarian 3D power Doppler flow indices than their overweight counterparts.[36] Higher age, obesity and amenorrhea as compared to young age, normal weight and oligomenorrhea show higher uterine artery resistance and increased ovarian stromal flow. These are the patients who also have higher LH and higher androstenedione levels and higher ovarian volumes. Uterine artery resistance has also been found to be higher in obese than in lean patients and is also associated with hyperinsulinemia, high triglycerides, low high density lipids and higher heamtocrit values. Oligoanovulatory patients with PCO but without hyperandrogenism have mild endocrine and metabolic features of PCOS.[37]

The results were different when 3D and 3D power Doppler were used. Women with PCOS had higher AFC (median 16.3 v/s 5.5 per ovary), ovarian volume (12.56 v/s 5.6 mL), stromal volume (10.79 v/s 4.69 mL) and stromal vascularization (VI 3.85 v/s 2.79%, VFI 1.27 v/s 0.85). Ovarian stromal FI is higher (33.94 v/s 29.30) in hirsutes than in normoandrogenic PCOS women. But in PCOS women with obesity the vascularity was lower than in normal weight women (VI 3.25 v/s 4.51%, VFI 1.22 v/s 1.56).[38] Though VI, FI and VFI were significantly higher in normal weight PCOS than in obese PCOS women.[36] This explains excessive response to gonadotrophins in PCOS females.

Endometrium in Polycystic Ovarian Syndrome

Normal endometrial growth and regeneration after shedding off is a result of balanced estrogen followed by progesterone exposure and ultimately withdrawal of both. In patients with polycystic ovarian syndrome, the endometrial behavior is also typical. This is because of persistent exposure to estrogen. Chronic anovulation and prolonged exposure to estrogen leads to increase androgen and low progesterone levels these together lead to persistent increase in endometrial thickness. Because of cumulative estrogen of several medium and large antral follicles and few dominant follicles, endometrium grows and becomes multilayered early in the cycle. This does not correspond with the follicular status. When the follicles grow further towards maturity the total estrogen level (cumulative of all follicles), rises much higher than that for one mature follicle, leading to homogeneous isoechoic endometrium. High estrogen levels lead to a positive feedback to the pituitary for LH. This leads to progesterone production from the theca cells of the ovary even before the follicle ruptures and therefore a hyperechogenecity of the endometrium starts from the periphery of its margins even before the follicular rupture. This is typically described as out of phase endometrium or advancement of endometrium.

Subendometrial and endometrial blood flow is significantly impaired in women with PCOS who have clinical signs of hyperandrogenism. Hyperandrogenism leads to increased smooth muscle tone, increased tone in the muscularis of uterine artery and increased uterine artery resistance, which is being carried forward to its branches. Endometrial blood flow is impaired in women with polycystic ovarian syndrome who are clinically hyperandrogenic. This ultimately results into bad endometrial receptivity, implantation failure or early abortions in PCOS patients.[39]

Persistent estrogen exposure may result into unopposed endometrial growth and proliferation of endometrial glands. This is described as endometrial hyperplasia. It may be cystic glandular hyperplasia in 0.4%, and adenomatous hyperplasia in 18% of the women with PCOS. Endometrial thickness of >14 mm in a premenopausal woman is considered endometrial hyperplasia.[40] This endometrial is echogenic and shows multiple small anechoic areas **(Figs 4.13A and B)**. Peripheral distribution of regularly separated vessels is typical of endometrial hyperplasia. These vessels have a mean RI of 0.5.[41] But the vascular distribution is not very dense. Insulin resistance and hyperinsulinemia in PCOS patients adds to mitogenic effect in the endometrium and higher risk of endometrial carcinoma at earlier age. IGF I modulate the effect of estrogen and progesterone on the endometrium. Endometrial carcinoma though a seriously dreaded late complication. On ultrasound, it is suspected when a thick endometrium has heterogeneous echogenicity, interrupted endometrio-myometrial junction, a dense irregular vascular distribution and the vessels showing very low resistance flow **(Figs 4.14A and B)**.

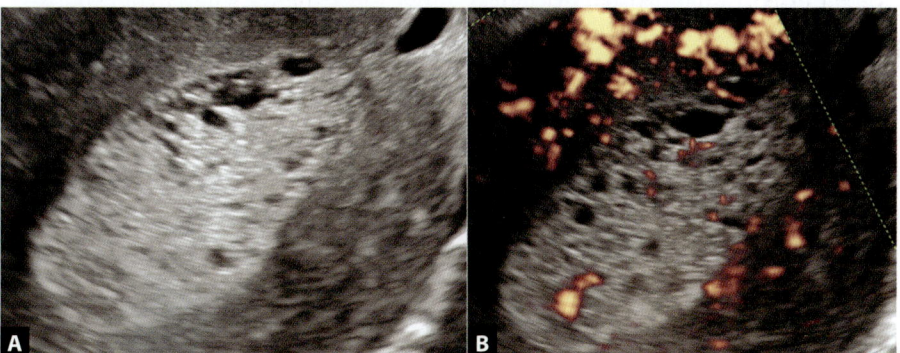

Figs 4.13A and B (A) Endometrial hyperplasia of PCOS on b mode; (B) Power Doppler assessment showing vascular distribution in endometrial hyperplasia

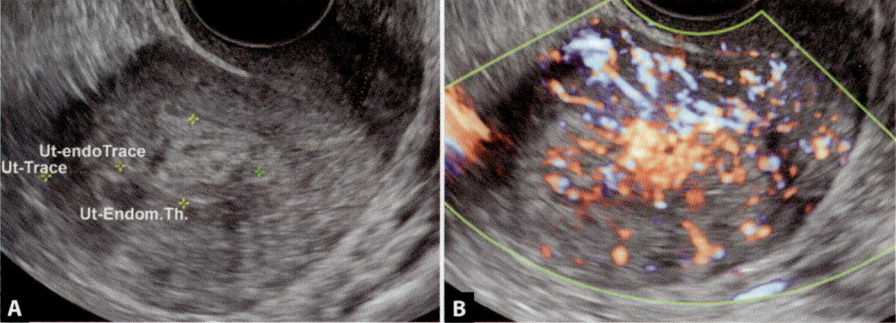

Figs 4.14A and B (A) B mode ultrasound image of endometrial carcinoma showing heterogeneous, thick endometrium with interrupted junctional zone; (B) On power Doppler, the endometrium shows dense irregularly distributed vessels

CONCLUSION

Though large ovary and multiple antral follicles are generally considered as diagnostic features of PCO, these are not the most consistent ones. Stromal abundance and increased stromal vascularity are the most consistent features and these can be explained by the pathophysiology of PCOS. All the ultrasound features of PCO can be correlated with and explained by the hormonal derangement occurring in PCO.

KEY POINTS

- Ovulatory dysfunction and androgen excess are cardinal features of PCO.
- Antral follicle count and stromal characteristics are found to be better discriminators than ovarian volume.
- Average value of 26 or more follicles per ovary is a reliable threshold for detecting polycystic ovaries
- Stromal abundance is the most consistent ultrasound feature of PCOS and that can be established by stromal echogenicity, stromal area or stromal volume.
- Stromal abundance can be correlated with the high LH and high insulin levels.
- PCO ovaries also show hypervascularity due to high LH and VEGF.

REFERENCES

1. Aziz R, Carmina E, Dewailly D, Diamanti-Kandaraakis E, Escobar-Morreale HF, Futterweit W, et al. The androgen excess and PCOS society criteria for polycystic ovarian syndrome: the complete task force report. Fertil Steril. 2009;91:456-88.
2. Norman RJ, Dewailly D, Legros RS, Hickey TE. Polycystic ovarian syndrome. Lancet. 2007;370:685-97.
3. Dr. Thatcher: Defining PCOS- a perspective: The American Infertility Association News letter, February 2001.
4. Balen A, Bouchard Ph, Dahlgren E, Devoto L, Diamanti E, Dunaif A, Filicori M, Homburg R, Ibanez L, Laven J, Magoffin D, Nestler J, Norman R, Pasquali R, Pugeat M, Strauss J, Tan S, Taylor A, Wild R, Wild S. The Rotterdam ESHRE/ASRM-Sponsored PCOS Consensus Workshop Group. Revised 2003 consensus on diagnostic criteria and long-term health risks related to polycystic ovarian syndrome. Fertil Steril. 2004;81(1):19-25.
5. Po-Mui Lam, N.Raine-Fenning, The role of three-dimensional ultrasonography in polycystic ovarian syndrome. Hum Reprod. 2006;21(9):2209-15.
6. Takahashi K, Eda Y, Abu Musa A, Okada S, et al. Transvaginal ultrasound imaging, histopathology and endocrinopathy in patients with polycystic ovarian syndrome. Hum Reprod. 1994;9:1231-6.
7. Kyei-Mensah A et al, Relationship of ovarian stromal volume to serum androgen concentrations in patients with PCOS. Hum Reprod. 1998;13:1437-41.

8. Wu M-H, Tang H-H, Hsu C-C, Wang S-T, Huang KE. The role of three-dimensional ultrasonographic images in ovarian measurement. Fertil Steril. 1998;69:1152-5.
9. Legro RS, Gnatuk CL, Kunselman AR, Dunaif A. Changes in glucose tolerance over time in women with polycystic ovarian syndrome: a controlled study. J Clin Endocrinol Metab. 2005;90:3236-42.
10. Jonard S, Robert Y, Cortet-Rudelli C, Decanter C, Dewailly D. Ultrasound examination of polycystic ovaries: is it worth counting the follicles? Hum Reprod. 2003;18:598-603.
11. Jonard S, Robert Y, Cortet-Rudelli C, Pigny P, Decanter C, Dewailly D. Ultrasound examination of polycystic ovaries: is it worth counting the follicles? Oxford Journals, Medicine & Health Human Reproduction. 2003;18(3):598-603.
12. Mei-Jou Chen, Wei-Shiung Yang, Chi-ling Chen, Ming-Yih Wu, Yu-Shih Yang, Hong-Nerng Ho.The relationship between anti-Müllerian hormones, androgen and insulin resistance on the number of antral follicles in women with polycystic ovarian syndrome Hum Reprod. 2008;23(4):952-7.
13. Dewailly D, Gronier H, Poncelet E, Robin G, Leroy M, Pigny P, et al. Diagnosis of polycystic ovarian syndrome (PCOS): revisiting the threshold values of follicle count on ultrasound and of the serum AMH level for the definition of polycystic ovaries. Hum Reprod. 2011;26(11):3123-9.
14. Lujan ME, Jarrett BY, Brooks ED, Reines JK, Peppin AK, Muhn N, et al. Updated ultrasound criteria for polycystic ovarian syndrome: reliable thresholds for elevated follicle population and ovarian volume. Hum Reprod. 2013;28(5):1361-8.
15. Polson DW, Wadsworth J, Adams J, Franks S. Polycystic ovaries—a common finding in normal women. The Lancet. 1988;331:870-2.
16. Jonard S, Robert Y, Cortet-Rudelli C, Decanter C, Dewailly D. Ultrasound examination of polycystic ovaries: is it worth counting the follicles? Hum Reprod 2003;18:598-603
17. Pache TD, Wladimiroff JW, Hop WC, Fauser BCJM. How to discriminate between normal and polycystic ovaries - TVS study. Radiology. 1992;183:421-3.
18. Buckett WM, Bouzayen R, Watkin KL, Tulandi T, Tan SL.Ovarian stromal echogenicity in women with normal and polycystic ovaries. Hum Reprod. 1999;14:618-21.
19. Dewailly D, Robert Y, Helin I, et al. Ovarian stromal hypertrophy in hyperandrogenic women. Clin Endocrinol (Oxf). 1994;41:557-62.
20. Belosi C, Selvaggi L, Apa R, Guido M, Romualdi D, Fulghesu AM, Lanzone A. PCOS diagnosis solved by ESHRE/ASRM 2003 consensus or could it include ultrasound examination of the ovarian stroma? Hum Reprod. 2006;21:3108-15.
21. Wu M-H, Tang H-H, Hsu C-C, Wang S-T, Huang KE. The role of three-dimensional ultrasonographic images in ovarian measurement. Fertil Steril. 1998;69:1152-5.
22. Fulghesu AM, Ciampelli M, Belosi C, Apa R, Pavone V, Lanzone A. A new ultrasound criterion for the diagnosis of polycystic ovarian syndrome: the ovarian stroma/total area ratio. Fertil Steril. 2001;76:326-31.
23. Fulghesu AM, Angioni S, Frau E, et al. Ultrasound in polycystic ovarian syndrome—the measuring of ovarian stroma and relationship with circulating androgens: results of multicentric study. Hum Reprod. 2007;22:2501-8.
24. Jonard S, Robert Y, Dewailly D. Revisint the ovarian volume as diagnostic criterion for polycystic ovaries. Hum Reprod. 2005;20:2893-8.
25. Ardaens Y, Robert Y, Lemaitre L, Fossati P, Dewailly D. Polycystic ovarian disease: contribution of transvaginal endosonography and reassessment of ultrsonographic diagnosis. Fertil Steril. 1991;55:1062-8.
26. Balen A, et al. Polycystic ovarian syndrome: A guide to clinical management, Taylor & Francis Group, 2005.
27. Pache TD, et al. Association between ovarian changes assessed by TVS & clinical & endocrine signs of PCOS. Feril Steril. 1993,59:544-9.
28. Nagori CB, Panchal SY. Assessing correlation between ovarian & stromal volumes and fasting & postprandial insulin levels in PCOS patients. Presented at ISUOG 2008, Chicago.

29. Pache, et al. Association between ovarian changes assessed by transvaginal sonography and clinical and endocrine signs of polycystic ovarian syndrome. Fertil Steril. 1993;59:544-9.
30. Matsunaga I, Hata T, Kitao M. Ultrasonographic identification of polycystic ovary. Asia Oceania J Obstet Gynecol. 1985;11:227-32.
31. Takahashi K, Ozaki T, Okada M, Uchida A, Kitao M. Relationship between ultrasonography and histopathological changes in polycystic ovarian syndrome. Hum Reprod. 1994;9:2255-8.
32. Robert Y, Dubrulle F, Gailandre L, et al. Ultrasound assessment of ovarian stroma hypertrophy in hyperandrogenism and ovulation disorders: visual analysis versus computerized quantification. Fertil Steril. 1995;64:307-12.
33. Battalgia C, Artini PG, D'Ambrogio G, Genazzani A, D Genazzani AR. The role of colour Doppler imaging in the diagnosis of polycystic ovarian syndrome. Am J Obstet Gynecol. 1995;172:108-13.
34. Battalgia C, Artini PG, Salvatori M, Giulini S, Petraglia F, Maxia N, Volpe A. Ultrasonographic patterns of polycystic ovaries; colour Doppler and hormonal correlations. Ultrasound Obstet Gynecol. 1998;11:332-6.
35. Ozkan S, Vural B, Caliskan E, Bodur H, Turkoz E, Vural F. Colour Doppler sonographic analysis of uterine and ovarian artery blood flow in women with PCOS. J Clin Ultrasound. 2007;35:305-13.
36. Ng EH, Chan CC, Yeung WS, Ho PC. Comparison of ovarian stromal blood flow between fertile women with normal ovaries and infertile women with polycystic ovarian syndrome. Hum Reprod. 2005;20:1881-6.
37. Dewailly D, Jonard SC, Reyss AC, Leroy M, Pigny P. Oligoanovulation with polycystic ovaries but not overt hyperandrogenism JCEM, 91(10).
38. Lam PM, Jhonson IR, Rainne-Fenning NJ. Three dimensional ultrasound features of the polycystic ovary and the effect of different phenotypic expressions on these parameters. Hum Reprod. 2007;22:3116-23.
39. Lam P, Johnson I, Rainne-Fenning N. Endometrial blood flow is impaired in women with polycystic ovarian syndrome who are clinically hyperandrogenic. Ultrasound Obstet Gynecol. 2009;34:326-34.
40. Kurjak A, Kupesic S, Zalud I, Predanic M. Transvaginal colour Doppler: In: Dodson MG (Ed). Transvaginal ultrasound. New York: Churchill Livingstone. 1995. pp. 325-39.
41. Kupesic-Urek S, Shalan H, Kurjak A. Early detection of endometrial cancer by transvaginal colour Doppler. EUROBS. 1993;49:46-9.

SECTION 3

POLYCYSTIC OVARIAN SYNDROME AND FERTILITY

5. Infertility in Polycystic Ovarian Syndrome
6. Ovulation Inductions in Polycystic Ovarian Syndrome
7. Assisted Reproductive Technology in Polycystic Ovarian Syndrome
8. Complications in Assisted Reproductive Technique
9. Embryology in Polycystic Ovarian Syndrome

SECTION 2

CHAPTER 5

Infertility in Polycystic Ovarian Syndrome

Asha Baxi, Dhaval Baxi

INTRODUCTION

Polycystic ovarian syndrome (PCOS), characterized by anovulatory cycles and hyperandrogenism is one of the common causes of infertility in women and the most common endocrinopathy in women.[1] The classic syndrome was originally described by Stein and Leventhal as the association of amenorrhea, hirsutism and obesity with ovaries containing multiple cysts. It has now been recognized that the syndrome comprises of a spectrum of features: hyperandrogenism, menstrual dysfunction, central obesity and polycystic ovaries. The cause of PCOS is not yet known and has a multifactorial etiology linked to lifestyle and environmental factors. It has also been found to run in families, suggesting a possible genetic component.[2] Women with PCOS usually present to the gynecologist with complaints of menstrual dysfunction, hyperandrogenic features and reproductive problems, either due to subfertility or early pregnancy loss.

EPIDEMIOLOGY AND DIAGNOSIS

In 1990, the National Institute of Health (NIH) in its conference on PCOS defined PCOS as a chronic syndrome with menstrual dysfunction and hyperandrogenism (clinical/biochemical) after excluding secondary causes.[3] In 2003, European Society for Human Reproduction and Embryology (ESHRE) and American Society for Reproductive Medicine (ASRM) cosponsored the Rotterdam Polycystic ovarian syndrome Consensus Workshop Group to revise the guidelines for diagnosis and management of PCOS, where they added an additional finding of polycystic ovaries to the diagnostic criteria.[4] To be diagnosed with PCOS by the Rotterdam criteria, a woman must have two of the following three manifestations: irregular or absent ovulation, elevated levels of androgenic hormones, and/or enlarged ovaries containing at least 12 follicles each. Other conditions with similar signs, such as androgen-secreting tumors or Cushing's syndrome, must be ruled out. The prevalence of PCOS in women using the NIH/NICHD criteria was reported to be 4-8%[5,6] but the prevalence almost doubled when the Rotterdam criteria was used.[7]

PATHOPHYSIOLOGY OF PCOS-ASSOCIATED INFERTILITY

Polycystic ovaries have been reported in up to 75% of women with anovulatory infertility.[8] A high prevalence has also been reported in women with multiple miscarriages.[9] Ovarian function in women with PCOS associated infertility is characterized by abnormal steroidogenesis and disordered folliculogenesis. There is acceleration of gonadotropin-releasing hormone (GnRH) pulsatile activity, hypersecretion of luteinizing hormone (LH), theca stroma cell hyperactivity and hypofunction of the follicular stimulating hormone (FSH) granuloma cell axis. This results in follicular arrest, disruption of ovarian cyclicity and excessive androgen production with or without hirsutism. Ovaries of women with PCOS contain excessive number of primary and secondary follicles[10] and follicular arrest between 5–8 mm.[11]

ETIOLOGY OF EXCESSIVE FOLLICULAR GROWTH

While the numbers of primary and secondary follicles are up to 6 times than that in the normal ovaries, the pool of primordial follicles remains the same. This may indicate that there may be an intrinsic ovarian abnormality leading to increased recruitment of follicles. Studies have linked the increased number of follicles in polycystic ovaries to high serum levels of testosterone and androstenedione suggesting that intra-ovarian hyperandrogenism plays an important role, although other factors may also be involved.[12] Extraovarian factors such as excessive LH were thought to be the cause of hyperandrogenism but recent data suggests LH hypersecretion to be a consequence of impaired feedback due to ovarian dysfunction rather than the cause.[13] Hyperinsulinemia and insulin resistance also contribute to hyperandrogenism by amplifying the action of LH on steroid production.[14] Inhibin produced by granulosa cells is thought to enhance basal and LH-induced androgen production by theca cells through a paracrine effect from granulosa cells.[12] Women with PCOS have higher levels of anti-Müllerian hormone (AMH) which has been significantly linked with higher serum testosterone and androstenedione levels suggesting a possible paracrine effect on theca cells. A possible protection of follicles from atresia has been proposed via the hypersecretion of growth factors such as EGF and TNF-α leading to multiple small follicles in the ovaries.

ETIOLOGY OF FOLLICULAR ARREST

Follicular arrest accounts for anovulation by hampering the development of a single dominant follicle. The low and constant levels of FSH levels in PCOS may be the critical abnormality leading to follicular arrest. The lack of rise of FSH in the cycle may be due to the result of feedback from the hypothalamic pituitary ovarian (HPO) axis due to excessive ovarian steroid production or due to increased inhibin production. Inhibin is secreted in a pulsatile manner in normal ovulating women but in women with anovulation due to PCOS, no such pattern is seen, though it may reappear after laparoscopic ovarian drilling.[15]

Local growth factors such as EGF, TFG-α and β and cytokines such as TNF alpha have been demonstrated to have an inhibitory activity on FSH activity. They have inhibitory effects on local estrogen production from granuloma cells and correlate inversely with follicular size.[16] Recently, the role of anti-Müllerian hormone has also gained importance. Women with PCOS have higher AMH levels and an inverse AMH-E2 level relationship.[17] In a recent study, the levels of AMH correlated positively with the number of follicles between 2–5 mm in normal as well as in women with PCOS, but not with 6–9 mm follicles and were also negatively related to FSH levels. AMH levels were positively related with serum testosterone and androstenedione levels in PCOS only. Also, the ratio of AMH/number of follicles was not increased. These findings suggest that AMH may play a role in the disordered folliculogenesis in PCOS by modulation of ovarian E2 synthesis and that the inhibitory effect of AMH is not due to an intrafollicular excess but due to an excessive amount of AMH within the ovarian micro-environment of the selected follicles.

In women with PCOS, there is an increased responsiveness of theca tissue to LH versus normal ovaries. Granulosa cells have also been shown to acquire LH receptors prematurely and in a higher number compared to normal ovaries. This premature response to LH indicates an advanced stage of development triggering premature luteinization and arrest of follicular growth.[18]

Insulin resistance in PCOS is frequently seen in obese women. Anovulatory women have higher body mass index (BMI) than women with regular ovulation. Insulin and Insulin such as growth factors act as co-gonadotropins in the ovary. In theca cells, they act synergistically with LH to increase androgen production, whereas in granulosa cells, they increase FSH-mediated estradiol production. Also, acting with LH, hyperinsulinemia may induce premature maturation of granuloma cells and may cause follicular arrest.[19]

The heterogeneity of PCOS may very well reflect multiple pathophysiologic mechanisms, and the disorder itself can be initiated at any one of many entry points. Based on our current understanding of PCOS, the underlying pathogenetic mechanisms can be categorized as follows: (1) Insulin resistance and hyperinsulinemia, (2) Disruption of the hypothalamic-pituitary-gonadal axis, (3) Dysregulation of ovarian steroidogenesis, (4) Abnormalities of adrenal steroidogenesis, and (5) Genetic factors.

INSULIN RESISTANCE AND HYPERINSULINEMIA

Greater than normal amount of insulin is required to elicit a quantitatively normal response is called insulin resistance. Insulin resistance is a common feature of the syndrome, and both obese and nonobese women with the syndrome are more insulin resistant and hyperinsulinemic than age- and weight-matched normal women.[20] In PCOS patients, secretory function of pancreatic β-cell is effected along with the decrease in insulin sensitivity. The clinical expression is directly proportional to the severity of hyperinsulinemia.[21]

The mechanism of insulin signaling to define the pathogenesis of insulin resistance in PCOS, Insulin action is mediated through a protein tyrosine kinase receptor. Tyrosine autophosphorylation increases the insulin receptors tyrosine kinase activity, whereas serine phosphorylation inhibits it. A potential mechanism of insulin resistance in women with PCOS appears to be related to excessive serine phosphorylation of insulin receptors. Interestingly, serine phosphorylation of insulin receptor substrate-1 appears to be the mechanism of the tumor necrosis factor (TNF)-α-mediated insulin resistance of obesity. Serine phosphorylation has also been shown to increase P450cl7 enzyme activity, leading to higher androgen biosynthesis.[22] It is therefore possible that a single defect—serine phosphorylation—produces both insulin resistance and hyperandrogenism in a subgroup of women with PCOS.

Ovaries and the Effect of Insulin

PCOS causes the ovaries to produce the cluster of small cysts filled with fluid and contain immature eggs. The effect of PCOS and its expression is different in all. Some are less sensitive to insulin while some are hypersensitive. Depending on the severity of the disease, insulin causes production and imbalance of hormones. Increased levels of Insulin and androgen affect the ovulation cycle leading to delayed menses, irregularity in menses or anovulation. Some women conceive naturally without any medications, while some faces miss abortion and other needs medical assistance. Insulin affects the FSH, and induces the production of estradiol by granulosa cells. Insulin acts like gonadotropin in steroidogenesis of theca cells. Excess of Insulin increases LH stimulated androgen secretion by the proliferation of theca cells. At genetic levels, it increases P450c17 messenger RNA levels, up-regulate LH receptors, and up-regulate ovarian insulin-like growth factor-1 (IGF-1) receptors.[23]

Gonadotropins and the Effect of Insulin

Hypothalamus and pituitary glands contains insulin receptors which in presence of high insulin enhances the amplitude of LH pulses in obese women with PCOS. Insulin also stimulates GnRH, increasing release of LH and FSH in pituitary cells but still it is not clarified. Insulin sensitizing agents, which reduces insulin levels also helps in reduction of basal levels of LH and LH response to GnRH.[24]

Insulin, IGF, and Sex Hormone-binding Globulins

Insulin binds to the IGF-1 receptors with an affinity 50–500 times less than that of IGF-1. The crossover effect of insulin with IGF-1 receptors on ovarian theca cells is therefore an important consideration at high insulin concentrations, leading to hyperandrogenism.[25] There is a significant increase in the IGF-1 to IGF binding protein-1 ratio in women with PCOS, leading to increased bioavailability of IGF-1 for theca cells steroidogeneis.[26] A reduction in hyperinsulinemia in PCOS patients causes a significant increase in circulating levels of SHBG, leading to improvement in hyperandrogenism because of an inverse relationship between insulinemia and SHBG plasma levels.

Insulin and the Adrenal Glands

Physiologic concentrations of insulin and IGF-1 were found to increase messenger RNA levels irrespective of adrenocorticotropic hormone leading to higher production of adrenal steroids.[27] When circulating levels of insulin were reduced by the administration of metformin, a significant reduction in the response of 17-hydroxyprogesterone, androstenedione, and testosterone to adrenocorticotropic hormone is noted.[28]

Insulin Resistance and Obesity

It is universally accepted that obesity and insulin resistance are correlated. Insulin resistance is observed more in obese PCOS as compare to lean PCOS because central obesity is considered to have a major role in induction of insulin resistance. Increased production of free-fatty acids in obesity may inhibit insulin clearance and induce defects in cell uptake of glucose and glycogen synthesis.[29] Expression of cytokine TNF-α is greater in adipose tissues and muscle of obese animals. TNF-α, as mentioned earlier, exerts a direct effect on insulin signaling by stimulating serine phosphorylation of insulin receptor substrate, with consequent impairment of the cellular response to insulin.[30] Interestingly, higher levels of TNF-α have been reported even in PCOS patients of normal weight, implying its central role in the induction of insulin resistance in PCOS patients.

Insulin Resistance, Glucose Intolerance, and Diabetes Mellitus

PCOS women are at increased risk for Type 2 Diabetes Mellitus compare to normal women as studied by Dunaif et al. Around 40% of PCOS women have impaired glucose tolerance (IGT) or T2DM women with PCOS are at significantly increased risk for IGT (31.1%) and T2DM (7.5% undiagnosed). Even non-obese women with PCOS also have a higher incidence of IGT and T2DM. The incidence of gestational diabetes mellitus is higher in women with PCOS.

DISRUPTION OF HYPOTHALAMIC-PITUITARY-GONADAL AXIS IN PCOS

Hypersecretion of LH is one of the typical syndromes of PCOS. Increased secretion of LH both from basally and in response to GNRH is observed in PCOS from hypothalamus and pituitary. In PCOS, LH/GnRH pulses are persistently rapid and favor LH synthesis, hyperandrogenemia, and impaired follicular maturation but the mechanism is still unclear. Insensitivity of the hypothalamus and pituitary to the negative feedback of hyperandrogenemia can also be the reason as suggested in some studies. The potential roles of hyperinsulinemia and hyperandrogenemia, in women with PCOS, in modifying ovarian steroid regulation of GnRH pulse generator in neuroendocrine system needs to be clarified, although an intrinsic abnormality of ovarian steroidogenesis also cannot be excluded.

DEREGULATION OF OVARIAN STEROIDOGENESIS

Multiple studies have proposed an alternate model of PCOS as a form of gonadotropin-dependent ovarian hyperandrogenism in which the central abnormality is an elevated intraovarian androgen concentration.[31] According to these studies, women with PCOS shows increased production of 17α-hydroxyprogesterone and androstenedione in response to LH. This is because of enzymatic dysregulation of ovarian steroidogenesis. Ovarian follicles show arrested granulosa cells and very active theca cells in PCOS patients due to FSH blockage or insensitivity of ovarian follicular cells. Factors such as inhibin, IGF system, and insulin have been incriminated in the etiology of follicular arrest in PCOS patients. Follicles are therefore unable to change their microenvironment from androgen dominance to estrogen dominance, a change that is essential for continued follicular growth and development.[32]

GENETIC FACTORS IN PCOS

Genetic factors have a strong role in PCOS. In a prospective study of first-degree female relatives of women with PCOS, of the 46% of sisters thus affected, one half had PCOS and one half had hyperandrogenemia with regular menstrual cycles. Insulin resistance also demonstrated familial aggregation consistent with a genetic trait. Twins of PCOS women have shown a high degree of concordance for both PCOS and insulin resistance.[33] From the results of both linkage and association studies, Frank, et al.[21] have demonstrated that the steroid synthesis gene *CYP11A*, which encodes for P450scc, and the insulin gene variable number of tandem repeats regulatory polymorphism are important factors underlying the genetic basis of PCOS and may explain the heterogeneity of the syndrome. PCOS appears to represent a quantitative trait in which a relatively small number of key genes contribute to the observed clinical and biochemical heterogeneity in conjunction with environmental factors.[34]

CONCLUSION

The pathophysiology of PCOS is poorly understand. PCOS is now clearly defined as a syndrome which causes a series of metabolic consequensces.[35] More than one organ is involved such as ovaries, liver, pancreas, cardiovascular system and the hypothalamopituary axis. The symptoms are produced due to the vicious cycle of hormonal disturbances, one of the most important symptoms being infertility. The pathophysiology of PCOS causing infertility has to be identified and the management focused should be indivialized, and also it should take care of future metabolic consequences. The management of infertility would be sucessful only, if the disturbed pathophysiology and all the areas which are affected are taken care of.

KEY POINTS

- PCOS is a spectrum of hyperandrogenism, hyperinsulinemia, menstrual dysfunction, obesity and polycystic ovaries.
- The pathophysiology of PCOS is multifactorial, has a genetic component but also linked to lifestyle and environmental factors.

- PCOS leads to disordered ovarian function and anovulation characterized by abnormal steroidogenesis and folliculogenesis.
- PCOS with increased androgen levels and abnormal hypothalamic pituitary axis leads to changes in microenvironment of the follicle causing follicular arrest and disruption of ovarian cycle contributing to infertility.

REFERENCES

1. Aziz R, Woods KS, Reyna R, Key TJ, Knochenhauer ES, Yildiz BO. The prevalence and features of the polycystic ovarian syndrome in an unselected population. J Clin Endocrinol Metab. 2004;89:2745-9.
2. Stein IF, Leventhal ML. Amenorrhoea associated with bilateral polycystic ovaries. Am J Obstet Gynecol. 1935;29(2):181-91.
3. Azziz R. PCOS: a diagnostic challenge. Reprod Biomed Online. 2004;8(6):644-8.
4. The Rotterdam ESHRE/ASRM-sponsored PCOS consensus workshop group. Revised 2003 consensus on diagnostic criteria and long term health risks related to polycystic ovarian syndrome. Hum Reprod. 2004;19(1):41-7.
5. Asunción M, Calvo RM, San Millán JL, Sancho J, Avila S, Escobar-Morreale HF. A prospective study of the prevalence of the polycystic ovarian syndrome in unselected Caucasian women from Spain. J Clin Endocrinol Metab. 2000;85(7):2434-8.
6. Diamanti-Kandarakis E, Kouli CR, Bergiele AT, Filandra FA, Tsianateli TC, Spina GG, et al. A survey of the polycystic ovarian syndrome in the Greek island of Lesbos: hormonal and metabolic profile. J Clin Endocrinol Metab. 1999;84(11):4006-11.
7. March WA, Moore VM, Willson KJ, Phillips DI, Norman RJ, Davies MJ. The prevalence of polycystic ovarian syndrome in a community sample assessed under contrasting diagnostic criteria. Hum Reprod. 2010;25(2):544-51.
8. Polson DW, Adams J, Wadsworth J, Franks S. Polycystic ovaries: a common finding in normal women. Lancet. 1988;1(8590):870-2.
9. Kousta E, White DM, Cela E, McCarthy MI, Franks S. The prevalence of polycystic ovaries in women with infertility. Hum Reprod. 1999;14(11):2720-3.
10. Webber LJ, Stubbs S, Stark J, Trew GH, Margara R, Hardy K, et al. Formation and early development of follicles in the polycystic ovary. Lancet. 2003;362(9389):1017-21.
11. Pigny P, Merlen E, Robert Y, Cortet-Rudelli C, Decanter C, Jonard S, et al. Elevated serum level of anti-mullerian hormone in patients with polycystic ovarian syndrome: relationship to the ovarian follicle excess and to the follicular arrest. J Clin Endocrinol Metab. 2003;88(12):5957-62.
12. Jonard S, Dewailly D. The follicular excess in polycystic ovaries, due to intra-ovarian hyperandrogenism, may be the main culprit for the follicular arrest. Hum Reprod Update. 2004;10(2):107-17.
13. Van der Spuy ZM, Dyer SJ. The pathogenesis of infertility and early pregnancy loss in polycystic ovarian syndrome. Best Pract Res Clin Obstet Gynaecol. 2004;18(5):755-71.
14. de Niet JE, de Koning CM, Pastoor H, Duivenvoorden HJ, Valkenburg O, Ramakers MJ, et al. Psychological well-being and sexarche in women with polycystic ovarian syndrome. Hum Reprod. 2010;25(6):1497-503.
15. Dunaif A, Segal KR, Futterweit W et al. Profound peripheral insulin resistance, independent of obesity, in polycystic ovarian syndrome. Diabetes. 1989;38:1165–1174.
16. Benson S, Hahn S, Tan S, Mann K, Janssen OE, Schedlowski M, et al. Prevalence and implications of anxiety in polycystic ovarian syndrome: results of an internet-based survey in Germany. Hum Reprod. 2009;24(6):1446-51.

17. Dunaif A. Insulin resistance and the polycystic ovarian syndrome: mechanism and implications for pathogenesis. Endocr Rev. 1997;18:774-800.
18. Mansson M, Norstrom K, Holte J, Landin-Wilhelmsen K, Dahlgren E, Landen M. Sexuality and psychological wellbeing in women with polycystic ovarian syndrome compared with healthy controls. Eur J Obstet Gynecol Reprod Biol. 2011;155(2):161-5.
19. Ohno S, et al. Serine phosphorylation of human P450cl7 increases 17,20-lyase activity: implications for adrenarche and the polycystic ovarian syndrome. Proc Natl Acad Sci USA. 1995;92:10619-23.
20. Eftekhar T, Sohrabvand F, Zabandan N, Shariat M, Haghollahi F, Ghahghaei-Nezamabadi A. Sexual dysfunction in patients with polycystic ovarian syndrome and its affected domains. Iran J Reprod Med. 2014;12(8):539-46.
21. Romualdi D, Guido M, Ciampelli M, et al. Selective effects of pioglitazone on insulin and androgen abnormalities in normo–and hyperinsulinaemic obese patients with polycystic ovarian syndrome. Hum Reprod. 2003;18:1210-8.
22. Thalheimer J. Ketosis fad diet alert: skip low-carb diets; instead focus on nutrient-rich choices like whole grains, fruits and vegetables. Environmental Nutrition. 2015;38(9):3.
23. Khademi A, Alleyassin A, Aghahosseini M, Tabatabaeefar L, Amini M. The effect of exercise in PCOS women who exercise regularly. Asian J Sports Med. 2010;1(1):35-40.
24. Malik SM, Traub ML. Defining the role of bariatric surgery in polycystic ovarian syndrome patients. World J Diabetes. 2012;3(4):71-9.
25. Bergh C, Carlsson B, Olsson JH, et al. Regulation of androgen production in cultured human thecal cells by insulin-like growth factor I and insulin. Fertil Steril. 1993;59:323-31.
26. van der Linden M, Buckingham K, Farquhar C, Kremer JAM, Metwally M. Luteal phase support for assisted reproduction cycles. Cochrane Database Syst Rev. 2015; (7):CD009154.
27. Bhandari S, Ganguly I, Bhandari M, Agarwal P, Singh A, Gupta N, et al. Effect of sleeve gastrectomy bariatric surgery-induced weight loss on serum AMH levels in reproductive aged women. Gynecol Endocrinol. 2016;17:1-4.
28. La Marca A, Morgante G, Paglia T, et al. Effects of metformin on adrenal steroidogenesis in women with polycystic ovarian syndrome. Fertil Steril. 1999;72:985-9.
29. Boden G, Chen X, Ruiz J, et al. Mechanisms of fatty acid-induced inhibition of glucose uptake. J Clin Invest. 1994;93:2438-46.
30. Barnes RB, Rosenfield RL, Burstein S, et al. Pituitary-ovarian responses to nafarelin testing in the polycystic ovarian syndrome. N Engl J Med. 1989;320:559-65.
31. Al-Inany HG, Youssef MA, Ayeleke R, Brown J, Lam W, Broekmans FJ. Gonadotrophin-releasing hormone antagonists for assisted reproductive technology. Cochrane Database Syst Rev. 2016;4:CD001750.
32. Walls ML, Hunter T, Ryan JP, Keelan JA, Nathan E, Hart RJ. In vitro maturation as an alternative to standard in vitro fertilization for patients diagnosed with polycystic ovaries: a comparative analysis of fresh, frozen and cumulative cycle outcomes. Hum Reprod. 2015;30(1):88-96.
33. Seok HH, Song H, Lyu SW, Kim YS, Lee DR, Lee WS, Yoon TK. Application of serum anti-Mullerian hormone levels in selecting patients with polycystic ovarian syndrome for in vitro maturation treatment. Clin Exp Reprod Med. 2016;43(2):126-32.
34. Chang JR. A practical approach to the diagnosis of polycystic ovarian syndrome. Am J Obstet Gynecol. 2004;191:713-7.
35. Siristatidis C, Sergentanis TN, Vogiatzi P, Kanavidis P, Chrelias C, Papantoniou N, et al. In vitro maturation in women with versus without polycystic ovarian syndrome: a systematic review and meta-analysis. PLoS One. 2015;10(8):e0134696.

CHAPTER 6

Ovulation Inductions in Polycystic Ovarian Syndrome

Kanthi Bansal

INTRODUCTION

Polycystic ovarian syndrome (PCOS) is one of the most common reproductive disorders. PCOS is a heterogeneous disorder which seems to be increasing in incidence worldwide. PCOS was described in 1935 by Irving F Stein and Michael L Leventhal as a syndrome complex of oligomenorrhea, hirsutism and obesity together with a demonstration of enlarged polycystic ovaries. Infertility is one of the major impacts of PCOS, which is due to anovulation. Ovulation is induced to manage ovulatory dysfunction by various modes of treatment which includes oral medicines, injections and surgery.

Polycystic ovarian syndrome (PCOS) is a syndrome which comprises hyperandrogenism, chronic anovulation, polycystic ovaries linked by hyperinsulinemia and insulin resistance. About 75% of anovulatory women of any cause have PCOS. The elevated androgen levels compound the problem through the process of extraglandular conversion as well as suppression of sex hormone-binding globulin (SHBG) synthesis resulting in elevated estrogen levels and associated increase in free testosterone. This prevents the normal follicular development and induces premature atresia.[1]

HISTORY OF OVARIAN STIMULATION

Infertility has been a condition known and studied for thousands of years. However, it was not until this past century that effective treatments were developed. With the advancement of knowledge of the hypothalamic-pituitary axis, therapies utilizing gonadotropins were developed to stimulate ovulation. Not only anovulatory infertility is treated but superovulation also be induced for IVF. In 1970 Clomiphene/hMG was used, later after ten years, i.e. in 1980s GnRH-agonist/hMG came into existence and was used. The latest in this era, newer forms of gonadotropins were developed by research and they were recombinant FSH, GnRH antagonist/hMG in 1990 and long acting FSH in 2000.[2]

PATHOPHYSIOLOGY OF OVULATION

In normal women, the menstrual cycle is of 28 days where a mature follicle develops up to size 18–22 mm diameter, and normally the follicle ovulates around the 14th day of the cycle. If the oocyte does not fertilize, then she will get her menses and the same cycle continues regularly.

In PCOS women, the ovaries develop multiple follicles because of hormonal imbalance, all small in size; they do not develop and mature properly to one dominant follicle capable of fertilization, which leads to anovulation.[3] The pathophysiology of PCOS is still not very clear, but hormonal and biochemical imbalance can be considered as the cause of PCOS. Around 50–70% of PCOS patients suffer from hyperinsulinemia, which impairs the action of insulin and leads to hyperandrogenemia. Because of high levels of insulin circulating in the blood, the thecal cells of ovaries respond to it and increases androgen production. Insulin and androgen suppresses the production of SHBG from hepatic glands and leads to increases in testosterone. Insulin also effects the production of LH from granulosa cells and all this leads to abnormal differentiation and premature arrest of follicular growth and hence anovulation. Increased levels of LH signal to produce more androgen which in turn produces more insulin and the cycle continues and the syndrome becomes more severe.

MANAGEMENT OF OVULATION INDUCTION

Polycystic ovarian syndrome (PCOS) is an endocrine metabolic syndrome which occasionally ameliorates spontaneously, but usually needs individualized approach to the treatment. The treatment has to be multidimensional and the aim should be:
- To correct metabolic dysfunction
- To achieve ovulation
- Optimum ovulation not requiring too many gonadotropins, making it simple and cost-efficient
- Avoiding ovarian hyperstimulation
- Improving implantation and avoiding miscarriage.

Treatment initially includes preconceptional counseling for lifestyle changes especially for weight loss. If the women with PCOS have been trying to conceive for 6 months, then evaluation should be started (ASRM). Semen analysis and tubal patency test should be done before starting the treatment. Overall the choice of the most appropriate treatment depends on the age of patient, the associated factors of infertility, experience and duration of previous treatment and the anxiety of couple.[4,5]

Lifestyle Modification

Weight loss is recommended first line treatment in obese women with PCOS. The treatment of obesity is multifaceted and involves behavioral counseling, lifestyle therapy (diet and exercise), pharmacological treatment and bariatric surgery.[6] If there is no great rush in conceiving and one can wait for some time, then weight reduction by lifestyle modification is worth trying. If there is not much time then concomitantly during ovulation induction also various strategies, which are not harmful to pregnancy, can be tried.

These strategies help women conceive naturally with lot of satisfaction. But it works only in those women who are thoroughly counseled, willing to follow the instructions and wait, as it is a slow process. Weight loss also leads to improvement in multiple other conditions like diabetes and cardiovascular diseases. Multiple studies have shown that losing as little as 5% of initial body weight have improved spontaneous ovulation rates.[7] The main pillars of lifestyle modification are counseling, dietary changes and exercise.

Counseling

There are several studies assessing the impact of symptoms and treatment of PCOS patients on their quality of life.[8] Women with PCOS and their partners are less satisfied with their sex life.[9] Due to hirsutism, the patients 'body image' is affected which leads to impairment in desire and decreased libido which contributes to the infertility. Affected women could be referred for a consult with psychologist or sexologist who could improve their quality of life with simple interventions. Prospective clinical studies are suggested to evaluate possible targeted treatments in order to regain normal sexual function in PCOS patients.[10]

Proper counseling regarding different methods available for induction of ovulation including dosage, methods of administration complications and side effects like OHSS and multiple pregnancies to be advised.

Diet

Reduction in weight by 5–10 kg the effect is tremendous or 5% decrease of body weight might be clinically meaningful and will increase the chances of spontaneous regulation and menstruation cycle. It is well known that calorie restriction is required for weight loss. But PCOS women who are on strict diet may have nutritional deficiencies. So, it may be worth giving them some multivitamin supplements.[11] Patients should be advised to take a diet which has:
- Nutrient dense, high fiber carbohydrates
- High protein foods (legumes, beans, meat, etc.)
- Healthy fats—olive oil, nuts, fish, etc.

Various modified diets have been proposed for PCOS women. The Atkins diet is a low-carbohydrate fad diet.[12] In a pilot study, a low carbohydrate led to significant improvement in weight, percent free testosterone, LH/FSH ratio, and fasting insulin in women with obesity and PCOS over a 24 week period.[13] Various other diets have been proposed including the general motors diet, but there are no studies proving their efficacy. Gluten free diet is a new talked about diet in PCOS patients to reduce unhealthy carb intake and reduce weight. But there is a lack of significant evidence to support a gluten-free diet in all women with PCOS. The main goal of women with PCOS should be to significantly restrict energy intake through carbohydrates and fats in order to maintain a normal weight.[14] Patient should be counseled to eat to live and not live to eat. Binge eating, purging and stowing to be avoided. Omega 3 has been shown to reduce testosterone in women with PCOS. A big breakfast diet (subsequently followed by progressively smaller meals) has been proposed to boost fertility for PCOS women.

Exercise

Inadequate exercise or physical activity may lead to overweight or obesity in PCOS women. Baseline activity levels by self-reporting were less in women with PCOS when compared with controls.[15] Randeva et al showed that exercise, such as regular walking, reduces waist-to-hip ratio, in overweight PCOS women.[16] The effect of exercise in long-term could be less efficient in obese patients. Various exercise regimes comprising of a mixture of cardiovascular as well as weight bearing exercises should be followed for optimum results. However, any form of exercise requires motivation from within and support from the husband. A good strategy could be to involve the husband to also exercise with the patient to keep her mentally motivated.

For PCOS subjects trying to conceive, best option would be to combine diet control along with exercise, which in turn reduces the weight and helps in conception.

Pharmacotherapy for Weight Loss

Metformin

Women with PCOS have a higher risk of developing diabetes compared with women of similar age and weight. Metformin has been used off label in PCOS to prevent diabetes and increase ovulation through weight loss.[17] In a recent randomized controlled trial comparing metformin, oral contraceptive pills (OCPs), and the combination of the two in patients with PCOS without T2D, metformin alone or with OCPs decreased weight and BMI. The median decrease in weight with metformin at 12 months was 3 kg (25th and 75th quartiles; -10.3, 0.6). OCP use was associated with increased weight changes of 1.2 kg (25th and 75th quartiles; -0.8, 3.0), and the combination decreased weight by 1.9 kg (25th and 75th quartiles; -4.9, 0.1).[18]

In a systematic review that included 12 randomized controlled trials in women with PCOS, metformin produced a significant decrease in BMI when compared with placebo; however, many of the studies were not adequately powered. So, metformin is known to cause some weight loss, improve ovulation and pregnancy rate in women with PCOS, but more adequately powered trials are required for the same as well as to determine the dose, duration and long-term effects.

Thiazolidinediones

Rosiglitazone and pioglitazone are shown to improve insulin resistance but their effect on weight is unclear. They should be used with contraception and therefore have no role in women trying to conceive.

Flutamide

Antiandrogen which helps in losing weight in obese PCOS. It can be given alone or with metformin.

Statins

Statins as lipid-lowering agents with pleiotropic actions, are likely not only has to improve had the dyslipidemia associated with polycystic ovarian syndrome but may also exerted other beneficial metabolic and endocrine effects. However, there is no evidence that statins improve resumption of menstrual regularity or spontaneous ovulation, nor is there any improvement of hirsutism or acne. In patients with PCOS, 3 months of treatment with atorvastatin resulted in a significant reduction in inflammatory markers, insulin resistance and hyperandrogenemia, in addition to the expected improvement in the lipid profile.[19]

Bariatric Surgery

Bariatric surgery can be effective in achieving significant weight loss, restoration of the hypothalamic pituitary axis, reduction of cardiovascular risk and even in improving pregnancy outcomes. Ultimately, bariatric surgery should be considered part of the treatment in PCOS women, especially in those with metabolic syndrome. Bariatric surgery in reproductive age women has been shown to decrease menstrual irregularities. Surgery has been shown to decrease the levels of androgens and increase the level of sex hormone binding globulin. LH and FSH levels have been reported to increase after surgery. On a more functional level, ovulatory function measured by luteal LH and progesterone secretion improved postoperatively, although levels were still below normal expected values. Additionally, leptin levels decrease after bariatric surgery, reflecting improved reproductive metabolic status. Many of these women (10-25%) have subclinical hypothyroidism which was significantly reduced following bariatric surgery. These changes certainly would suggest improved reproductive function and more studies are certainly needed to gain a better understanding. Bariatric surgery has also been reported to decrease the levels of AMH in women postoperatively and may benefit women with PCOS and high AMH levels.[20]

PRINCIPLES OF OVULATION INDUCTION

- To induce ovulation, follicle-stimulating hormone (FSH) is necessary in early phase of cycle to recruit and select follicles.
- For growth and maturation both FSH and LH are necessary and usually takes 4–6 days.
- Daily increase in follicular diameter, during the active phase is by 1.5–2 mm/day
- Serum estradiol levels should be about 200–300 pg/mL per growing follicle of 16 mm or more.[5]

OVULATION INDUCTION BY ORAL OVULOGENS

Clomiphene Citrate

The first clinical trial of clomiphene citrate (CC) was performed in 1960 by Kisther and Smith and soon afterwards, Greenblatt and colleagues reported ovulation in nearly 80% of amenorrheic anovulatory women. Since that time, it has remained the first choice in the treatment of anovulatory PCOS. It exhibits both estrogen agonist as well as antagonist properties depending on levels of endogenous estrogens. Estrogen agonist properties are exhibited when endogenous estrogens are very low otherwise it mainly acts as antiestrogen. It is a racemic mixture of two distinct stereoisomers enclomiphene and zuclomiphene having different properties. Enclomiphene is more potent isomer and is primarily responsible for ovulation-inducing action. Levels of enclomiphene rise rapidly and fall soon after the administration. Zuclomiphene is cleared slowly. CC binds to nuclear endoplasmic reticulum (ER) for extended period of time, weeks rather than hours. The mechanism of action is most likely due to blockade of negative feedback mechanism that results in increased secretion of FSH.[21]

Dose

Starting dose should be as low as 50 mg daily for 5 days from days 2–5 of the cycle. Recommended maximum dose is 150 mg because beyond this dose, no clear evidence of efficacy has been recommended. Approximately 75–80% of PCOS patients will ovulate with CC. Adverse effects—hot flushes, headache, visual complaints, multiple pregnancy (<10%), hyperstimulation and antiestrogenic effects on cervical mucus and endometrium.

Combination Therapy

There is now clear evidence that addition of metformin or dexamethasone to CC as primary therapy for induction of ovulation has no clear benefit.

Clomiphene Citrate/Gonadotropin

Clomiphene citrate remains the first line treatment for ovulation induction in infertile PCOS women. Second line treatment interventions include either exogenous gonadotropins or laparoscopic ovarian surgery. Failure of ovulation with clomiphene is termed "clomiphene resistance", whereas failure of pregnancy despite ovulation with clomiphene is considered as "clomiphene-failure". It had been estimated that between 20 and 25% of PCOS women are resistant to CC.[22] CC co-administered with low dose FSH to CC-resistant PCOS would improve ovarian response. It significantly reduces the duration and total dose of uFSH. Furthermore, CC co-treatment with uFSH is associated with significantly lower number of medium sized follicles and higher ovulation rates. Endometrial thickness is also not compromised. In early days of gonadotropin therapy, combined use of hMG/Clomiphene modality is advocated, the main reason for it being a reduction in cost. Clomiphene, acting on the hypothalamus could increase the endogenous FSH secretion and hence, the combined therapy required smaller hMG doses.

- Clomiphene citrate is given in the dose of 100 mg from the day 2 till the day 6 and then gonadotropins added from the day 5 or day 6 onwards.
- This is particularly helpful in PCOS patients, who have shown no response with CC alone and will show response with the use of combined therapy.
- All these patients need proper monitoring to avoid the risk of OHSS and decrease the incidence of multiple pregnancies.

Aromatase Inhibitors

Aromatase inhibitors have been used for the last decade as adjunctive treatments in breast cancer. They block the conversion of testosterone and androstenedione to estradiol and estrone, respectively, and hence inhibit the estrogen-negative feedback on the hypothalamic–pituitary axis. This leads to increased gonadotropin secretion, which in turn leads to ovarian follicular growth and development. The use of aromatase inhibitors in ovulation induction was first introduced in 2001. Ovulation and pregnancy rates with aromatase inhibitors such as letrozole and anastrozole appear to be promising, and these agents appear to have less anti-estrogen effect on the endometrium, but the evidence on endometrial effects is conflicting, and most studies show equivalence with clomiphene citrate. The aromatase inhibitor, letrozole, is typically administered on days 3–7 of the menstrual cycle at doses of 2.5–7.5 mg/day in 2.5 mg increments. Adverse effects include gastrointestinal disturbances, asthenia, hot flushes, headache and back pain. Initially, there was concern that the use of letrozole for infertility treatment may be associated with teratogenic effects and has led to the drug being banned for ovulation induction in various countries including India. However, later publications did not find an association with fetal anomalies. Given that aromatase inhibitors have recently been used in the treatment of infertile women with PCOS, it is important to evaluate their effectiveness in improving fertility outcomes in this group of women.[23]

Ovulation Induction by Gonadotropins

Principles of Gonadotropin Therapy

The basic principles were suggested by Insler and Lunenfeld in 1974 and are still followed till today.[24]

Effective Daily Dose (Threshold Principle)

Ovarian response can be elicited only when a certain dose of FSH is applied. Administrations of dose of gonadotropins below that threshold will not evoke a response, even over a prolonged period of time.

Latent Phase (FSH Window)

The number of days the FSH level is above threshold will decide the number of follicles to be activated. As the sensitivity to FSH of the growing follicles increases with development, the required amount of FSH for a follicle will decrease. The method of ovulation induction using gonadotropin therapy is based on the physiological concept that initiation and maintenance of follicle growth may be achieved by a transient increase in FSH above a threshold dose for sufficient duration to generate a limited number of developing follicles. Application of this concept is essential when ovulation induction is conducted in women with PCOS, because they are especially prone to excessive multiple follicle development.[25] For IVF, more number of eggs is required. So, gonadotropins can be used as step-up, step-down or constant dose protocols with low or ultra-low dose. Starting doses

TABLE 6.1 Comparison of dose of gonadotropins to be administered in PCOS, normal, and poor responders

Age	PCOS-FSH hyper-responder	Normal responder	Poor responder
<30 years	75 IU	75 IU	225 IU
30–35 years	75 IU	150 IU	300 IU
>35 years	150 IU	225 IU	300–450 IU

Abbreviations: PCOS, polycystic ovarian syndrome

of daily 150 IU FSH are no longer recommended in women with PCOS and have been replaced by low-dose FSH protocols.

Factors Determining the Dose of Gonadotropins

To determine the dose of gonadotropin first of all ovarian reserve is checked by performing baseline TVS to know the antral follicle count. Other determining factors are BMI, age and previous response of ovaries to gonadotropin treatment. The dose of gonadotropin administered in PCOS, normal and poor responders with reference to age, is shown in **Table 6.1**.

Different Regimes for Gonadotropin Therapy Used in PCOS

- Step-up protocol
- Combined therapy with other drugs.

Different Regimes for Gonadotropin Therapy not to be Used in PCOS

- Fixed dose regime
- Individually adjusted regimes
- Step-down protocol.

In the conventional step-up or low dose step-up protocols for gonadotropin induction of ovulation, administered doses are kept constant once an 'adequate' ovarian response is observed, resulting in high FSH serum levels in the late follicular phase and a broad FSH window.

Step-up Protocol

Low-dose administration of FSH/hMG in step-up regimen is a safe and convenient treatment protocol, and many studies have confirmed its effectiveness and safety.

The step-up regimen is as follows:
- It consists of administering a starting dose of 75 IU per day of FSH/hMG from day 2.
- If there is no evidence of follicular development after 5 days, (maximum follicular diameter <12 mm), the daily dose is increased by an ampoule (75 IU).
- If the leading follicle reaches 12 mm in diameter, the same dose of FSH/hMG is maintained until follicular maturation is achieved.

- Follicular development is monitored by serum estradiol assays and vaginal ultrasound scans.
- Serum LH is assayed daily to rule out a LH surge when the dominant follicle is at least 17 mm in diameter and serum estradiol was >250 pg/mL, 5000 IU human chorionic gonadotropin (hCG) is administered.

It is now widely accepted that the efficacy of ovulation induction combined with intrauterine insemination (IUI) has been demonstrated to be superior to human menopausal gonadotropin (hMG) treatment or IUI alone. Thus, gonadotropin with IUI has been advocated as a treatment for unexplained infertility to produce more oocytes and improve pregnancy rates.

Chronic Low Dose Protocol

Gonadotropin treatment in clomiphene citrate resistant polycystic ovarian syndrome (PCOS) patients using chronic low dose step-up protocol is highly effective to achieve singleton live births. There is need for optimization of starting dose in this protocol; such optimization will prevent hyperstimulation due to a starting dose far above the FSH threshold.

The chronic low-dose step-up regimen is administered as follows:
- Starting 75 IU of FSH from day 2.
- Dose is increased by 75 IU, after 7 days, if no follicle is ≥ 10 mm and E_2 <200.
- Weekly increment by 75 IU is done till adequate response and then the same dose is maintained till hCG.
- This protocol is extremely safe and effective in IUI since it results in development of 2-4 follicles.[35]

In PCOS patients chronic low dose protocol is started with 37.5-50 IU and it is increased after 14 days, increment dose is also kept low i.e., 25-37.5 IU. In PCOS, patients may require more than standard 10-12 days of stimulation. Art of ovarian stimulation in PCOS is to get optimum number of eggs (7-14) and at the same time, avoid OHSS.

Recombinant vs hMG

Ovarian stimulation performed with hMG in PCOS patients treated with a long GnRH agonist protocol results in the same clinical pregnancy and take baby home rates compared to ovarian stimulation with rFSH. However, for the consideration of other important factors such as the need of coasting and safety in particular, hMG has major advantages over rFSH. This results warrant further evaluation in larger prospective series. In patients who over-responded to FSH during ovulation induction, administration of rLH in the late follicular phase appeared to increase the proportion of patients who developed a single dominant follicle. Thus, according to these researchers, the use of LH-containing preparations such as hMG in ovulation induction might be advantageous in the protection from OHSS.[26]

Induced Controlled Ovulation Stimulation (ICOS) for IUI / IVF

The aim of ICOS in PCOS is to restore fertility and achieve a singleton live birth. For timed intercourse and IUI, first line of treatment should be clomiphene citrate, letrozole or anastrozole. This should be combined with ovulation monitoring using transvaginal sonography.

The mechanism of action of CC involves the blockade of the negative feedback mechanism that results in increased secretion of FSH. The starting dose of CC generally should be 50 mg/day for 5 days from days 2–5, with maximum dose being 150 mg/day. Approximately 75–80% patients with PCOS will ovulate after CC, with a conception rate of 22% per cycle. Treatment should be generally limited to six cycles.[27] Sometimes, there is no response to CC and in such cases; addition of adjuvants and gonadotropins might help. With gonadotropins, hyper-response may occur, so it is very important to use low doses. The method of ovulation induction using gonadotropin therapy is based on initiation and maintenance of follicular growth may be achieved by transient increase in FSH above a threshold dose for sufficient time. The recommended starting dose of gonadotropin is 37.5–50 IU/day. Small dose increment of about 50% from the initial dose is less likely to result in OHSS. Ultrasound assessment can be performed at baseline followed by serial assessment of follicular growth. Before starting, patients should be counseled regarding the associated risks and should be agreed upon to strict cancelation criteria. Recent data stress the need for taking into account the overall number of follicles and cycle cancelation may be considered in the presence of more than three follicles >14 mm. If there are more than 3 follicles or risk of OHSS, there either the cycle is canceled or converted to IVF using antagonist control with GnRH analog for trigger.

Use of GnRH Analog versus Antagonist and Trigger hCG versus Agonist

Recently, most of the clinics have shifted to antagonist cycles in case of PCOS because of reduced risk of OHSS, as GnRH analog can be used as a trigger for the cycle. In a Cochrane review and a recent meta-analysis of nine RCTs examining PCOS patients undergoing IVF/ICSI, clinical pregnancy rate was found to be similar in both the groups. However, they found reduced incidence of severe OHSS with antagonist protocol. Hence concluded that for severe OHSS, a GnRH antagonist protocol is significantly better in PCOS patients. Therefore, antagonist protocol seems to have an edge over agonist protocol.

Adjuvants to Ovarian Stimulation

Metformin

In women with PCOS, metformin appears to lower the fasting insulin level, but does not appear to result in consistent significant changes in BMI or waist-to-hip ratio.[28] Although oligomenorrhea improves in some women with PCOS, significant numbers remain anovulatory and at risk for menorrhagia and endometrial hyperplasia. The degree of improvement in ovulation frequency is the same as is achieved with weight reduction through lifestyle medication with no difference between metformin and placebo in this regard, and has been estimated to represent one extraovulation every five woman-months. With regard to the use of metformin for induction of ovulation, two RCTs indicate that metformin does not increase live birth rates above those observed with CC alone, in either obese or normal weight women with PCOS. The larger of these two trials demonstrated a selective disadvantage to metformin compared with CC and no apparent advantage to adding metformin to CC, except perhaps in women with BMI >35 kg/m² and as an adjunct in those patients with CC resistance. Metformin used as a single agent to induce ovulation is not cost effective and therefore at present, metformin should be used for patients with PCOS having glucose intolerance or CC resistance, after careful evaluation of risks and benefits.[29]

Myo-inositol and D-chiro-inositol

Inositol belongs to the vitamin B complex. Epimerization of the six hydroxyl groups of inositol leads to the formation of up to nine stereoisomers, including myo-inositol (MYO) and D-chiro-inositol (DCI); both stereoisomers were used, as insulin sensitizer drugs, in the treatment of PCOS treatments. Gerli et al. demonstrated a significant reduction in weight in the patients treated with MYO, in contrast to the placebo group where the BMI increased. Associated with the weight loss, it was possible to observe a significant reduction in circulating leptin and an increase in HDL concentrations, while LDL showed a trend toward reduction.[30] A recent clinical trial aiming to compare the effect of MYO or DCI supplementation on oocyte quality of PCOS patients showed that only MYO rather than DCI is able to improve oocyte quality. In conclusion, by analyzing different studies focused on MYO supplementation to improve several of the hormonal disturbances of PCOS, the study provides a level Ia evidence of MYO effectiveness. MYO mechanism of action appears to be mainly based on improving insulin sensitivity of target tissues, resulting in a positive effect on the reproductive axis (MYO restores ovulation and improves oocyte quality) and hormonal functions (MYO reduces clinical and biochemical hyperandrogenism and dyslipidemia) through the reduction of insulin plasma levels.

N-Acetylcysteine

N-acetyl cysteine (NAC) is the acetylated variant of the amino acid L-cysteine. It is an excellent source of sulfhydryl groups and is converted *in vivo* into metabolites that stimulate glutathione production, promote detoxification, and act directly as free-radical scavengers.

It is primarily a powerful antioxidant; it has activity on insulin secretion in pancreatic cells and on insulin receptors on human erythrocytes. NAC has antiapoptotic effects; it can preserve vascular integrity and has immunological functions. Reports in the literature have discussed the possible beneficial effects of NAC on ovulation in CC-resistant PCOS patients. Rizk et al. have noted that the combination of CC and NAC increases ovulation and pregnancy rates in CC-resistant PCOS patients who also suffer from infertility. In 2007, Badawy et al. noted that the addition of NAC to a CC regimen in patients with PCOS would increase ovulation rates significantly. A recent randomized controlled trial by Abu Hashim et al. showed that the efficacy of metformin-CC combination therapy is higher than that of NAC-CC for inducing ovulation and achieving pregnancy among CC-resistant PCOS patients. The level of serum estrogen, the endometrial thickness on the day of human chorionic gonadotropin administration, and the serum progesterone level on cycle days 21–23 were all significantly higher for women in metformin-CC group than for those in NAC-CC group. Additionally, a lower miscarriage rate was observed among women in metformin-CC group than among those in NAC-CC group.[31] However, studies regarding its utility in PCOS have shown inconsistent results; further randomized clinical trials with large number of CC-resistant PCOS women are still needed to shed more light on this topic.

Melatonin

The role of melatonin (N–acetyl-5- methoxytryptamine), a small lipophilic indoleamine, in human reproduction is still unknown. Melatonin, as well as its metabolites, are claimed to be broad-spectrum antioxidants and free radical scavengers, and their role is to quench reactive oxygen species (ROS) as well as reactive nitrogen species. There may be a reduction in the uptake of melatonin from circulation into the ovarian follicles of PCOS cases due to anovulation and increased number of atretic follicles and consequently serum melatonin concentration may increase in PCOS as a feedback response to decreased follicular concentration. Similarly, the raised serum melatonin level seen in PCOS cases was then found to be positively associated with serum testosterone level ($P < 0.001$). However, it has been seen that melatonin gets decreased in ovarian follicular fluid of PCOS patients and this intrafollicular decrease in melatonin is responsible for follicular atresia because of increased oxidative stress and consequent follicular damage in PCOS. These atretic follicles escape full maturation and lead to formation of multiple small follicular cysts, surrounded by hyperplastic theca cells. Atretic follicles ultimately contribute to an expanding stroma that increases in volume over time cellular mass producing androgens, sets in another self-propagating cycle that predisposes to chronic anovulation and leads to increased concentration of androgens.[32] High level of melatonin in the follicular fluid is essential for follicle growth, ovulation, and oocyte quality, whereas reduced follicular melatonin concentration may be responsible for anovulation and poor oocyte quality in PCOS. Follicles fail to mature fully and become atretic. Small follicles respond poorly to gonadotropins and undergo atresia. However, this needs further research and validation from larger studies.

Berberine

Berberine, the major active component of rhizoma coptidis, exists in a number of medicinal plants and displays a broad array of pharmacological effects. In Chinese medicine, berberine has long been used for its antidiabetic effects. Recently, berberine has been shown to have positive effects on type 2 diabetes mellitus, insulin resistance, lipid metabolism, nitric oxide production, and metabolic syndrome greater reductions in total testosterone, free androgen index, fasting glucose, fasting insulin and HOMA-IR, and increases in SHBG, were observed in the berberine and metformin groups. Three months of treatment with berberine or metformin before the IVF cycle increased the pregnancy rate and reduced the incidence of severe ovarian hyperstimulation syndrome. Furthermore, treatment with berberine, in comparison with metformin, was associated with decreases in BMI, lipid parameters and total FSH requirement, and an increase in live birth rate with fewer gastrointestinal adverse events. Berberine and metformin treatments prior to IVF improved the pregnancy outcome by normalizing the clinical, endocrine and metabolic parameters in PCOS women. Berberine has a more pronounced therapeutic effect and achieved more live births with fewer side effects than metformin. The mechanisms of berberine in treating PCOS are still unclear. Berberine was found to improve insulin resistance in theca cells and granulosa cells in a way similar to metformin. Therefore, berberine could also have the same androgen production regulation effects as metformin within PCOS.[33]

Combined Oral Contraceptives

Combined oral contraceptive (COC) therapy has long been a cornerstone of care for women with PCOS. COC therapy often provides clinical improvement in the areas of excessive hair growth, unpredictable menses, acne, and weight gain. PCOS patients with significant endocrine disorders had reduced implantation and pregnancy rates and increased miscarriage rate. OCP pretreatment, significantly improved the implantation and pregnancy rates, and reduced the incidence of small-for-gestational age infants, which was accompanied by remarkably decreased hyperandrogenism and antral follicles.[34]

Dexamethasone

Some women with PCOS have elevated adrenal androgen levels, although their contribution to ovulatory dysfunction appears modest. Glucocorticoids suppress adrenal androgen secretion and have been used in patients with adrenal hyperandrogenism. Unless a woman with PCOS has marked adrenal androgen excess, prolonged use of glucocorticoids is not advised.

SURGICAL MANAGEMENT OF OVULATION INDUCTION BY LAPAROSCOPIC OVARIAN DRILLING

Historically, Stein and Leventhal reported wedge resection of the ovary as the mode of surgical management of PCOS with 80% of their patients resuming regular menstruation. The procedure however was associated with high percentage of ovarian and adnexal adhesions and also with substantial tissue loss which may in turn lead to infertility. This technique has now been replaced by ovarian drilling. Ovarian drilling involves making multiple punctures over the surface of the ovary. It can be done either by laparotomy or laparoscopy, the latter being the preferred route. This is usually performed with the help of a needle point monopolar electrode. Various energy sources have been used to perform ovarian drilling, which include use of a monopolar hook electrode, harmonic scalpel and CO_2 laser, amongst which electrocautery seems to be the energy source of choice which may be attributed to the reduced rate of adhesion formation when compared with laser energy. The exact mechanism of action by which laparoscopic ovarian drilling works is not clear. The beneficial effect is apparently due to destruction of the stroma leading to a decrease in androgen production. The reduction in total and free testosterone concentration is approximately 50 percent. There is also a reduction in serum LH concentration and a rapid increase in serum FSH levels and thereafter demonstrates a cyclical pattern. These changes are sustained for a long period of time and result in restoration of ovulation in most subjects.[35]

Usually surgeons stick to the 'Rule of 4" i.e. 4 punctures in each ovary with 40 W of current to be delivered for 4 seconds, leading to a total dosage of 640 J which has been reported to be the lowest effective dosage. Titrating the dosage of energy depending upon the ovarian volume (60 J/cc) has been reported to have better reproductive outcomes when compared with delivery of a fixed dosage of 600 J/ovary. According to a recent Cochrane review, comparing gonadotropin therapy with ovarian drilling, found no difference in pregnancy rates, however, the rates of multiple pregnancies were less in the ovarian drilling group.[36] The role of a repeat LOD was assessed by Amer et al who concluded that repeat ovarian drilling was effective only in people who had previously responded to ovarian drilling. Complications associated with ovarian drilling may be associated with anesthesia, establishment of the surgical access and the procedure itself. Procedure related complications include bleeding from the drilling sites, laceration of the utero-ovarian ligament, destruction of a large number of follicles leading to decrease in the ovarian reserve and formation of post-operative adhesions. Use of an insulated needle and abdominal lavage may help in reducing cautery related complications and adhesion formation respectively. The procedure must be performed in a meticulous manner to obtain good results and simultaneously avoiding complications.

Luteal Phase Support

Luteal phase support using progesterone intravaginally or intramuscularly or orally has been used instead of hCG. A Cochrane review concluded that progesterone during the luteal phase is associated with higher rates of live birth or ongoing pregnancy than placebo. There is no conclusive evidence that hCG is more effective than placebo or no treatment. The addition of GnRH-a to progesterone appears to improve outcomes. hCG may increase the risk of OHSS compared to placebo.[37]

COMPLICATIONS

Overhyperstimulation syndrome (OHSS) is one of the most common complications faced during the stimulation in case of PCOS. OHSS can be avoided using individualized protocols. If OHSS is still impending, segmentation using freeze all policy can be done. Multiple pregnancies are a complication which is inevitable in cases of PCOS with COS.Ovarian torsion is another complication that can be encountered during ovarian stimulation. Patients complaining of pain should be evaluated with a color Doppler study to rule out the same.

CONCLUSION

Polycystic ovarian syndrome (PCOS) is increasingly being encountered as a major cause for infertility. Lifestyle modification and weight loss should be the first line of management if the couple is young and can wait for a few more months. Ovarian stimulation with clomiphene citrate as an ovulogen has stood the test of time. In cases with clomiphene resistance use of adjuvants, ovarian drilling or gonadotropins is advocated. Ovarian stimulation should be done with soft protocols to avoid OHSS, multiple gestation and ovarian torsion. There is a definite role of metformin in cases with insulin resistance. An individualized multifaceted, multidisciplinary approach can successfully treat infertility in women with polycystic ovarian syndrome.

KEY POINTS

- Semen analysis and tubal patency test should be done before starting ovulation induction.
- Weight loss is recommended as the first line of treatment in obese women with PCOS.
- Losing as little as 5% of initial body weight improves spontaneous ovulation rates.
- The main pillars of lifestyle modification are counseling, dietary changes and exercise.
- Proper counseling regarding different methods for ovulation induction, dosage, methods of administration, complications and side effects to be advised.
- For the PCOS subjects trying to conceive, best option would be to combine diet control along with exercise, which in turn reduces the weight and helps in conception.
- Bariatric surgery during the reproductive age has shown to decrease menstrual irregularities.
- Clomiphene citrate remains the first line of treatment for ovulation induction in infertile PCOS women.
- Second line of treatment includes either exogenous gonadotropins or laparoscopic ovarian surgery.
- Failure of ovulation with clomiphene is termed as clomiphene resistance.
- Failure of pregnancy despite ovulation with clomiphene is considered as clomiphene-failure.
- Factors determining the dose of gonadotropin are antral follicle count, BMI, age and previous response of ovaries to gonadotropin treatment.
- Art of ovarian stimulation in PCOS is to get optimum number of oocytes (7 to 14) and at the same time, avoid OHSS.
- Antagonist protocol seems to have an edge over agonist protocol.
- Metformin should be used for patients with PCOS having glucose intolerance or CC resistance, after careful evaluation of risks and benefits.
- Myo-inositol improves insulin sensitivity of target tissues, resulting in a positive effect on the reproductive axis and hormonal functions through the reduction of insulin plasma levels.
- OCP pretreatment improves the implantation and pregnancy rates, reduces the incidence of small-for-gestational age infants, which is accompanied by decreased hyperandrogenism and antral follicles.
- Soft and individualized protocol can be used to avoid OHSS, multiple gestation and ovarian torsion.

REFERENCES

1. Kanthi Bansal," PCOS: The Recent Management", Practical Approach to Infertility Management. 2004. pp. 298-301.
2. Ref Shaw RJ, Lamia KA, Vasquez D, Koo SH, Bardeesy N, Depinho RA, Montminy M, Cantley LC. The kinase LKB1 mediates glucose homeostasis in liver and therapeutic effects of metformin. Science. 2005;310:1642-6.
3. Nestler JE, Jakubowicz DJ. Decreases in ovarian cytochrome P-450c17 alpha activity and serum free testosterone after reduction of insulin secretion in polycystic ovarian syndrome. N Engl J Med. 1996;335:617-23.
4. Lord JM, Flight IHK, Norman RJ. Metformin in polycystic ovarian syndrome: systematic review and meta-analysis. BMJ. 2003;327:951-3.
5. Asunción M, Calvo RM, San Millán JL, Sancho J, Avila S, Escobar-Morreale HF. A prospective study of the prevalence of the polycystic ovarian syndrome in unselected Caucasian women from Spain. J Clin Endocrinol Metab. 2000;85(7):2434-8.
6. Eftekhar T, Sohrabvand F, Zabandan N, Shariat M, Haghollahi F, Ghahghaei-Nezamabadi A. Sexual dysfunction in patients with polycystic ovarian syndrome and its affected domains. Iran J Reprod Med. 2014;12(8):539-46.
7. Romualdi D, Guido M, Ciampelli M, et al. Selective effects of pioglitazone on insulin and androgen abnormalities in normo–and hyperinsulinaemic obese patients with polycystic ovarian syndrome. Hum Reprod. 2003;18:1210-8.
8. Webber LJ, Stubbs S, Stark J, Trew GH, Margara R, Hardy K, et al. Formation and early development of follicles in the polycystic ovary. Lancet. 2003;362(9389):1017-21.
9. Thalheimer J. Ketosis fad diet alert: skip low-carb diets; instead focus on nutrient-rich choices like whole grains, fruits and vegetables. Environmental Nutrition. 2015; 38(9):3.
10. Khademi A, Alleyassin A, Aghahosseini M, Tabatabaeefar L, Amini M. The effect of exercise in PCOS women who exercise regularly. Asian J Sports Med. 2010;1(1):35-40.
11. Malik SM, Traub ML. Defining the role of bariatric surgery in polycystic ovarian syndrome patients. World J Diabetes. 2012;3(4):71-9.
12. Bergh C, Carlsson B, Olsson JH, et al. Regulation of androgen production in cultured human thecal cells by insulin-like growth factor I and insulin. Fertil Steril. 1993;59: 323-31.
13. van der Linden M, Buckingham K, Farquhar C, Kremer JAM, Metwally M. Luteal phase support for assisted reproduction cycles. Cochrane Database Syst Rev. 2015;7; (7):CD009154.
14. Bhandari S, Ganguly I, Bhandari M, Agarwal P, Singh A, Gupta N, et al. Effect of sleeve gastrectomy bariatric surgery-induced weight loss on serum AMH levels in reproductive aged women. Gynecol Endocrinol. 2016. pp. 1-4.
15. La Marca A, Morgante G, Paglia T, et al. Effects of metformin on adrenal steroidogenesis in women with polycystic ovarian syndrome. Fertil Steril. 1999;72:985-9.
16. Boden G, Chen X, Ruiz J, et al. Mechanisms of fatty acid-induced inhibition of glucose uptake. J Clin Invest. 1994;93:2438-46.
17. Barnes RB, Rosenfield RL, Burstein S, et al. Pituitary-ovarian responses to nafarelin testing in the polycystic ovarian syndrome. N Engl J Med. 1989;320:559-65.
18. Al-Inany HG, Youssef MA, Ayeleke R, Brown J, Lam W, Broekmans FJ. Gonadotrophin-releasing hormone antagonists for assisted reproductive technology. Cochrane Database Syst Rev. 2016;4:CD001750.
19. Walls ML, Hunter T, Ryan JP, Keelan JA, Nathan E, Hart RJ. In vitro maturation as an alternative to standard in vitro fertilization for patients diagnosed with polycystic ovaries: a comparative analysis of fresh, frozen and cumulative cycle outcomes. Hum Reprod. 2015;30(1):88-96.

20. Seok HH, Song H, Lyu SW, Kim YS, Lee DR, Lee WS, Yoon TK. Application of serum anti-Mullerian hormone levels in selecting patients with polycystic ovarian syndrome for in vitro maturation treatment. Clin Exp Reprod Med. 2016;43(2):126-32.
21. Carmina E, Lobo RA. Polycystic ovarian syndrome (PCOS): Arguably the most common endocrinopathy is associated with significant morbidity in women. J Clin Endocrinol Metab. 1999;84:1897-99.
22. Ron-EI R, Raziel A, Schachter M, Strassburger D, Kasterstein E, Friedler S. Induction of ovulation after GnRH antagonists. Human Rep Update. 2000;6(4):318-21.
23. Felberbaum R, Diedrich K. The use of GnRH antagonist in IVF. In: Shoham Z, Howles CM, Jacobs HS (Eds). Female Infertility Therapy, London, Martin Dunitz. 1999. pp. 203-11.
24. Fluker M, Grifo J, Leader A, Levy M, Meldrum D, Muasher SJ, et al. Efficacy and safety of ganirelix acetate versus leuprolide acetate in women undergoing controlled ovarian hyperstimulation. Fertil Steril. 2001;75(1):38-45.
25. Barros Del Gadillo JC, Siebzehnrubl E, Dittrich R, Wildt L, Lang N. Comparison of GnRH agonists and antagonist in unselected IVF/ICSI patients treated with different controlled ovarian hyperstimulation protocols: a matched study. Europ J of Obs and Gynecol and Reprod Biol. 2002;102(2):179-83.
26. The European and Middle East Orgalutran study group. Comparable Clinical outcome using The GnRH antagonist ganirelix or a long protocol of the GnRH agonist triptorelin for the prevention of premature LH surges in women undergoing ovarian stimulation. Hum Reprod. 2001;16(4):644-51.
27. Hwang JL, Seow KM, Lin YH, Huang LW, Hsieh BC, Tsai YL, et al. Ovarian stimulation by concomitant administration of cetrorelix acetate and hMG following Diane -35 pretreatment for patients with polycystic ovarian syndrome: a prospective randomized study. Hum Reprod. 2004;19(9):1993-2000.
28. Azziz R, Woods KS, Reyna R, Key TJ, Knochenhauer ES, Yildiz BO. The prevalence and features of the polycystic ovarian syndrome in an unselected population. J Clin Endocrinol Metab. 2004;89:2745-9.
29. Stein IF, Leventhal ML. Amenorrhoea associated with bilateral polycystic ovaries. Am J Obstet Gynecol. 1935;29(2):181-91.
30. Azziz R. PCOS: A diagnostic challenge. Reprod Biomed Online. 2004;8(6):644-8.
31. The Rotterdam ESHRE/ASRM-sponsored PCOS consensus workshop group. Revised 2003 consensus on diagnostic criteria and long term health risks related to polycystic ovarian syndrome. Hum Reprod. 2004;19(1):41-7.
32. Diamanti-Kandarakis E, Kouli CR, Bergiele AT, Filandra FA, Tsianateli TC, Spina GG, et al. A survey of the polycystic ovarian syndrome in the Greek island of Lesbos: hormonal and metabolic profile. J Clin Endocrinol Metab. 1999;84(11):4006-11.
33. March WA, Moore VM, Willson KJ, Phillips DI, Norman RJ, Davies MJ. The prevalence of polycystic ovarian syndrome in a community sample assessed under contrasting diagnostic criteria. Hum Reprod. 2010;25(2):544-51.
34. Polson DW, Adams J, Wadsworth J, Franks S. Polycystic ovaries—a common finding in normal women. Lancet. 1988;1(8590):870-2.
35. Kousta E, White DM, Cela E, McCarthy MI, Franks S. The prevalence of polycystic ovaries in women with infertility. Hum Reprod. 1999;14(11):2720-3.
36. Chang JR. A practical approach to the diagnosis of polycystic ovarian syndrome. Am J Obstet Gynecol. 2004;191:713-7.
37. Siristatidis C, Sergentanis TN, Vogiatzi P, Kanavidis P, Chrelias C, Papantoniou N, et al. In Vitro Maturation in Women with vs. without Polycystic ovarian syndrome: A Systematic Review and Meta-Analysis. PLoS One. 2015;10(8):e0134696.

CHAPTER 7

Assisted Reproductive Technology in Polycystic Ovarian Syndrome

Manish Banker, Reena Gupta

INTRODUCTION

Polycystic ovarian syndrome (PCOS) is the most common endocrinopathy affecting 5–10% of women in their reproductive age. Its importance in infertility management is reflected by the fact that it accounts for 70–80% of anovulatory disorders causing infertility. According to National assisted reproductive technology assisted reproductive technology (ART) registry of India 2012 data, PCOS is the culprit in 19.92% of patients undergoing IVF.

Besides infertility, PCOS is associated with many other health problems such as marked insulin resistance, increased risk for type 2 diabetes mellitus, coronary heart disease, atherogenic dyslipidemia, cerebrovascular morbidity, anxiety and depression. If pregnant, these women have substantially increased odds for miscarriage, development of gestational diabetes, pre-eclampsia, fetal macrosomia, small-for-gestational age infants, and perinatal mortality.[1-3]

INDICATIONS FOR ART IN PCOS

In principle, anovulation is not an indication for *in vitro* fertilization (IVF). The logical therapy for women with PCOS is induction of ovulation. First line therapy is clomiphene citrate, and in case of failure with clomiphene citrate, the second line is gondotropins. However, the major complication of ovulation induction is the occurrence of multiple pregnancies (about 10% incidence), especially after the use of gonadotropin therapy. For this reason, use of gonadotropins has been questioned by many. Further, many authors find it more difficult to induce ovulation in patients with more severe PCOS (overweight, hyperandrogenemia and with polycystic ovaries) and a follicle-stimulating hormone (FSH) starting dose >50 ± 75 IU may result in ovarian hyperstimulation in at least 30% of an unselected PCOS population.[4] Hence, after failure of weight reduction, antiestrogen therapy and laparoscopic ovarian drilling, it has been argued that induction of ovulation with exogenous gonadotropin therapy can be omitted and replaced by ovarian stimulation and IVF.[5]

In vitro fertilization (IVF) and embryo transfer (ET) is an effective therapy for PCOS patients, and results in pregnancy rates that are comparable with those for women with tubal factor infertility.[6,7] Moreover, because the number of multiple pregnancies can be kept to a minimum by transferring less number of embryos, IVF-ET becomes a reasonable option for PCOS patients who are refractory to conventional infertility modalities or who have coexisting infertility factors.[2,6] IVF is indicated in women with PCOS who do have associated pathologies, such as in cases of tubal damage, severe endometriosis, preimplantation genetic diagnosis and male factor infertility.

The recommended indications for IVF in PCOS by Thessaloniki ESHRE/ASRM-Sponsored PCOS Consensus Workshop Group 2007 are given in **Box 7.1**.

CHALLENGES IN OVULATION INDUCTION IN PCOS FOR ART

Ovulation induction for ART in women with polycystic ovaries needs a different approach from that for women with normal ovaries. These women respond slowly but once the follicle-stimulating hormone (FSH) threshold is crossed they can blow up rapidly resulting in ovarian hyperstimulation syndrome.[6,7] In these patients, there is a thin line between no response and hyper-response. Theoretically one would expect an altered response in the multifollicular recruitment required for conventional IVF and indeed this has been illustrated in several studies.[7]

There are several explanations for the excessive response of the polycystic ovary to ovarian stimulation:

- Women with PCOS have an increased number of antral follicles.[8,9] Contrary to earlier theories, these follicles are not atretic but rather there is an increased cohort of selectable antral follicles sensitive to exogenous gonadotropins. An increase in number of antral follicles is contributed to by an increase in recruitment of primordial follicles from the resting pool.[10,11]
- Anti-Müllerian hormone (AMH), a dimeric glycoprotein produced from the granulosa cells of the preantral and antral follicles, is elevated in PCOS. Serum AMH is 2 to 4-folds higher in women with PCOS than in healthy women.[12,13] There is a spectrum of response, with some responding easily to treatment while others with higher AMH levels are difficult to respond with ovulation regimes and exhibit more symptoms such as amenorrhea and insulin resistance.[14]

BOX 7.1 Indications for assisted reproductive technology in polycystic ovarian syndrome

Women who remain refractory to ovulation induction
Who do not conceive despite ovulation
Who have other co-existing pathologies such as tubal factor, male factor, severe endometriosis
Advanced age/infertility of prolonged duration
Need for preimplantation genetic screening/preimplantation genetic diagnosis

Circulating insulin, insulin-like growth factor (IGF), and androgen concentrations are all implicated in the higher rate of recruitment.[15-17]

PROTOCOLS FOR STIMULATION

Two protocols are mostly used:
1. Long/agonist protocol.
2. Antagonist protocol.

Long Protocol/Agonist Protocol

In the typical long protocol, gonadotropin-releasing hormone (GnRH) agonist treatment begins during the midluteal phase, generally on the 21st day of cycle at a time when endogenous gonadotropin levels are at or near their nadir and the acute release of stored pituitary gonadotropins in response to the agonist, known as the "flare" effect, is least likely to stimulate a new wave of follicular development. In women who do not cycle predictably, oral contraceptives (OC) can be used, starting GnRH agonist treatment 1 week before the discontinuation of pills. Leuprolide acetate (administered subcutaneously) is the most commonly used human chorionic gonadotropins (GnRH) agonist. The usual regimen begins with 1.0 mg daily for approximately 10 days or until onset of menses or gonadotropin stimulation, decreasing to 0.5 mg daily thereafter until human chorionic gonadotropin (hCG) is administered. A single dose of a longer-acting depot form of GnRH agonist (leuprolide, goserelin, triptorelin) can also be given. Gonadotropin stimulation is started after confirming the effective pituitary down-regulation (serum estradiol level <30–40 pg/mL, no follicles >10 mm in diameter). The initial dose of exogenous gonadotropins must be individualized depending upon age, ovarian reserve, BMI and response in previous cycles. These patients particularly require lower dose. Typical starting doses range between 150 and 225 IU of recombinant FSH (rFSH) or urinary FSH (uFSH).

Theoretically, it seems that recombinant FSH would work better in these patients as they have high luteinizing hormone (LH)/FSH ratio. But a Cochrane database review in 2015 found no evidence of a difference in live birth and OHSS rates between urinary-derived gonadotropins and rFSH or HMG/highly purified-human menopausal gonadotropin (HP-HMG).[18] This review included 14 trials with 1726 women. They could not find any difference in live births (OR 1.26, 95% CI 0.80 to 1.99) or clinical pregnancy rate (OR 1.08, 95% CI 0.83 to 1.39) between rFSH versus urinary-derived gonadotropins. Even for the comparison between HMG or HP-HMG versus FSH-P, there was no significant difference in live birth rate (OR 1.36, 95% CI 0.58 to 3.18). Similarly, regarding OHSS there was no evidence of any difference between rFSH versus urinary-derived gonadotropins and between HMG or HP-HMG versus FSH-P.

Either a 'step-up' (beginning with a low dose, increasing as necessary based on response) or a 'step-down' (beginning with a higher dose, decreasing as necessary based on response) can be used. The response to stimulation is monitored with serial measurements of serum estradiol and transvaginal ultrasonography. In general, stimulation continues until at least two follicles measure 17–18 mm in mean diameter, while other follicles typically measure 14–16 mm, endometrial thickness more than 7 mm and the serum estradiol concentration reflects the overall size and maturity of the cohort. Most women require a total of 8–12 days of stimulation. When the cohort of ovarian follicles reaches maturity, recombinant hCG 250 μg is administered to stimulate the final stages of follicular development. The advantage of using a long protocol is correction of hormonal milieu by suppressing endogenous LH and androgens.[18]

About 40% of patients with PCOS have elevated LH/FSH ratio. In women with PCOS, high endogenous levels of LH were associated with lower pregnancy rates and higher rate of miscarriage as compared to those who had lower LH levels. A higher likelihood of pregnancy was observed when the LH level was <10 IU/L and the miscarriage rate was significantly higher in women with LH levels >10 IU/L.[19] Poor fertilization, oocyte quality and embryo quality have all been previously attributed to high LH in these patients.

So, it seems logical that suppressing endogenous LH levels by using long protocol or OCP pretreatment should improve the IVF outcome in these patients. However, recently Ganor-Paz et al. compared the long protocol, antagonist protocol and *in vitro* maturation in women with PCOS with high LH/FSH ratio on day 3 and concluded that High LH/FSH ratio had no adverse effect on pregnancy rates and embryo quality in all the three treatment modes.[20]

GnRH Antagonist Protocols

The two GnRH antagonists available for clinical use are Ganirelix and Cetrorelix. Both are equally potent and effective. For both, the minimum effective dose to prevent a premature LH surge is 0.25 mg daily, administered subcutaneously. The treatment protocol may be fixed and may begin after 5–6 days of gonadotropin stimulation or may be kept flexible to the response of the individual, starting the treatment when the lead follicle reaches approximately 13–14 mm in diameter (flexible protocol). Alternatively, a single larger dose of cetrorelix (3.0 mg) can also be used to prevent LH surge for 96 hours.

Advantage of antagonist protocol as compared to long protocol:[21,22]
- Shorter duration of treatment
- Reduced gonadotropin dosage requirement
- Reduced risk of ovarian hyperstimulation syndrome (OHSS)
- Avoidance of cyst formation
- More patient-friendly
- Use of GnRH agonist trigger in place of hCG for ovulation trigger to avoid OHSS.

Recently Haiyan Lin, et al.[21] conducted a meta-analysis on whether GnRH antagonist protocol is better in PCOS patients. Nine RCTs examining PCOS patients undergoing IVF/ICSI were included, with 588 women who underwent long agonist protocols and 554 women who underwent GnRH antagonist protocols. The clinical pregnancy rate per-embryo transferred was similar in the two groups (relative risk: 0.97, 95% confidence interval: 0.85–1.10). They found that a GnRH antagonist protocol was better than an agonist long protocol to reduce the rate of severe OHSS (odds ratio: 1.56, 95% CI: 0.29–8.51).

The major advantage of antagonist protocol in these patients is that final oocyte maturation can be triggered by using GnRH agonist (leuprolide 1 mg/1.5 mg, triptorelin 0.2 mg, buserelin 0.5 mg). Agonist trigger is potentially more physiological with a lower risk of OHSS, due to shorter half-life of LH (60 minutes vs 32–34 hours). Agonist trigger has been found to be comparable with hCG number of oocytes retrieved, quality of embryos, implantation and pregnancy rates.[23-25] However, the Cochrane review by Youssef et al. reported significantly lower live birth rates following agonist trigger. Later, it became clear that the poor pregnancy rate seen in agonist group was not due to detrimental effect on oocyte quality or embryo quality, but was a result of luteolysis and thus luteal phase insufficiency. Because of this luteal phase insufficiency in cycles triggered with agonist, 'freeze all' policy came into limelight and has been found to be the most successful way of almost eliminating the risk of OHSS, and with better pregnancy rates.

To conclude, literature as well as our personal experience favors antagonist protocol in PCOS.

PCOS AND OHSS

Women with PCOS undergoing IVF are at a higher risk of ovarian hyper-stimulation syndrome but the incidence varies in different studies, ranging from 10 to 18%.[26,27] Those who develop OHSS have higher estradiol concentrations, more number of follicles, especially medium size follicles (12–14 mm) at the time of trigger, and more oocyte number.[28-30] The cardinal feature of the pathogenesis of OHSS is an increased capillary permeability leading to increase in third space volume. hCG is the main triggering agent in pathogenesis of OHSS, whether it is exogenous in the form of trigger or luteal support or endogenous (pregnancy) as is the case in late OHSS. Vascular endothelial growth factor (VEGF), a potent angiogenic endothelial cell mitogen is the key mediator in the pathogenesis of OHSS.[31] Serum and follicular levels of VEGF are higher in PCOS subjects and those who develop OHSS on the day of egg collection.[32] Furthermore, OHSS is more common in a successful pregnancy cycle, i.e. late OHSS and in IVF cycle where hCG is used for luteal support. Herr, et al. had demonstrated the direct effect of hCG on the expression of VEGF mRNA within human luteinized granulosa cells.[33]

So, to prevent this dreaded complication, it is safe to use antagonist protocol with GnRH agonist trigger, freeze all the embryos and transfer in the subsequent cycle.[34-38] Borges et al. recently compared fresh transfers with frozen embryo transfers in patients at risk of OHSS and found that 'freeze all' does not just decrease the risk of hyper-stimulation but the clinical pregnancy rate, implantation and cumulative pregnancy rates all were higher with the 'freeze all'.[36]

In the present era, the main strategies to prevent OHSS in PCOS are:
- Using the lesser dose of gonadotropins for ovarian stimulation (150–225 IU).
- Antagonist protocol.
- Triggering final oocyte maturation with GnRH agonist, freezing all the embryos and transferring in subsequent frozen embryo transfer cycle.

ART OUTCOMES IN PCOS

There have been controversies regarding IVF outcomes in PCO patients with respect to oocyte quality, fertilization rates, embryo quality, cancellation rates, implantation rates and pregnancy rates.

A Meta-analysis by Heijnen et al. compared the IVF outcomes in PCOS patient's versus Non-PCO patients.[39] They concluded that:
- Significantly more oocytes per oocyte retrieval were obtained in PCOS patients compared with controls
- Cycle cancellation rate is significantly increased in patients with PCOS (12.8% vs 4.1%; OR 0.5, 95% CI 0.2–1.0).
- Duration of stimulation is significantly longer in patients with PCOS, even when the daily dose of FSH is like that in women without PCOS.
- Significantly more cumulus-oocyte complexes (2.9, 95% CI 2.2-3.6) were retrieved in women with PCOS, but fertilization rates were similar as compared with women without PCOS.[39]
- Clinical pregnancy rate per started cycle was similar (35%) between PCOS and non-PCOS patients. The same was true for pregnancy rates per oocyte retrieval and embryo transfer (ET).
- Overall, PCOS and control patients achieved similar pregnancy and live birth rates per cycle.

Though this meta-analysis has shown comparable fertilization rates amongst PCO and non–PCO patients other authors have found reduced fertilization rates in PCO group.[29,40]

Even if the pregnancy rates are comparable, the miscarriage rate in women with PCOS following IVF remains high compared with women with normal ovaries (35.8% vs 23.6%, p = 0.0038).[41] This unwanted outcome has been found to be proportional to BMI, increased waist-hip ratio, and insulin resistance. Fedorcsak et al. reported a relative risk of 1.77 for miscarriage for women with a BMI over 25 kg/m^2 in early pregnancy.[42] This could be related to obesity, hyperinsulinemia, high LH, or poor endometrial receptivity.

There has always been a debate on whether PCO has a poor impact on oocyte and embryo quality, but this remains a controversial issue. However, most recent studies refute that oocyte quality is poor in PCOS.[43,44]

Corrective Strategies to Improve ART Outcome

- Weight reduction
- Role of metformin
- Role of OCP pre-treatment
- Role of laparoscopic ovarian drilling (LOD)
- Role of adjunctive therapies such as myoinositol.

Weight Reduction

Obesity is common in women with PCOS, seen in 38–66% of women with diagnosis of PCO and is directly related to failure or delayed response to the various treatments proposed, such as administration of CC, gonadotropins and laparoscopic ovarian diathermy. Weight loss is recommended as a first-line therapy in obese women with PCOS seeking pregnancy.

Clinical pregnancy rates (CPRs) are found to be significantly lower in the obese women in both natural and assisted conception cycles.[45-47] Morbidly obese patients show reduced fertilization rate, fewer oocytes, and reduced peak estradiol level indicating an impaired follicular and oocyte response in them after stimulation.

Other problems related to obesity include high miscarriage rate and cancellation of assisted reproductive cycles, as mentioned before.[48] These patients require higher doses of gondotropins, but once the FSH threshold is crossed they show a hyper-response and are at risk of OHSS.[49,50] These patients need pre-conceptional counseling as even after conceiving both obesity and PCO are at increased risk of obstetric complications such as GDM, Pre-eclampsia, increased risk of operative delivery, wound infection and thromboembolism.

Multiple observational studies have shown that weight loss is associated with improved spontaneous ovulation rates in women with PCOS with pregnancies being reported after losing as little as 5% of initial body weight.[51] So, these patients are recommended to lose 5–10% of their initial body weight by diet and exercise aiming the BMI of <27 kg/m^2.

Role of Metformin

As hyperinsulinemia is a key factor in the pathophysiology of PCOS and hyperandrogenism seen in these patients, one can assume that use of insulin sensitizing agents should improve metabolic and reproductive outcome in these Patients. Metformin, an oral biguanide, a category B drug is mostly tried for the same. Metformin reduces hepatic gluconeogenesis, increases peripheral glucose utilization and mediates receptor kinase activity within granulosa and theca cells.

Regarding the use of metformin for induction of ovulation, two RCTs have reported that metformin does not increase live birth rates above those observed with CC alone, in either obese or normal weight women with PCOS.[52,53] Those patients with clomiphene resistance however did benefit from addition of metformin.

Fleming, et al.[54] demonstrated that metformin given over four months before IVF may decrease the antral follicle count and AMH levels; however, this was not shown to improve the number of oocytes retrieved or fertilization rates.[55] Kjotred et al. suggested that the live birth rate may be improved in lean women with PCOS.[56]

A recent Cochrane review on use of metformin in IVF including nine randomized controlled trials involving a total of 816 women with PCOS concluded that when metformin was compared with placebo there was no clear evidence of a difference between the groups in live birth rates though the clinical pregnancy rate was higher in metformin group.[57] The most consistent and beneficial effect was reduction in the risk of ovarian hyper stimulation in metformin group. The review suggested that for a woman with a 27% risk of having OHSS without metformin, the corresponding chance using metformin treatment would be between 6% and 15%.

Pretreatment with Oral Contraceptive Pills

Oral contraceptive pills (OCP) pretreatment in IVF has been widely used in agonist and antagonist protocols for avoiding ovarian cysts formation, LH surge and for cycle scheduling purposes. Damario et al. used OCP's in conjunction with long protocol in PCO patients and reported significant improvements in oocyte fertilization rates, embryo implantation rates and clinical/ongoing pregnancy rates.[58] The proposed mechanism may be through an improved luteinizing hormone/follicle-stimulating hormone ratio following dual suppression. An additional feature of this dual method of suppression was significantly lower serum androgen concentrations, particularly dehydroepiandrosterone sulphate which might also help in correcting the hormonal milieu. Pan JX et al. also supported the above findings and in addition concluded that successive pretreatment with pills improves the pregnancy outcomes by decreasing hyperandrogenism and antral follicle excess.[59] On the contrary, Decanter et al. in their nonrandomized prospective trial, concluded that extended duration of OCP pretreatment, as a first intention IVF protocol for PCO patients, neither improves the pattern of follicular growth nor the oocyte and embryo quality.[60] In fact, clinical and ongoing pregnancy rates were significantly lower in the OCP group despite same oocyte and embryo quality. Nevertheless, the cumulative pregnancy rate did not differ between the two groups. This difference could be attributed to poor endometrial receptivity in OCP group. So, whether OCP pretreatment can be detrimental on the COH outcome regarding likelihood of pregnancy through adverse endometrial effects needs to be confirmed through a randomized controlled study in a large and well-defined population.

Role of Laparoscopic Ovarian Drilling

The ASRM has recommended laparoscopic ovarian drilling as a second line method for ovulation induction in comparison to gonadotropins for PCOS patients who remain refractory to clomiphene citrate. Women who have normal weight and high LH concentrations and who need laparoscopy for other reasons are the most suitable candidates for laparoscopic ovarian drilling (LOD). The mechanism involved in restoration of ovulation is the dramatic decrease in LH and androgen concentrations followed by an increase in FSH levels.

Very few studies have compared the effect of LOD on IVF in PCOS patients. The clinical pregnancy rates and ongoing pregnancy rates have been found to be similar in LOD versus non-LOD patients undergoing IVF, though the number of oocytes retrieved and number of embryos obtained per oocyte retrieval were lower in LOD group. The consistent finding in these studies was a significantly lower incidence of OHSS in LOD group.[61,62] However, as there are concerns regarding long term effects of LOD (such as ovarian adhesions, premature ovarian failure), this technique cannot be recommended before IVF as a measure for reducing OHSS.

Role of Myoinositol

Myoinositol and D–chiroinositol are isoforms of inositol and belong to vitamin B complex. In IVF techniques, the supplementation with myoinositol is positively correlated to a meiotic progression of mouse germinal vesicle oocytes, enhancing intracellular Ca^{2+} oscillations.[63] In human follicular fluids, higher concentrations of myoinositol represent a marker of good-quality oocytes.[64] Myoinositol in combination with folic acid is found to significantly lower the total dose of gonadotropins used, number of days of stimulation, peak estradiol levels at trigger, the mean number of germinal vesicles, an increase in percentage of metaphase II oocytes and better fertilization rates in patients undergoing IVF.[65,66] Though the initial data seems promising, we need to have larger studies before incorporating myoinsitol in PCOS patients in clinical practice.

IN VITRO MATURATION

In vitro maturation (IVM) refers to transvaginal retrieval of immature oocytes from antral follicles either without or with minimal stimulation of ovaries with exogenous gonadotropins and then culturing these immature germinal vesicle oocytes *in vitro* till metaphase II oocytes, before fertilizing them through ICSI.

Theoretically, IVM seems a promising technique in PCOS as it eliminates the risk of OHSS which is the most dreadful complication of IVF in PCOS. However, the results of IVM as compared to conventional IVF have been disappointing as IVM yields significantly lesser oocytes, lesser embryos, decreased implantation rates and decreased live birth rates.[67]

In addition, the developmental outcome of children conceived with IVM has been studied in small numbers and though the results so far reported are found to be no different from the children born through traditional IVF or ICSI,[68,69] the small number of children conceived through IVM limits the accuracy of malformation and anomaly rates, and developmental outcomes cannot be assessed accurately. A Cochrane review in 2013 concluded that though promising data on the IVM technique have been published in a few recent studies, no RCT's exist to base practice recommendations regarding IVM in PCOS.[70] In our opinion, *in vitro* maturation should only be performed as an experimental procedure and in specialized centers with expertise. Further, since now we have effective means of preventing OHSS in PCOS by agonist trigger and 'freeze all' policy, the role of IVM appears limited.

CONCLUSION

Women with PCOS require ART when other treatments for ovulation induction fail or when associated infertility factors are present. PCOS patients exhibit a less predictable response to stimulation due to higher sensitivity to gonadotropins and there is a thin demarcation between no response and hyper-response. GnRH antagonist protocol with agonist trigger, 'freeze all' and transferring embryos in subsequent cycle is the preferred approach as it gives better results and eliminates the risk of OHSS.

KEY POINTS

- Ovarian stimulation and IVF is indicated in women with PCOS when other treatments for ovulation induction fail or other infertility factors coexist.
- Ovulation induction in ART should be carefully monitored due to unpredictable response of the polycystic ovary to stimulation.
- Antagonist protocol is preferred over the long agonist protocol in PCOS patients.
- OHSS prevention in PCOS includes using lower dose of gonadotropins, antagonist protocol with GnRH agonist (instead of hCG), freezing all the embryos and transfer in subsequent cycle.
- Role of metformin, myoinositol and IVM (in vitro maturation) is unclear and requires further research

REFERENCES

1. Boomsma CM, Eijkemans MJC, Hughes EG, Visser GHA, Fauser BCJM, Macklon NS. A meta-analysis of pregnancy outcomes in women with polycystic ovarian syndrome. Hum Reprod Update. 2006;12(6):673-83.
2. Kjerulff LE, Sanchez-Ramos L, Duffy D. Pregnancy outcomes in women with polycystic ovarian syndrome: a metaanalysis. Am J Obstet Gynecol. 2011;204(6):558.e1-6.
3. Qin JZ, Pang LH, Li MJ, Fan XJ, Huang RD, Chen HY. Obstetric complications in women with polycystic ovarian syndrome: a systematic review and meta-analysis. Reprod Biol Endocrinol. 2013;26:11:56.
4. van Santbrink EJP, Fauser BCJM. Is there a future for ovulation induction in the current era of assisted reproduction? Hum Reprod. 2003;18(12):2499-502.
5. Eijkemans MJC, Polinder S, Mulders AGMGJ, Laven JSE, Habbema JDF, Fauser BCJM. Individualized cost-effective conventional ovulation induction treatment in normogonadotrophic anovulatory infertility (WHO group 2). Hum Reprod. 2005;20(10):2830-7.
6. Balen A. The effects of ovulation induction with gonadotrophins on the ovary and uterus and implications for assisted reproduction. Hum Reprod. 1995;10(9):2233-7.
7. Shoham Z, Conway GS, Patel A, Jacobs HS. Polycystic ovaries in patients with hypogonadotropic hypogonadism: similarity of ovarian response to gonadotropin stimulation in patients with polycystic ovarian syndrome. Fertil Steril. 1992;58(1):37-45.
8. Dewailly D, Catteau-Jonard S, Reyss A-C, Maunoury-Lefebvre C, Poncelet E, Pigny P. The excess in 2-5 mm follicles seen at ovarian ultrasonography is tightly associated to the follicular arrest of the polycystic ovarian syndrome. Hum Reprod. 2007;22(6):1562-6.
9. Jonard S, Dewailly D. The follicular excess in polycystic ovaries, due to intra-ovarian hyperandrogenism, may be the main culprit for the follicular arrest. Hum Reprod Update. 2004;10(2):107-17.
10. Webber LJ, Stubbs S, Stark J, Trew GH, Margara R, Hardy K, et al. Formation and early development of follicles in the polycystic ovary. Lancet. 2003;27;362(9389):1017-21.
11. Webber LJ, Stubbs SA, Stark J, Margara RA, Trew GH, Lavery SA, et al. Prolonged survival in culture of preantral follicles from polycystic ovaries. J Clin Endocrinol Metab. 2007;92(5):1975-8.

12. Pigny P, Merlen E, Robert Y, Cortet-Rudelli C, Decanter C, Jonard S, et al. Elevated serum level of anti-mullerian hormone in patients with polycystic ovarian syndrome: relationship to the ovarian follicle excess and to the follicular arrest. J Clin Endocrinol Metab. 2003;88(12):5957-62.
13. Lie Fong S, Schipper I, de Jong FH, Themmen APN, Visser JA, Laven JSE. Serum anti-Müllerian hormone and inhibin B concentrations are not useful predictors of ovarian response during ovulation induction treatment with recombinant follicle-stimulating hormone in women with polycystic ovarian syndrome. Fertil Steril. 2011;96(2):459-63.
14. Pellatt L, Rice S, Mason HD. Anti-Müllerian hormone and polycystic ovary syndrome: a mountain too high? Reproduction. 2010;139(5):825-33.
15. Kezele PR, Nilsson EE, Skinner MK. Insulin but not insulin-like growth factor-1 promotes the primordial to primary follicle transition. Mol Cell Endocrinol. 2002;28;192(1-2):37-43.
16. Otala M, Mäkinen S, Tuuri T, Sjöberg J, Pentikäinen V, Matikainen T, et al. Effects of testosterone, dihydrotestosterone, and 17beta-estradiol on human ovarian tissue survival in culture. Fertil Steril. 2004;82 (Suppl 3):1077-85.
17. Vendola K, Zhou J, Wang J, Bondy CA. Androgens promote insulin-like growth factor-I and insulin-like growth factor-I receptor gene expression in the primate ovary. Hum Reprod. 1999;14(9):2328-32.
18. Weiss NS, Nahuis M, Bayram N, Mol BWJ, Van der Veen F, van Wely M. Gonadotrophins for ovulation induction in women with polycystic ovarian syndrome. Cochrane Database Syst Rev. 2015 ;9;(9):CD010290.
19. Homburg R, Armar NA, Eshel A, Adams J, Jacobs HS. Influence of serum luteinising hormone concentrations on ovulation, conception, and early pregnancy loss in polycystic ovarian syndrome. BMJ. 1988(22);297(6655):1024-6.
20. Ganor-Paz Y, Friedler-Mashiach Y, Ghetler Y, Hershko-Klement A, Berkovitz A, Gonen O, et al. What is the best treatment for women with polycystic ovarian syndrome and high LH/FSH ratio? A comparison among in vitro fertilization with GnRH agonist, GnRH antagonist and in vitro maturation. J Endocrinol Invest. 2016;39(7): 799-803.
21. Lin H, Li Y, Li L, Wang W, Yang D, Zhang Q. Is a GnRH antagonist protocol better in PCOS patients? A meta-analysis of RCTs. PLoS ONE. 2014;9(3):e91796.
22. Lainas TG, Sfontouris IA, Zorzovilis IZ, Petsas GK, Lainas GT, Alexopoulou E, et al. Flexible GnRH antagonist protocol versus GnRH agonist long protocol in patients with polycystic ovarian syndrome treated for IVF: a prospective randomised controlled trial (RCT). Hum Reprod. 2010;25(3):683-9.
23. Fauser BC, de Jong D, Olivennes F, Wramsby H, Tay C, Itskovitz-Eldor J, et al. Endocrine profiles after triggering of final oocyte maturation with GnRH agonist after cotreatment with the GnRH antagonist ganirelix during ovarian hyperstimulation for *in vitro* fertilization. J Clin Endocrinol Metab. 2002;87(2):709-15.
24. Acevedo B, Gomez-Palomares JL, Ricciarelli E, Hernández ER. Triggering ovulation with gonadotropin-releasing hormone agonists does not compromise embryo implantation rates. Fertil Steril. 2006;86(6):1682-7.
25. Babayof R, Margalioth EJ, Huleihel M, Amash A, Zylber-Haran E, Gal M, et al. Serum inhibin A, VEGF and TNFalpha levels after triggering oocyte maturation with GnRH agonist compared with HCG in women with polycystic ovaries undergoing IVF treatment: a prospective randomized trial. Hum Reprod. 2006;21(5):1260-5.
26. Kodama H, Fukuda J, Karube H, Matsui T, Shimizu Y, Tanaka T. High incidence of embryo transfer cancellations in patients with polycystic ovarian syndrome. Hum Reprod. 1995;10(8):1962-7.
27. MacDougall MJ, Tan SL, Balen A, Jacobs HS. A controlled study comparing patients with and without polycystic ovaries undergoing in-vitro fertilization. Hum Reprod. 1993;8(2):233-7.

28. Agrawal R, Conway G, Sladkevicius P, Tan SL, Engmann L, Payne N, et al. Serum vascular endothelial growth factor and Doppler blood flow velocities in in vitro fertilization: relevance to ovarian hyperstimulation syndrome and polycystic ovaries. Fertil Steril. 1998;70(4):651-8.
29. Humaidan P, Quartarolo J, Papanikolaou EG. Preventing ovarian hyperstimulation syndrome: guidance for the clinician. Fertil Steril. 2010;94(2):389-400.
30. Lee T-H, Liu C-H, Huang C-C, Wu Y-L, Shih Y-T, Ho H-N, et al. Serum anti-Müllerian hormone and estradiol levels as predictors of ovarian hyperstimulation syndrome in assisted reproduction technology cycles. Hum Reprod. 2008;23(1):160-7.
31. Pellicer A, Albert C, Mercader A, Bonilla-Musoles F, Remohí J, Simón C. The pathogenesis of ovarian hyperstimulation syndrome: in vivo studies investigating the role of interleukin-1beta, interleukin-6, and vascular endothelial growth factor. Fertil Steril. 1999;71(3):482-9.
32. Artini PG, Monti M, Matteucci C, Valentino V, Cristello F, Genazzani AR. Vascular endothelial growth factor and basic fibroblast growth factor in polycystic ovary syndrome during controlled ovarian hyperstimulation. Gynecol Endocrinol. 2006;22(8):465-70.
33. Herr F, Baal N, Reisinger K, Lorenz A, McKinnon T, Preissner KT, et al. HCG in the regulation of placental angiogenesis. Results of an in vitro study. Placenta. 2007;28 (Suppl A):S85-93.
34. Youssef MA, Van der Veen F, Al-Inany HG, Griesinger G, Mochtar MH, Aboulfoutouh I, et al. Gonadotropin-releasing hormone agonist versus hCG for oocyte triggering in antagonist assisted reproductive technology cycles. Cochrane Database Syst Rev. 2011;19;(1):CD008046.
35. Youssef MAFM, Van der Veen F, Al-Inany HG, Mochtar MH, Griesinger G, Nagi Mohesen M, et al. Gonadotropin-releasing hormone agonist versus hCG for oocyte triggering in antagonist-assisted reproductive technology. Cochrane Database Syst Rev. 2014;31;(10):CD008046.
36. Borges E, Braga DPAF, Setti AS, Vingris LS, Figueira RCS, Iaconelli A. Strategies for the management of OHSS: Results from freezing-all cycles. JBRA Assist Reprod. 2016(1);20(1):8-12.
37. Boothroyd C, Karia S, Andreadis N, Rombauts L, Johnson N, Chapman M; Australasian CREI Consensus Expert Panel on Trial evidence (ACCEPT) group. Consensus statement on prevention and detection of ovarian hyperstimulation syndrome. Aust N Z J Obstet Gynaecol. 2015;55(6):523-34.
38. Krishna D, Dhoble S, Praneesh G, Rathore S, Upadhaya A, Rao K. Gonadotropin-releasing hormone agonist trigger is a better alternative than human chorionic gonadotropin in PCOS undergoing IVF cycles for an OHSS Free Clinic: A Randomized control trial. J Hum Reprod Sci. 2016;9(3):164-172.
39. Heijnen EMEW, Eijkemans MJC, Hughes EG, Laven JSE, Macklon NS, Fauser BCJM. A meta-analysis of outcomes of conventional IVF in women with polycystic ovarian syndrome. Hum Reprod Update. 2006;12(1):13-21.
40. Dor J, Shulman A, Levran D, Ben-Rafael Z, Rudak E, Mashiach S. The treatment of patients with polycystic ovarian syndrome by in-vitro fertilization and embryo transfer: a comparison of results with those of patients with tubal infertility. Hum Reprod. 1990;5(7):816-8.
41. Balen AH, Tan SL, MacDougall J, Jacobs HS. Miscarriage rates following in-vitro fertilization are increased in women with polycystic ovaries and reduced by pituitary desensitization with buserelin. Hum Reprod. 1993;8(6):959-64.
42. Fedorcsák P, Storeng R, Dale PO, Tanbo T, Abyholm T. Obesity is a risk factor for early pregnancy loss after IVF or ICSI. Acta Obstet Gynecol Scand. 2000;79(1):43-8.
43. Sahu B, Ozturk O, Ranierri M, Serhal P. Comparison of oocyte quality and intracytoplasmic sperm injection outcome in women with isolated polycystic ovaries or polycystic ovarian syndrome. Arch Gynecol Obstet. 2008;277(3):239-44.

44. Sigala J, Sifer C, Dewailly D, Robin G, Bruyneel A, Ramdane N, et al. Is polycystic ovarian morphology related to a poor oocyte quality after controlled ovarian hyperstimulation for intracytoplasmic sperm injection? Results from a prospective, comparative study. Fertil Steril. 2015;103(1):112-8.
45. Fedorcsák P, Dale PO, Storeng R, Tanbo T, Abyholm T. The impact of obesity and insulin resistance on the outcome of IVF or ICSI in women with polycystic ovarian syndrome. Hum Reprod. 2001;16(6):1086-91.
46. Pasquali R, Pelusi C, Genghini S, Cacciari M, Gambineri A. Obesity and reproductive disorders in women. Hum Reprod Update. 2003;9(4):359-72.
47. Wass P, Waldenström U, Rössner S, Hellberg D. An android body fat distribution in females impairs the pregnancy rate of in-vitro fertilization-embryo transfer. Hum Reprod. 1997;12(9):2057-60.
48. Brewer CJ, Balen AH. The adverse effects of obesity on conception and implantation. Reproduction. 2010;140(3):347-64.
49. Dale PO, Tanbo T, Haug E, Abyholm T. The impact of insulin resistance on the outcome of ovulation induction with low-dose follicle stimulating hormone in women with polycystic ovarian syndrome. Hum Reprod. 1998;13(3):567-70.
50. Loveland JB, McClamrock HD, Malinow AM, Sharara FI. Increased body mass index has a deleterious effect on in vitro fertilization outcome. J Assist Reprod Genet. 2001;18(7):382-6.
51. Hamilton-Fairley D, Kiddy D, Watson H, Paterson C, Franks S. Association of moderate obesity with a poor pregnancy outcome in women with polycystic ovarian syndrome treated with low dose gonadotrophin. Br J Obstet Gynaecol. 1992;99(2):128-31.
52. Legro RS, Barnhart HX, Schlaff WD, Carr BR, Diamond MP, Carson SA, et al. Clomiphene, metformin, or both for infertility in the polycystic ovarian syndrome. N Engl J Med. 2007;8;356(6):551-66.
53. Moll E, Bossuyt PMM, Korevaar JC, Lambalk CB, van der Veen F. Effect of clomifene citrate plus metformin and clomifene citrate plus placebo on induction of ovulation in women with newly diagnosed polycystic ovarian syndrome: randomised double blind clinical trial. BMJ. 2006;24;332(7556):1485.
54. Fleming R, Harborne L, MacLaughlin DT, Ling D, Norman J, Sattar N, et al. Metformin reduces serum mullerian-inhibiting substance levels in women with polycystic ovarian syndrome after protracted treatment. Fertil Steril. 2005;83(1):130-6.
55. Fedorcsák P, Dale PO, Storeng R, Abyholm T, Tanbo T. The effect of metformin on ovarian stimulation and in vitro fertilization in insulin-resistant women with polycystic ovarian syndrome: an open-label randomized cross-over trial. Gynecol Endocrinol. 2003;17(3):207-14.
56. Kjøtrød SB, Carlsen SM, Rasmussen PE, Holst-Larsen T, Mellembakken J, Thurin-Kjellberg A, et al. Use of metformin before and during assisted reproductive technology in non-obese young infertile women with polycystic ovarian syndrome: a prospective, randomized, double-blind, multi-centre study. Hum Reprod. 2011;26(8):2045-53.
57. Tso LO, Costello MF, Albuquerque LET, Andriolo RB, Macedo CR. Metformin treatment before and during IVF or ICSI in women with polycystic ovarian syndrome. Cochrane Database Syst Rev. 2014;18;(11):CD006105.
58. Damario MA, Barmat L, Liu HC, Davis OK, Rosenwaks Z. Dual suppression with oral contraceptives and gonadotrophin releasing-hormone agonists improves in-vitro fertilization outcome in high responder patients. Hum Reprod. 1997;12(11):2359-65.
59. Pan J-X, Liu Y, Ke Z-H, Zhou C-L, Meng Q, Ding G-L, et al. Successive and cyclic oral contraceptive pill pretreatment improves IVF/ICSI outcomes of PCOS patients and ameliorates hyperandrogenism and antral follicle excess. Gynecol Endocrinol. 2015;31(4):332-6.
60. Decanter C, Robin G, Thomas P, Leroy M, Lefebvre C, Soudan B, et al. First intention IVF protocol for polycystic ovaries: does oral contraceptive pill pretreatment influence COH outcome? Reprod Biol Endocrinol. 2013(19);11:54.

61. Eftekhar M, Deghani Firoozabadi R, Khani P, Ziaei Bideh E, Forghani H. Effect of Laparoscopic Ovarian Drilling on Outcomes of In Vitro Fertilization in Clomiphene-Resistant Women with Polycystic ovarian syndrome. Int J Fertil Steril. 2016;10(1):42-7.
62. Tozer AJ, Al-Shawaf T, Zosmer A, Hussain S, Wilson C, Lower AM, et al. Does laparoscopic ovarian diathermy affect the outcome of IVF-embryo transfer in women with polycystic ovarian syndrome? A retrospective comparative study. Hum Reprod. 2001;16(1):91-5.
63. Chiu TTY, Rogers MS, Briton-Jones C, Haines C. Effects of myo-inositol on the in-vitro maturation and subsequent development of mouse oocytes. Hum Reprod. 2003;18(2):408-16.
64. Chiu TTY, Rogers MS, Law ELK, Briton-Jones CM, Cheung LP, Haines CJ. Follicular fluid and serum concentrations of myo-inositol in patients undergoing IVF: relationship with oocyte quality. Hum Reprod. 2002;17(6):1591-6.
65. Lesoine B, Regidor P-A. Prospective Randomized Study on the Influence of Myoinositol in PCOS Women Undergoing IVF in the Improvement of Oocyte Quality, Fertilization Rate, and Embryo Quality. Int J Endocrinol. 2016;2016:4378507.
66. Papaleo E, Unfer V, Baillargeon J-P, Fusi F, Occhi F, De Santis L. Myo-inositol may improve oocyte quality in intracytoplasmic sperm injection cycles. A prospective, controlled, randomized trial. Fertil Steril. 2009;91(5):1750-4.
67. Das M, Son W-Y, Buckett W, Tulandi T, Holzer H. In-vitro maturation versus IVF with GnRH antagonist for women with polycystic ovarian syndrome: treatment outcome and rates of ovarian hyperstimulation syndrome. Reprod Biomed Online. 2014;29(5):545-51.
68. Söderström-Anttila V, Salokorpi T, Pihlaja M, Serenius-Sirve S, Suikkari A-M. Obstetric and perinatal outcome and preliminary results of development of children born after in vitro maturation of oocytes. Hum Reprod. 2006;21(6):1508-13.
69. Buckett WM, Chian R-C, Holzer H, Dean N, Usher R, Tan SL. Obstetric outcomes and congenital abnormalities after in vitro maturation, in vitro fertilization, and intracytoplasmic sperm injection. Obstet Gynecol. 2007;110(4):885-91.
70. Siristatidis CS, Vrachnis N, Creatsa M, Maheshwari A, Bhattacharya S. In vitro maturation in subfertile women with polycystic ovarian syndrome undergoing assisted reproduction. Cochrane Database Syst Rev. 2013;8;(10):CD006606.

CHAPTER 8

Complications in Assisted Reproductive Technique

Kedar Ganla

INTRODUCTION

Global infertility prevalence rates are difficult to determine. As per the World Health Organization (WHO), one in every four couples in developing countries had been found to be affected by infertility and is ever increasing.[1] A WHO study (2012), has shown that the number of cycles performed in many developed countries has grown by 5–10% per annum over the last few years.[1,2]

Transvaginal oocyte retrieval (TVOR) was first described by Wickland et al. in 1985, and has now become the technique of choice for obtaining oocytes for IVF, owing to its good oocyte retrieval yield, minimal invasiveness, and light sedation required.[3,4] Although TVOR is less invasive than oocyte retrieval through laparoscopy, it should not be considered to be a risk-free procedure. Various complications, from minor complications such as bleeding from the vaginal wall to major life threatening complications such as injury to pelvic vessels, pelvic abscess, and direct lesion to the bowel or ureter, have been reported.[3,5,6] However, there is very little systematic data about these complications during TVOR. Although these complications may be rare, both fertility specialist and general gynecologist need to be aware of them so that they can counsel their patients better, and can provide proper treatment as well.

There is a wide variation in the way this common procedure of TVOR is performed by different centers, with room for improvement through guidelines. This chapter reviews the most common complications reported in literature, summarizes the recommendations made to minimize their occurrence, and raises some of the controversial issues related to the procedure especially that of pelvic infection. The complications related to ovulation induction are described in relevant chapters.

ANESTHESIA-RELATED COMPLICATIONS

The TVOR can be done under intravenous sedation, local anesthesia, or total intravenous anesthesia (TIVA). In TIVA there is no control on the abdominal muscle movements. These may create problem in difficult retrieval, especially in hyperstimulated ovaries and obese patients. Such cases may require low dose

BOX 8.1 Procedure-related complications

Immediate	Delayed

• Bleeding
  – Vaginal vault bleeding
  – Retroperitoneal hematoma
  – Injury to major vessels in pelvis
  – Ovarian surface bleeding
• Urinary tract injury
• Bowel injury
	• Pelvic Abscess
	• Infection
	• Fistula
	• Infertility

BOX 8.2 High-risk factors for these complications

- Obesity
- Difficult retrieval
- Hyper-responders, >10 oocytes
    - Hyperstimulated large fragile ovaries
    - Repeated punctures
- Frozen pelvis
    - Endometriosis
    - PID
- Medical issues
    - Hypertension/diabetes mellitus

scoline or even intubation. There can be additional drug requirement in certain women. Pre-existent medical conditions will increase the risk.

PROCEDURE-RELATED COMPLICATIONS

Oocyte retrieval is associated with complications which may be early or delayed **(Box 8.1)**. The incidence of complications is higher in high risk cases and additional precautions are warranted if these cases are identified **(Box 8.2)**.

Hemorrhage

Case

A 32-year-old woman with primary infertility underwent IVF (PCOS and male factor infertility). There was no other relevant medical history and coagulation profile was normal. Ovarian stimulation was done using antagonist regimen. Trigger for ovulation was given with injection Decapeptyl 0.2 mg after 11 days of GnRH treatment. The peak serum estradiol at that time was 3800 pg/mL. Oocyte retrieval was done by USG-guided transvaginal follicular puncture under GA. 26 oocytes were retrieved and the patient discharged after 3 hours of pick up. She was called back the next day for a pelvic sonography. She was stable, except for a little tachycardia (Pulse—100/min). The sonography showed free fluid in pelvis, pouch of Douglas and abdomen, with bulky enlarged ovaries. There was a suspicion of hemoperitoneum. An emergency laparoscopy was performed after adequate counseling and consent. On laparoscopy, hemoperitoneum was confirmed. There was slow oozing of blood from a single puncture site from the right ovarian surface **(Fig. 8.1)**. This was cauterized and abdominal wash given **(Fig. 8.2)**. She recovered well and was discharged on third postoperative day. All embryos were frozen and transferred in the later cycle.

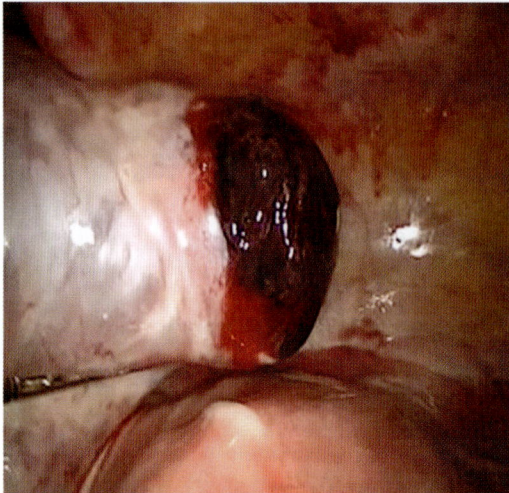

Fig. 8.1 Bleeding from ovarian surface

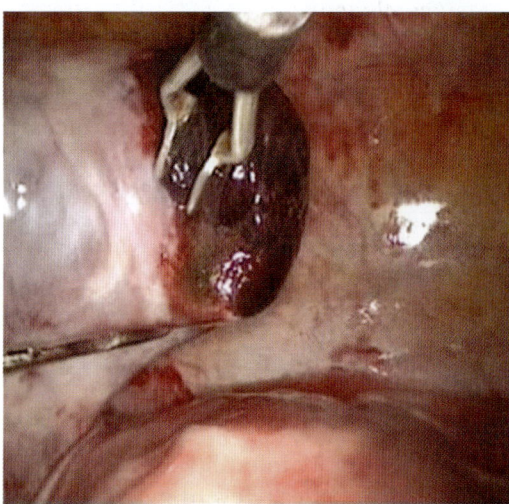

Fig. 8.2 Laparoscopic cauterization of bleeding from ovarian surface

The common problem associated with TVOR is undoubtedly minor vaginal hemorrhage because of trauma to vaginal vessels occurring in 1.4–18.4%.[7] The other major complication could arise by injury to major vessels or bleeding from the highly fragile ovarian surface. In the previously discussed case, there was bleeding from the punctured ovarian surface in the highly stimulated and fragile ovaries.

A major complication could be averted in the above case due to the follow-up of the patient on the very next day, even before she was symptomatic. These complications can be avoided or minimized by careful visualization of the vessels before advancing the needle and avoiding movement of the needle in the vaginal wall, particularly laterally, which can cause vaginal tear.[8] Aspiration of all the follicle without withdrawing the needle tip from the ovary (thereby leaving only a single puncture in the capsule) will also reduce the risk of hemorrhage from ovarian surface, whereas multiple punctures increase the likelihood of further damage to the ovarian surface.[9]

Treatment of minimal vaginal hemorrhage or nonexpanding hematoma in great majority is local pressure, topical hemostatic agents or suture of the lesion.[10] It is important to avoid stretching of the vaginal walls while applying local pressure.[9] The number of follicles aspirated, number of oocytes retrieved and preovulatory estradiol levels, duration of procedure does not correlate with the amount of blood loss.[11]

More serious hemorrhage can occur in 0.07–0.08%.[9,12] This can be due to direct trauma to the pelvic vessels or pelvic organs. Injuries to pelvic vessels have been described in literature.[13] These major complications can be avoided if the operator carefully visualizes all structures in both longitudinal and transverse axis before the follicular puncture. Some studies suggest the use of color Doppler to avoid puncturing of vessels. The pelvis should always be inspected before withdrawing the USG probe to ensure that there is no excessive collection of fluid or blood in the pouch of Douglas.[8] It has also been suggested that reducing the size of the needle significantly reduces the patient's postoperative pain without affecting the number of oocytes retrieved, or the subsequent fertilization of oocytes and clinical pregnancy rates.[14,15]

Hemoperitoneum can also occur due to bleeding from injury to ovary or due to necrotizing vasculitis.[16] Massive retroperitoneal bleeding has been described in literature due to puncture of the mid-sacral vein.[17] This women presented with pain and tenesmus and hence one needs to be aware of the possibility of retroperitoneal bleeding as a differential of abrupt pain after TVOR. Battaglia et al. 2001 reported a case of massive hemoperitoneum due to deficit of coagulation factor XI which was not detected preoperatively.[18] This highlights the importance of diagnosis and specific management of women with coagulation disorders. A positive family history or an occurrence of unusual bleeding or an abnormal coagulation tests helps in its diagnosis. A multidisciplinary approach with close and early liasion with the hematologist prior to initiation of IVF therapy in cases of myeloproliferation, essential thrombocytopenia, etc. is a must.[5] Sometimes the ovaries are inaccessible and it may be necessary to pass the needle through the myometrium or even endometrium or use transabdominal route for these high-fixed ovaries. This increases the risk of hemorrhage and can lead to intrauterine infection and low implantation rates if the endometrium is traversed.[19] A study by Licciardi (1995) talks about using a tenaculum on the cervix to stabilize the uterus and ovary.[20] Management of hemoperitoneum is depicted in the following **Flow chart 8.1**.

Ovarian Torsion

Case

A 29-year-old woman, primary infertility underwent IVF in view of male factor infertility. There was no other relevant medical history. Ovarian stimulation was done with antagonist regime and trigger for ovulation was given with rhCG (Ovitrelle 500 µg). The peak serum estradiol levels at that time were

Flow chart 8.1 Management of hemoperitoneum

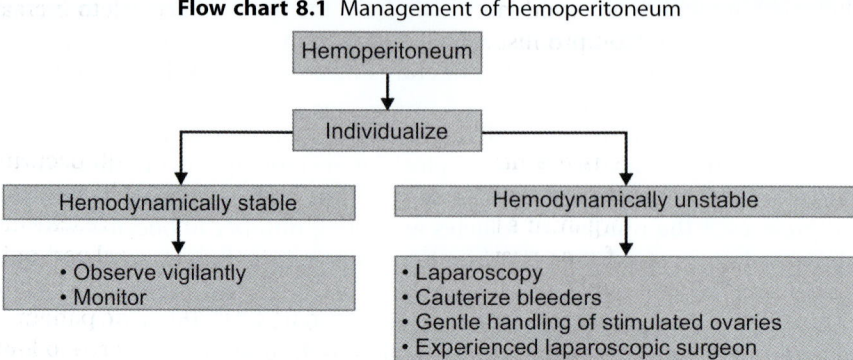

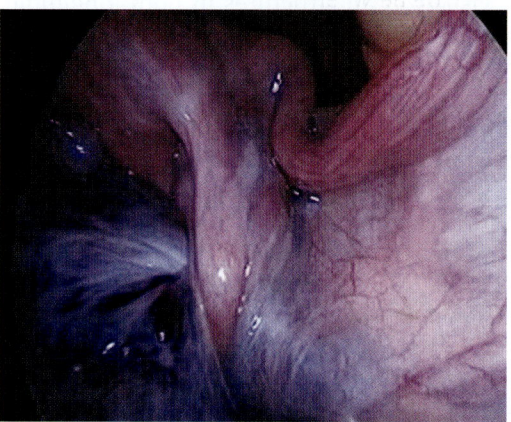

Fig. 8.3 Ovarian torsion

3900 pg/mL. TVOR was done and 28 oocytes were retrieved. There was no intraoperative complication and patient was discharged after 3 hours of pick up. She came back with complaints of severe colicky pain in abdomen, on the right side (on Day 5 of pick up) which was not relieved with antispasmodics. Her vital parameters were stable. A USG pelvis with Doppler showed torsion of right ovarian pedicle with minimum free fluid in POD. Patient was taken up for emergency laparoscopy after taking consent. On laparoscopy, the right ovary was congested and discolored. There was minimal free fluid in pelvis. Complete 360° torsion of the right ovary was noted **(Fig. 8.3)**. Laparoscopy right ovarian de-torsion was done and hence the ovary could be salvaged. She recovered well and was discharged on second postoperative day. All embryos were frozen and transferred later.

Although ovarian torsion is not a very common condition, this complication needs to be considered once a woman presents with severe pain in abdomen. Due to stimulation of the ovaries they become enlarged and hence can become abdominal organs and have plenty of space for rotation. Also as they are large and friable with a long infundibulopelvic ligament, they are predisposed to torsion. Laparoscopic de-rotation in early stages is the only way to salvage the ovary.

Some studies have used vasodilators like sildenafil; post de-torsion to increase the blood flow to the compromised tissues.[21]

Pelvic Infection

After hemorrhage, this is the next common complication of TVOR, occurring in 0.6–0.9%.[9] This can occur because of ascending infection (follicle aspiration needle carrying microorganisms from the vagina into the pelvis), by reactivating the dormant infection (from a previous PID) or very unlikely from fecal peritonitis secondary to bowel injury.[9] This theory is supported as microorganisms isolated from pelvic abscess were commonly encountered in the vagina of the patient.

Minimizing the number of repeated vaginal penetrations may serve to lower this risk and examining the USG probe covers for defects after TVOR, as well as disinfecting the probe between uses as necessary are important to avoid the risk of infection.[12,22] The use of sterile needles, covering the USG machine with sterile cover, which enables the operator to make any adjustments under sterile conditions and using sterile drapes to cover the patient's legs and perigenital areas are all necessary prophylactic measures.[23]

There is conflicting evidence on the use of antiseptics for vaginal cleaning prior to procedure. A prospective randomized study by Van Os et al., reported no significant difference in the fertilization and pelvic infection rates when normal saline (NS) was used compared with povidone iodine, but in fact reported a significantly increased pregnancy rate when normal saline was used.[24] However, a further prospective randomized study by Hannoun et al. 2008, identified that betadine did not affect the IVF outcome.[25] The risk of pelvic infection after TVOR seems to be related to history of PID. Reinfection may occur through puncture of chronic-infected adnexa. In a study by Dicker, out of 3656 IVF patients, nine developed tubo-ovarian and pelvic abscess, all of whom had previous history of pelvic inflammatory disease.[12]

The question of routine antibiotic prophylaxis is still open for debate, with some studies for it and few against it.[12,26] Egbase et al. reported that prophylactic antibiotics not only reduced the number of microbiology positive embryo catheter tips 48 hours after procedure, but also significantly increased implantation and clinical pregnancy rates.[27] Others support selected prophylaxis in increased risk cases with previous pelvic inflammatory disease or endometriosis. Still there is noconsensus on the type of antibiotic, timing, or duration of treatment.[28]

There is another interesting view point to these infections, with certain authors having claimed that PID complicating TVOR is mostly caused by infected semen and infection of endometrium correlated with positive semen culture.[29,30] On the other hand some authors believe that routine bacterial culture of semen followed by antibiotic treatment does not improve IVF outcome.[31] On the contrary, this may increase the likelihood of inoculation of pathogenic,antibiotic resistant bacteria from the vagina into the embryo culture system. These conflicting reports regarding whether antibiotic administration for the male partner is of benefit or not is another matter of concern.

Pelvic infections can occur within a few days to couple of weeks of procedure, but delayed pelvic infection in early and late pregnancy have also been reported.[32-34] Late manifestation of pelvic abscess supports the notion that presence of blood in an endometrioma provides a culture medium for bacteria to grow slowly after transvaginal inoculation. A broad spectrum or prolonged antibiotic should be considered in such high-risk cases. Aspiration of endometrioma during TVOR must be discouraged. One can consider treatment before superovulation by operative laparoscopy.[35]

Thirdly, though very rare, infection can occur by direct needle puncture of the bowel with an inflammatory or infectious spillage.[36] This needs to be managed as per the severity. Hospitalization and intravenous antibiotics with laparoscopy/laparotomy and even oophorectomy in selected cases may be warranted.[9,10] A variety of pelvic infections have been reported in literature such as ovarian abscess, uterine abscess and salpingitis.[9,36] In case of any infection or suspicion of infection, one must consider cryopreservation and embryo transfer in subsequent cycles.[19]

Pelvic Injury

During TVOR, anatomically related structures such as the bowel, ureters, pelvic blood vessel or nerves can be traumatized by the aspirating needle.[13] TVOR approach has reduced the risk of bowel injury. However, one must be vigilant especially in patients with previous history of pelvic surgery, infections like PID or tuberculosis and endometriosis which can lead to extensive adhesion formation. USG allows visualization of the bowel peristalsis and hence the injury to bowels can be avoided. However, despite this, injuries do occur. Trauma to the appendix during TVOR has been reported in literature.[37,38]

The **Flow chart 8.2** depicts general management strategies following pelvic injury.

Case

A 28-year-old woman, with history of previous two spontaneous pregnancies, consented to participate in an anonymous voluntary oocyte donation program. There was no other relevant medical history, especially endometriosis, previous history of PID, TB, previous surgery or renal pathology. Postretrieval, while doing a routine check sonography, a 4.5 cm × 4 cm collection was noted on the right side between the right ovary, bladder and vaginal vault **(Fig. 8.4)**. There was minimal fluid collection in the POD. Abdominal USG was done, which did not reveal any intra-abdominal collection.

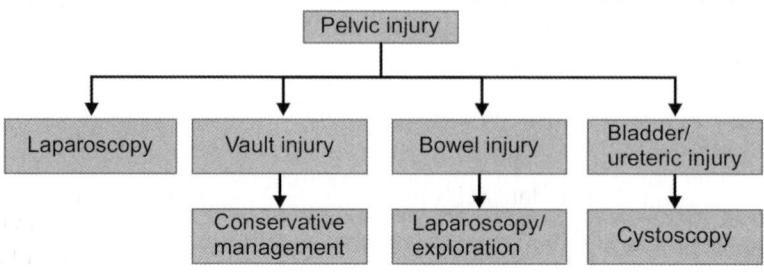

Flow chart 8.2 General management strategies following pelvic injury

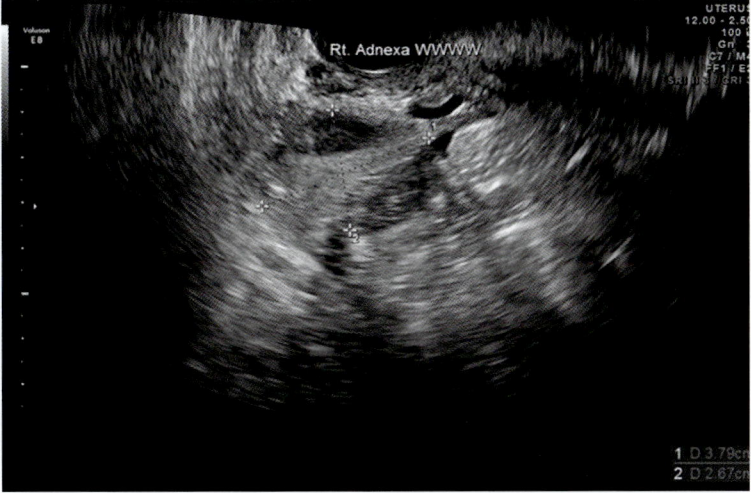

Fig. 8.4 Right adnexal hematoma on USG

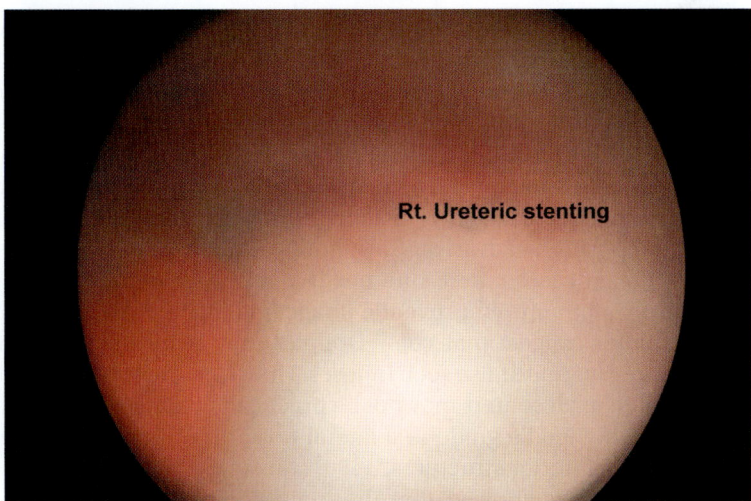

Fig. 8.5 Cystoscopic right ureteric stenting

Patient was catheterized immediately which revealed frank hematuria. Cystoscopy was performed to confirm the bladder/ureteric injury. Cystoscopy revealed bleeding from right ureteric orifice at the base of bladder, pointing to right ureteric injury. Right ureteral stenting was performed in the same sitting and patient started on intravenous antibiotics and analgesics **(Fig. 8.5)**. Continuous bladder irrigation was done to prevent blood clots.

After 24 hours urine routine microscopy revealed reduction in hematuria. There was no evidence of leucocytosis or infection. On third postoperative day, repeat urine examination showed only a few red blood cells and reduction in size of hematoma was observed on sonography. Ultrasound of abdomen and pelvis

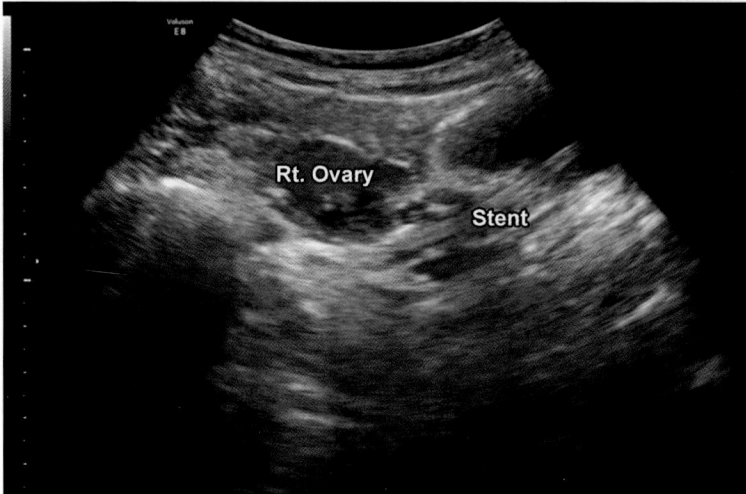

Fig. 8.6 Decrease in size of hematoma with the DJ stent *in situ*

was repeated after 7 days to look for the size of hematoma and any structural/anatomical aberrations, which showed decrease in size of hematoma (2.8 × 2.1 cm) and no structural or vascular abnormalities **(Fig. 8.6)**. The DJ stent was removed after 1 month.

As the ureter is located immediately anterolateral to the upper fornix of vagina, it is surprising that clinically recognizable ureteral injuries do not occur more often than that reported. This distance varies considerably depending on patient's size and position of ovaries. The identification of this structure becomes extremely difficult in cases where one needs to apply inward pressure to the vaginal USG probe, either to improve the image quality or stabilize the targeted ovary. Some studies suggest that color Doppler may help in identification of structures and prevent/minimise such injuries. However, the feasibility of having a Doppler machine in all centers may not be practically possible. Studies suggest that maintaining the needle guide in a lateral position prior to puncture, away from the dangerous anterior structures.[4]

A review of literature showed that the main complications of TVOR were hemorrhage (0.08%), pelvic abscess (0.6%), injuries of bowel, bladder and pelvic vessels occasionally.[6] Puncture in infertile women,[3-5,7,8] very few were diagnosed in the immediate postoperative period.[4] Acute or persistent abdominal pain immediately after oocyte pick up, suggestive of hemoperitoneum, confirmed by presence of free peritoneal fluid on USG. If this latter sign is absent, and patient has digestive and/or urinary disorders, differentials include damage to retroperitoneal anatomical structures such as a vessel or ureter.

In IVF setting, TVS is hindered by changes in ovarian volume and structure due to superovulation and follicular puncture. In most cases reported in literature,[3,7,8] diagnosis of ureteral injury was made between 5 days and 4 months. Urinary irritation, leukocytosis and negative urine culture was suggestive of urinary tract injury. In addition to renal sonography, CT-urography and MRI can help. Immediate conservative management is by ureteral stenting. Late diagnosis can lead to infection and renal dysfunction. More extensive surgery (ureteral reimplantation into bladder/nephrectomy) may be required.[3,7,8]

In a case reported of a ureteral lesion secondary to vaginal ultrasound follicular puncture for oocyte recovery in *in-vitro* fertilization by B.Coroleu, despite the surgical procedure to reimplant the ureter, the patient achieved a twin pregnancy which is ongoing uneventfully.[3] In that case, severe abdominal pain located in right iliac fossa, later spreading to right lumbar fossa, began 5 days after ET; it was accompanied by urinary symptoms (dysuria and vesical tenesmus) and digestive symptoms (nausea + vomiting). Transvaginal sonography revealed mild OHSS. Renal USG showed pyelo-calyceal hydronephrosis in right kidney with dilation of proximal ureter, left kidney was normal. A noticeable irregular enlargement of the right posterolateral wall of urinary bladder covering an area 57 mm in length was suggestive of hemorrhage resulting from an inflammatory pathology. Although it cannot be proved that the lesion was directly related to follicular puncture, facts suggest that it is highly probable that it occurred in this way either by direct lesion/by necrosis secondary to compression of a hematoma or abscess in the area. This case highlights the use of abdominal USG in cases of postpuncture pain since it can serve as a complementary diagnosis of extra pelvic pathology.[3]

There is another case report on ureteral stricture secondary to ultrasound-guided follicular puncture for oocyte retrieval that was corrected by a laparoscopic approach.[8] The first reported case of ureteral trauma immediately following seemingly uncomplicated oocyte retrieval was reported in 2002.[4] There is another case of with acute-onset uro-retroperitoneum in a volunteer oocyte donor, in which the patient recovered rapidly after ureteral stenting.[6] If these cases are not diagnosed immediately, they can lead to complications such as fistula, renal failure.[9] In most cases, the woman presented immediately (within a few hours) after TVOR with right lower abdominal pain with irradiation to the suprapubic area and vaginal discharge. A double-J catheter inserted under general anesthesia is the treatment of choice. In another such reported case, ureterovaginal fistula that formed approximately 7 days after oocyte retrieval. A percutaneous nephrostomy tube was placed using ultrasound guidance, and fistula was allowed to close secondarily.[10] Such complication could be prevented in our case due to timely diagnosis of the ureteric injury. Stenting of the ureters is most common therapeutic modality and should be used in subsequent retrievals to identify the ureters.[11]

Review of literature reveals a case of ureteric injury in women with past history of laparoscopic resection of endometriotic nodes of both sacro-uterine ligaments presenting with abdominal pain one day after oocyte retrieval. Four days after oocyte retrieval, she presented with massive hematuria. Monopolar coagulation with wire electrode and insertion of a double-J-stent was performed during operative cystoscopy. She recovered completely without signs of renal impairment after ureteric stent removal. This was the first report of ureteral injury after oocyte retrieval presenting itself with delayed massive hematuria and no signs of renal dysfunction or urinary leakage into retroperitoneal space.[12]

Ureteral trauma during transvaginal-guided oocyte retrieval is a rare complication with a variable clinical presentation. If ureteral injuries are not promptly recognized, significant morbidity may occur. This case demonstrates that early identification of injury and timely intervention result in favorable outcomes.[13]

LONG-TERM EFFECTS ON FERTILITY

There are two possible pathways by which oocyte retrieval might conceivably affect future fertility. The first pathway begins with the infection and bleeding that, as described above, are occasional side effects of retrieval surgery. These side effects sometimes lead to the need for surgery or to the formation of adhesions. Both could theoretically lead to fertility problems. However fortunately, there is little evidence to support this possibility. Furthermore, since women have two ovaries and fallopian tubes, and so they can remain fertile even if one set is damaged. There is no evidence that both might be threatened simultaneously by the side effects of retrieval surgery. As for adhesions, research has not found a higher rate of adhesions among women who have undergone TVOR.

The second potential pathway to fertility risk begins with the trauma applied to the ovary by having a needle thrust through its surface. It has been suggested that this trauma could lead to the development of anti-ovary antibodies, and, indeed, several studies have found that women who have undergone oocyte retrievals have a greater prevalence of antibodies to ovarian tissue than those who have not undergone the surgery.

Furthermore, antibodies to ovarian antigens have been shown to be associated with IVF failures and with women having multiple attempts at IVF—a situation that, again, implies that they have had previous failures. It is possible, that somehow these antibodies may interfere with sperm binding with or penetrating the oocyte and thus make it harder to fertilize the egg, but there is no evidence that this actually happens. It is difficult to know whether antibodies formed in one IVF cycle have anything to do with the failure of subsequent IVF attempts, or even if the antibodies play any role at all in infertility.

The complications of TVOR with preventive measures can be summarized in the following **Table 8.1**.

Recommendations suggested to increase the safety aspects of TVOR:
- Comprehensive preoperative evaluation of the patient before the procedure and a thorough anesthesia review of each patient.
- Multidisciplinary approach (as and when required).
- Development of clear guidelines especially for junior staff such as adequate supervision, continuous professional development and regular appraisal.
- Check list for identification of possible risk factors, e.g. history of PID, endometriosis, high/inaccessible ovaries, OHSS, obese patient, previous surgeries altering the course of ureter, bleeding and coagulation defects, etc.
- During procedure:
  - One must be more vigilant in a new setting/operation theater/place.
  - There may be equipment/instrument error, for example time lapse between USG probing and screen display must be noted before hand to avoid complications.
  - Highly placed ovary due to stimulation may require manual pressure from abdomen leading to compression of the vaginal vault vessels may cause difficulty in their visualization during oocyte retrieval and inadvertently lead to complications.

TABLE 8.1 Complications during TVOR

Complication	Incidence	Prevention/treatment
Infection	0.3–1.5%	Limit the number of vaginal punctures, preferably only two
		Antibiotic and/or antifungal prophylaxis (controversial), but especially in high-risk patients (history of pelvic inflammatory disease or endometriosis)
		Vaginal disinfection with povidone iodine then irrigate with saline (controversial)
		Be cognizant of peristaltic bowel on ultrasound to avoid bowel puncture and subsequent inflammation/infection
		Acute abdomen/peritonitis should be handled surgically and quickly. Stable patients can be handled medically only or also with radiologic assisted abscess drainage
Major bleeding	0.03–0.5%	Limit the number of vaginal punctures, preferably only two
		Visualize all structures by ultrasound in both the longitudinal and transverse axis before attempting puncture
		Inspect pelvis well to ensure that no significant fluid collection is forming
		Use color Doppler if available
		Hemodynamically unstable patients should be explored surgically and quickly
		Stable patients, even with large hematomas, may be observed and monitored with serial labs and CT scans
		Many hematomas reabsorb spontaneously
Torsion	0.1%	Aspirate all follicles to help decrease the size of the ovary
		Attempt early conservative management with laparoscopic untwisting of twisted adnexa
		Reserve salpingo-oophorectomy for cases of infarction

- Avoidance of repeated punctures of ovary and the vaginal wall to prevent intraperitoneal bleeding and postoperative pelvic infection, respectively.
- It is extremely important to do a USG (immediately and before discharge) in difficult cases like endometriosis, PID, past abdominal/pelvic surgeries, prolonged difficult oocyte retrieval.
- One must look for collection in both POD as well as anterior pouch and check Morrison's space if in doubt by transabdominal sonography.
• Documentation of such problems or complications during TVOR by a regional/central register.
• Use of Doppler, plastic modules for training in TVOR, etc.
• Further clinical research is needed in many areas of controversy like choice of solution for vaginal preparation prior to procedure, antibiotics prophylaxis, etc.

CONCLUSION

To conclude, the risk of rare but potentially severe complications of follicular puncture raises specific ethical and medicolegal issues. One must give proper information on the risks of such procedures to the patients as well as volunteer oocyte donors. Early identification of complications and prevention of complications is the need of hour.

KEY POINTS

- Complications of ART may be anesthesia or procedure-related
- Immediate problems (hemorrhage/organ injury) or delayed (pelvic infection/abscess) may complicate trans vaginal oocyte retrieval TVOR
- Obesity, difficult retrieval, hyperstimulated ovaries and pelvic adhesions may predispose to complications
- Severe hemorrhage with hemoperitoneum, ovarian torsion and injury during procedure will require laparoscopy
- Long-term effects on fertility are due to infection, postprocedure adhesions and anti-ovary antibodies due to trauma to ovary
- A comprehensive preprocedure evaluation, development of standard operative protocols and extreme vigilance during procedure is essential to prevent complications.

REFERENCES

1. National, regional, and global trends in infertility prevalence since 1990: A systematic analysis of 277 health surveys. 2012;12.
2. ART fact sheet (July 2014), ESHRE.
3. Coroleu B, Lopez Mourelle F, Hereter L, Veiga A, Calderon G, Martinez F, et al. Ureteral lesion secondary to vaginal ultrasound follicular puncture for oocyte recovery in in-vitro fertilization. Hum Reprod. 1997;12:948-50.
4. Miller PB, Price T, Nichols JE Jr, Hill L. Acute ureteral obstruction following transvaginal oocyte retrieval for IVF. Hum Reprod. 2002;17:137-8.
5. El-Shawarby S, Margara R, Trew G, Lavery S. A review of complications following transvaginal oocyte retrieval for in-vitro fertilization. Hum Fertil (Camb). 2004;7:127-33.
6. Fiori O, Cornet D, Darai V, Antoine JM, Bazot M. Uro-retroperitoneum after ultrasound-guided transvaginal follicle puncture in an oocyte donor: A Case Report. Human Reproduction. 2006;(21)11:2969-71. doi:10.1093/humrep/del252 Advance Access publication August 29, 2006.
7. Evers J, Larsen, Gnany Sieck. Complications and problems in transvaginal sector scan guided follicular aspiration, Fertility and Sterility. 1998;49:278-82.
8. Nugent, Smith, Balen. Ultrasound and the ovary, In: S Kupesic (Eds). Ultrasound and Infertility. London, New York: The Parthenon Publishing Group. 2000;2:23-43.
9. Waterstone B. Complications transvaginal ultrasound-directed follicle aspiration: a review of 2670 consecutive procedures, Journal of assisted reproduction and genetics. 1993;10:772-8.

10. Garcia T. Perioperative complications arising after transvaginal oocyte retrieval. Obstetrics and Gynaecology. 1193;81:590-3.
11. Rubattu D. Blood loss following non complicated transvaginal oocyte retrieval for IVF. Fertility and Sterility. 2001;76:205-6.
12. Ashkenazi D. Severe abdominal complications after transvaginal USG-guided retrieval of oocytes for IVF and ET. Fertility and Sterility. 1993;59:1313-5.
13. Lundkvist B. Clinical complications during IVF treatment. Human reproduction. 1992;7:625-6.
14. Biljain A. Effect of aspirating needle caliber on outcome of IVF. Human reproduction. 1993;8:1098-1000.
15. Waterstone A. Aprospective randomized study comparing needles of different diameters for transvaginal USG directed follicle aspiration. Fertility and Sterility. 1996;65:109-13.
16. Sundaresan I. Ovarian necrotizing vasculitis causing major intra abdominal haemorrhage after IVF case report and literature review. British journal of obstetrics and gynaecology. 1991;98:596-9.
17. Wolf A. Massive retroperitoneal retroperitoneal bleeding: a complication of transvaginal ultrasonographically guided oocyte retrieval for IVF –ET. Fertility and Sterility. 2000;74:405-6.
18. Regnani B. Severe intra-abdominal bleeding after transvaginal oocyte retrieval for IVF-ET and coagulation factor XI deficiency: A case report. Journal of Assisted Reproduction and Genetics. 2001;18:178-87.
19. Farhi A. Acute pelvic inflammatory disease after oocyte retrieval: adverse effects on the results of implantation. Fertility and Sterility. 1994;61:526-8.
20. Schwartz L. A tenaculum improves the ovarian accessibility during difficult transvaginal follicular aspiration: a novel but simple technique, Fertility and Sterility. 1995;63:677-9.
21. Incebiyik A, Seker A. Does sildenafil have protective effects against ovarian ischemia-reperfusion injury in rats? Arch Gynecol Obstet. 2015;291(6):1283-8.
22. Claman H. High rates of perforation are found in endovaginal ultrasound probe covers before and after oocyte retrieval for IVF-ET. Journal of assisted reproduction and Genetics. 1995;12:606-9.
23. Kurjak K. Interventional USG in human reproduction. In S Kupesic (Eds), USG and infertility. 2000;21:253-61. London, New York; The Parthenon Publishing group.
24. Van Os, Fetter. The influence of contamination of culture medium with hep B virus on the outcome of IVF pregnancies. American Journal of Obstetrics and Gynaecology. 1991;165(1):152-9.
25. Awwad H, et al. Effect of betadine vaginal preparation during oocyte aspiration in IVF cycles on pregnancy outcome. Gynecol Obstet Invest. 2008;66(4):274-8.
26. Meldrum. Antibiotics in vaginal oocyte aspiration. Journal of invitro fertilisation and embryo transfer. 1989;6:1-2.
27. Egbase PE, Udo EE, et al. Prophylactic antibiotics and endocervical microbial inoculation of the endometrium at embryo transfer. Lancet. 1999;354(9179):651-2.
28. Crutis, et al. Evaluation of the risk of pelvic infection following transvaginal oocyte retrieval. Human reproduction. 1991;7:1294-7.
29. Feichtinger, et al. Four years experience with USG-guided follicular aspiration. Annals of Newyork academic science. 1988;541:138-45.
30. Frydman T. Hysteroscopy and sperm infection. Contraception, Fertility and Sex. 1996;24:549-51.
31. Liversedge, et al. Antibiotic treatment based on seminal cultures for asympomatic male partners in IVF is unnecessary and may be detrimental. Human Reproduction. 1989;11:1227-31.
32. Sharpe K, et al. Transvaginal oocyte retrieval for IVFcomplicated by ovarian abscess during pregnancy. Fertility sterility. 2006:86(1):219.

33. Patounakis G, et al. Development of pelvic abscess during pregnancy following TVOR and in IVF. Eur J Obstet Gynecol Reprod Biol. 2012;164(1):116-7.
34. Kim JW, et al. Term delivery following tuboovarian abscess after IVF and ET. Am J Obstet Gynecol. 2013;208(5):e3-6.
35. Younis, et al. Late manifestations of pelvic abscess following oocyte retrieval for IVF in pts with severe endometriosis and endometrioma. Journal of assisted reproduction and genetics. 1997;14:343-46.
36. Peter Hecht, et al. Salphingitis or oophoritis: What causes fever following oocyte aspiration and ET? Obstetrics and Gynaecology. 1993;81:876-77.
37. Akam, et al. Perforated appendicitis and ectopic pregnancy following IVF. Human reproduction. 1995;10:3325-26.
38. Roest, et al. The incidence of major clinical complications in a Dutch transport IVF programme. Human Reproduction. 1996;2:345-53.

CHAPTER 9

Embryology in Polycystic Ovarian Syndrome

Keshav Malhotra, Dolly Sandhu Gill, Jaideep Malhotra, Narendra Malhotra

INTRODUCTION

In vitro fertilization (IVF) is the third line of treatment for polycystic ovarian syndrome (PCOS) patients. It is well established that PCOS is a complex multifaceted etiology characterized by hyperandrogenism, hyperinsulinemia, hypersecretion of luteinizing hormone (LH), menstrual dysfunction, hirsutism, infertility, and pregnancy and neonatal complications.[1-3] Women with PCOS undergoing IVF treatment have been well described in previous chapters.

The PCOS is typically marked by production of excessive number of oocytes, which are often of poor quality, which results in lower fertilization, cleavage and implantation rates; and consequently, higher miscarriage rates.[4-7] This manifestation of inferior oocyte and embryo quality may cause aneuploid embryos.[8,9] Recent literature suggests that despite high yield of oocytes and high production of euploid embryos in PCOS patients, lower pregnancy and higher miscarriage rates are prevalent. However, no causal genetic relation responsible for high-risk incidence of embryonic aneuploidy has been found.[6,10] Therefore, additional extrachromosomal factors such as abnormal endocrine or paracrine factors, metabolic dysfunction, and intrafollicular microenvironment disruptions during follicle maturation and folliculogenesis may play a significant role in this abnormally high risk of pregnancy loss in PCOS patients.[6,11-15]

Naturally, further research is warranted into investigating the intra- and extraovarian factors that disrupt the trajectory of normal oocyte development in PCOS. Exploring the consequences of these factors on granulose cell (GC)–oocyte interactions, oocyte maturation and potential embryonic developmental competence, are crucial areas of research that need to be actively pursued with the objective to optimize clinical stimulation, improve fertility and pregnancy outcomes in PCOS patients opting for IVF treatment.

EXTRAOVARIAN FACTORS

A mature oocyte is released by intricate developmental processes, starting from folliculogenesis and follicle maturation that produce several primordial follicles. One of these primordial follicles eventually yields a mature follicle, which is

released during ovulation. The abnormal extraovarian endocrine factors can lead to the disruption of these developmental processes resulting in ovarian dysfunction. Complex endocrine disorders include:
- FSH deficiency
- Hypersecretion of LH
- Hyperandrogenemia
- Hyperinsulinemia with insulin resistance

These disorders are responsible for pathogenetic effects of PCOS, which subsequently lead to high risks of impaired oocyte, developmental competence, implantation failure and miscarriage.[12,16-18]

Follicle-stimulating Hormone Deficiency

Follicular growth and recruitment of immature follicles from the ovary is stimulated by follicle-stimulating hormone (FSH). It is the prime survival factor during folliculogenesis, when there is a delicate balance between recruitment (one dominant follicle) and atresia of follicles (2–5 mm follicles). Human antral follicles between 2 and 5 mm depend on level of FSH, whereas slightly larger follicles between 6 and 8 mm become independent of FSH and acquire aromatase activity and possibly increase the estradiol (E2) levels.[12] With the collateral rise in E2 and inhibin B, FSH levels then decrease in the late follicular phase, and finally only the most advanced and mature follicle wins and progresses to ovulation,[19,20] whereas, PCOS patients exhibit lower serum FSH levels as compared with normal cycles.[21] Thus, there is increased accumulation of antral follicles between 2 and 8 mm due to FSH deficiency.[22] Undoubtedly, the large numbers of small follicles denotes that many have undergone premature arrest and were unsuccessful in transforming into the dominant follicle.[20,22]

The polycystic ovarian syndrome (PCOS) patients undertaking IVF commonly exhibit higher E2 levels, combined with a notably higher number of oocytes retrieved with significantly lower number of good quality oocytes, decreased fertilization rates, increased embryonic fragmentation, decreased percentage of blastocyst formation and lower implantation rates.[23,24] Increased E2 levels in PCOS patients may be damaging to oocyte maturation and embryonic development.[25] Furthermore, recovery of immature oocytes can be achieved by *in vitro* maturation (IVM), which is a potentially useful treatment option for women with PCOS-related infertility. IVM is discussed in detail in sections to follow.

Hypersecretion of Luteinizing Hormone

The polycystic ovarian syndrome (PCOS) women generally have tonic hypersecretion of LH during follicular phase of their cycles.[16,23,26] Increase in LH levels is inversely proportional to oocyte maturation, It also decreases fertilization rates and impairs the quality of the embryo, thereby decreasing the pregnancy rates and increasing miscarriage rates.[4,16,24,27-32] Hypersecretion of LH during folliculogenesis may downregulate FSH, leading to abnormal generative cell (GC) function by promoting premature GC luteinization and follicular atresia in small antral follicles from women with PCOS.[16,17,22] This causes premature oocyte maturation by impeding oocyte maturation inhibitors, affecting the quality of both oocyte and embryo.[33] LH-mediated processes may inflict oocyte nuclear damage catalyzing an apoptotic signal transduction cascade.[34] Loss of meiotic endocrine control may contribute to the embryonic aneuploidy, which is a possible consequence of compromised chromosomal normality in oocytes and impaired extrusion of the first polar body.[6] These embryogenic errors derived from a dysfunctional response to LH stimulation may help to explain the elevated spontaneous abortions in women with PCOS.[24,26]

Hyperandrogenemia

Hyperandrogenemia is a common comorbidity in PCOS. Elevated free circulating levels of bioactive androgen results from three possible mechanisms:
1. An intrinsic functional thecal defect
2. Hyperinsulinemia resulting in insulin resistance
3. Pituitary LH hypersecretion resulting in excessive thecal stimulation.[35-37]

Increased androgen concentrations in the follicular fluid (FF) are associated with high serum LH levels, which may block dominant follicle development and cause follicular arrest and degeneration.[34] It has been proposed that elevated levels of androgen may have a negative impact on oocyte developmental competence.[31,38] Oocyte incubation with androgen leads to lower oocyte maturation rates.[39] The reduction in calcium oscillations within the oocyte, a possible consequence of altered testosterone activity, may be responsible for inhibiting oocyte cytoplasmic maturation with emergent effects on meiotic maturation.[31,39] Besides, the premise that the androgens exact significant damage to folliculogenesis and endometrial function is supported by elevated testosterone concentrations in PCOS having been linked to higher miscarriage rates.[16,40,41]

Hyperinsulinemia

Polycystic ovarian syndrome is an endocrine–metabolic disorder, closely linked to insulin resistance and hyperinsulinemia. Insulin resistance has been associated with an increase in miscarriage rate.[42] Insulin has been implicated as an important mediator of oocyte developmental competence.[10,17,23] It may induce local androgen production resulting in poor quality of post-maturation oocytes.[23] Furthermore, insulin may also alter the gene expression of several genes involved in spindle dynamics[13] and centrosome function in PCOS oocytes by binding to receptors on GC and theca cells—an unintended consequence of stimulation for follicle recruitment.[33,43] Hyperinsulinemia may, therefore, impair developmental competence in oocytes, with the consequence of reduced fertilization rates, and error-prone embryonic development and implantation in PCOS patients with obesity.[10,18,23,31,44]

INTRAOVARIAN FACTORS

Oogenesis is immensely reliant on intraovarian factors, particularly follicle fluid factors (FFF).[20,45] Therefore, any disproportion or dysfunction between extra- and intraovarian factors may result in abnormal folliculogenesis and oogenesis.[11,22,46]

It has been proposed that the failure for selection of the dominant follicle in PCOS is due to the intrinsic alteration in folliculogenesis.[47] So these factors of GC origin like the transforming growth factor (TGF)-β superfamily such as anti-Müllerian hormone (AMH) and inhibins may play important roles in follicle recruitment, follicle selection and FSH responsiveness.[48] Disruption in their normal mechanisms can lead to thecal steroidogenic activity.[48] Proportions of other growth factors, derived from stromal ovarian cells, GCs, theca cells (TCs) and the oocyte itself, have been demonstrated for their normal folliculogenesis and their presumed role in PCOS **(Fig. 9.1)**. Selected intraovarian factors are listed in **Table 9.1**.

OOCYTE IN POLYCYSTIC OVARY

A typical PCOS patient has characteristic features of an increased production of oocytes with stimulation, poor oocyte quality, poor embryo quality, poor fertilization, cleavage and implantation rates when compared to non-PCOS stimulated patients and they also have a higher incidence of miscarriages. The extra- and intraovarian factors have already been discussed above. The question here is whether these factors have a direct influence on the follicle dynamics, oocyte maturity, fertilization, embryo quality and development and pregnancy or if these are a direct result of the endocrine imbalance in such patients, still need to be studied before any conclusion can be drawn. Many studies have compared all etiologies and outcomes of PCOS in view of endocrine, genetics, metabolism, etc. but the challenge still exists at the molecular level, where clinicians and scientists must correlate the oocyte competence with the different molecular mechanisms involved **(Fig. 9.2)**.

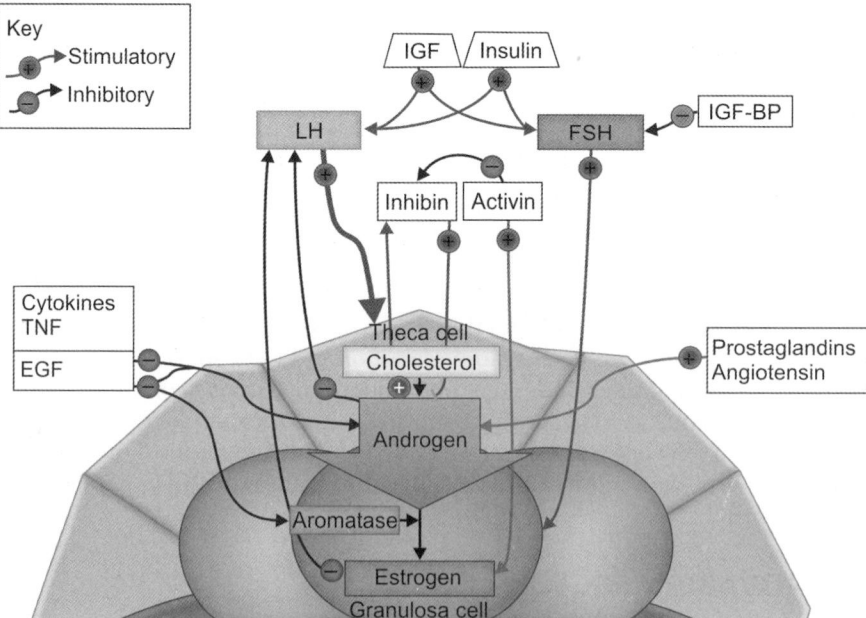

Fig. 9.1 Autocrine, paracrine and endocrine modulators of granulosa and theca cell function[48]

TABLE 9.1 Growth factors and their functions in normal ovulating women (NOW) and in PCOS women

Growth factor	Function in NOW	Function in PCOS	References
Anti-Müllerian Hormone	Expressed by GCs within ovaries of women of reproductive age, controlling the formation of primary follicles by inhibiting excessive follicular recruitment by FSH	AMH expression is reduced in early growing follicles, allowing entry into advanced follicular development. However, when the antral follicle stage is reached, there is an overall increase in AMH due to a larger number of follicles at this stage, and also a greater output per GC. AMH has also been shown to decrease ovarian aromatase expression, thus preventing premature aromatase expression in smaller follicles. Excess AMH may contribute to a defect in the selection of the dominant follicle in PCOS	(49-53)
Bone morphogenetic protein (BMPs) and growth differentiation factor (GDF)	Various BMPs are expressed in the ovary and display spatial and temporal changes throughout folliculogenesis	The expression of GDF-9 and BMP-15 has been shown to be reduced in the early follicular stage in PCOS ovarian tissues, thus contributing to the aberrant follicular development	(54, 55)
Insulin-like growth factors (IGF)	Important regulatory functions in ovarian follicular development. Circulating IGFs are produced in the liver, local IGF-I is secreted by theca cells, whereas IGF-II is synthesized by GCs	The FF IGF-I levels in PCOS women are elevated, although IGF-II and IGFBP-1 levels are lower than normally ovulation women. Affects the oocyte quality and maturity	(19, 33)
Fibroblast growth factor (FGF)	Expressed in GC and theca cells of growing follicles–physiological regulators of FSH action	Some say PCOS patients have increased FGF and others say it is decreased. Therefore, FGF alterations in the FF and serum remain controversial	(56, 57)
Epidermal growth factor (EGF)	Regulating follicular development and oocyte meiotic maturation competence via EGFR signaling transduction system in the cumulus cell (CCs)	Inhibits estrogen synthesis in GCs, which then blocks antral follicle growth and results in follicular arrest	(58-61)

Follicle Dynamics and Oocyte Maturity

Human reproductive medicine is advancing by leaps and bounds, and these advances have made one thing very clear, which is the fact that oocyte quality is one of the most important factors on which the further development of the embryo is based. There are a number of morphological characteristics available on which the prognosis of the cycle can be based but the reliability of these techniques is questionable.[62] We all know how complex the process of folliculogenesis really is, and there are many factors involved, these factors constantly change the intrafollicular environment, which leads to healthy oocyte development. The developmental competence of the egg is governed by the bidirectional cumulus-oocyte signal. So, the ability of an oocyte to undergo meiosis, subsequent fertilization and even embryo development is dependent on this signal. And the regulatory mechanisms of the follicle are definitely vulnerable in PCOS patients.[63] Numerous studies have reported a low percentage of maturity even though the number of oocytes retrieved in PCO patients were high.[64] The functioning of granulosa cells in anovulatory women with PCOS is also suboptimal. The follicles appear to be more heterogeneous when compared to normal ovaries and there is a conspicuous set of hypersecretory follicles. These estradiol and progesterone secreting follicles are prematurely receptive to LH. As mentioned above, one of the prime reasons for such a response is hyperinsulinemia. FSH though remains within normal limits but is not enough to allow for oocyte maturation and this can be supported by mathematically modeling the dynamics of follicles in women with PCOS, which suggests that high estradiol levels combined with normal regulation of Serum FSH results in maturation arrest of the antral follicles.[65]

SPINDLE ASSESSMENT AND REACTIVE OXYGEN SPECIES

The meiotic spindle is responsible for correct chromosome segregation during the process of oogenesis with disturbances in spindle assembly increasing the risk

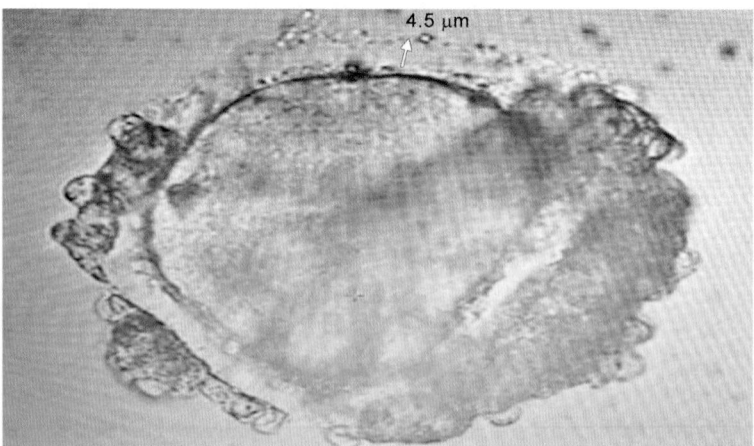

Fig. 9.2 Poor quality oocyte obtained from a PCOS patient at Rainbow IVF, Agra

of chromosome mal-segregation and aneuploidy in oocytes.[62,66] Aneuploidy is one of the most important reasons of abnormal fertilization, early embryo death, poor embryo development, and spontaneous abortion in humans.[67-69] Thus, oocytes possessing a birefringent spindle in polarized microscopy tend to have a better developmental potential compared to those without a spindle. Polarized light microscopy, in combination with imaging process software, allows imaging of non-invasively birefringent spindles in living cells.[66,70,71] Ovulated oocytes are arrested in metaphase II (MII), at which point a dense array of filaments and bundles forms the meiotic spindle. This molecular order is essential in cytoskeletal components for the optical property known as birefringence.[72]

Several studies in the literature suggest that the presence of a birefringent meiotic spindle predicts a higher embryonic developmental competence. A clear positive correlation between visualization of the meiotic spindle with fertilization rates, embryo development, and progression to blastocyst stage has been described in these studies **(Fig. 9.3)**.[62]

Importantly, detrimental effects on mouse oocyte and/or embryo development have been found after exposure to the polscope.[73] Although the number of oocytes retrieved was higher in women with PCOS (Group B) than the other two groups, they had a higher proportion of immature oocytes with only 56.42% oocytes graded as MII oocytes (as against 69.35% in endometriosis (Group A) and 66.27% in tubal block (Group C)). Meiotic spindles were visualized in 50.5% of mature (MII) oocytes retrieved from women in Group B, which was significantly lower than that in Group A (66%) (p < 0.001) as well as Group C (62.3%) (p <0.01) with spindle visibility comparable in the latter two groups (Groups A and C). Fertilization rate in Group B was also lower as compared to Groups A and C but this was not statistically significant **(Table 9.2)**. However, significant difference was observed in Grades I and II embryo formation in Group B (67.9%), which

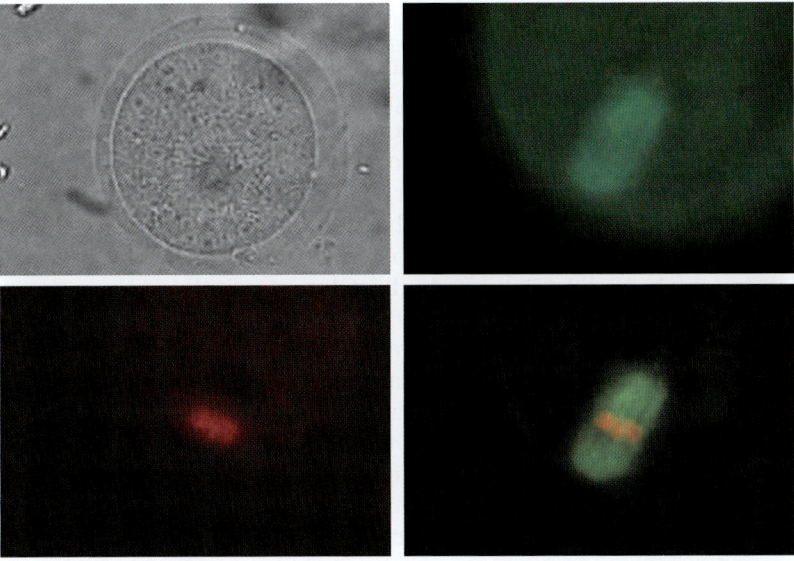

Fig. 9.3 Spindle assessment in mice oocytes

TABLE 9.2 Comparison of oocyte characteristics, ROS levels, and outcome parameters between the three groups

Outcome parameters	Group A (n = 56) endometriosis (mean ± SD)	Group B (n = 48) PCOS (mean ± SD)	Group C (n = 63) tubal factor (mean ± SD)	P value*
Number of oocytes retrieved (n)	5.54 ± 2.8	7.46 ± 3.9	5.27 ± 3.4	AB < 0.001 BC < 0.001 CA NS
Mature MII oocytes (%)	69.35 (215/310)	56.42 (202/358)	66.27 (220/332)	AB < 0.001 BC < 0.01 CA NS
Meiotic spindle present (%)	66 (142/215)	50.5 (102/202)	62.3 (137/220)	AB < 0.001 BC < 0.01 CANS
ROS (CPS)	64.59 ± 18.06	96.18 ± 75.75	98.28 ± 41.4	AB < 0.001 BC NS CA < 0.001
Fertilization rate (%)	81.4 (175/215)	78.7 (159/202)	81.4 (179/220)	AB NS BC NS CA NS
Grade I + Grade II Embryo formation (%)	80.6 (141/175)	67.9 (108/159)	76.5 (137/179)	AB < 0.01 BC NS CA NS
Endometrial thickness (mm)	9.39 ± 1.76	10.34 ± 1.92	9.47 ± 1.82	AB NS BC NS CA NS
Pregnancy rate (%)	32.1	39.58	43.75	AB NS BC NS CA NS

Abbreviations: MII, metaphase II; ROS, reactive oxygen species; CPS, counted photons per seconds; AB, comparison between Group A and Group B; BC, comparison between Group B and Group C; CA, comparison between Group C and Group A; NS, not significant *Statistically significant, p < 0.05 (ANOVA and post-hoc Bonferroni test)

was also low when compared with Group A (80.6%) and Group C (76.5%). The difference, however, was statistically significant (p < 0.01) when compared with Group A but not with Group C. Each group was then further analyzed based on presence or absence of MS and its association with fertilization rates, embryo grading, and ROS levels in the follicular fluid. Reactive oxygen species (ROS) in follicular fluid (FF) was significantly higher in the PCOS and tubal block group as compared to the endometriosis group (p < 0.001) **(Table 9.2)**. The absence of MS in each group (i.e. A2, B2, C2 versus A1, B1, C1, respectively) was associated with significantly higher ROS values (p < 0.001) **(Fig. 9.4)**.

Even with a higher oocyte yield in women with PCOS (Group B), the proportion of mature oocytes as well as MS visualization in these mature oocytes was lower. The relatively lower number of zygotes and embryos formed in Group B may be attributed to the higher number of oocytes lacking MS. In their meta-analysis,[74] similarly demonstrated a significantly higher number of oocytes retrieved with a lower fertilization rate and comparable number of good quality embryos in the PCOS than the control group (tubal factor). This has been confirmed by other authors.[75] It is suggested that a certain threshold level of ROS in FF is essential

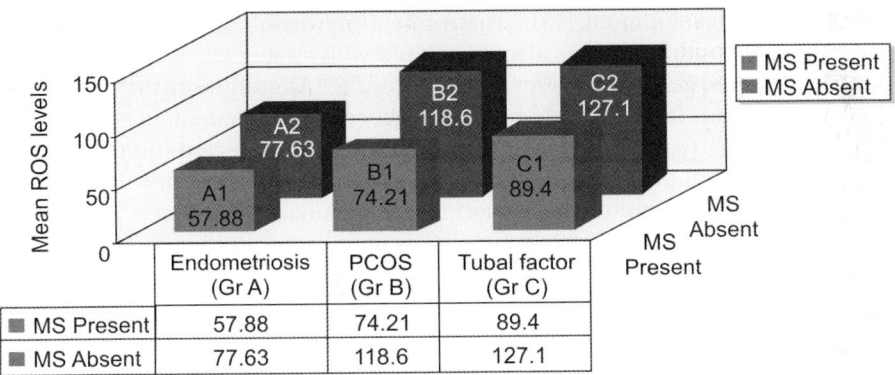

Fig. 9.4 MS imaging vs ROS levels

for several reproductive events,[76] and may be required for a better reproductive outcome in IVF/ICSI cycles.[77] While some studies suggest optimum level of follicular fluid ROS to be a marker for predicting success in IVF cycles,[78] others have demonstrated a toxic effect of high ROS levels in FF on oocytes and lower pregnancy rates.[79] A study by Das et al. also indicated that high FF ROS levels tend to decrease the fertilization potential of oocytes; furthermore, a higher percentage of good quality embryos was observed corresponding to ROS levels <100 CPS.[80] An association between adverse effects of OS on oocyte spindle assembly is suggested in mouse oocytes.[81] Irrespective of the cause of infertility, be it endometriosis, PCOS, or tubal infertility, the presence of MS and low ROS levels and lower OS is associated with an improved IVF outcome. Higher ROS levels and lower proportion of oocytes with MS in women with PCOS may thus contribute to a lower fertilization rate and lower good quality embryo formation. Though oxidative stress is postulated as one of the possible mechanisms of pathogenesis of endometriosis,[82] we found mean ROS follicular fluid levels to be lower in endometriosis as compared to PCOS and tubal factor controls.

High oxidative stress appears to inhibit meiotic spindle formation and subsequently affects embryo quality. Women with PCOS had less number of oocytes with meiotic spindle visualization and higher mean ROS levels in follicular fluid indicating a poorer oocyte and thus embryo quality in these women which may be attributed to an excessive generation of ROS and lipid peroxidation (LPO), and to an impaired antioxidant defense mechanism in FF of PCOS women.[83]

MITOCHONDRIAL ASSESSMENT AND METABOLISM

Polycystic ovary syndrome (PCOS) is associated with metabolic disturbances, which include impaired insulin signals and glucose metabolism in ovarian follicles. The oocyte is metabolically dependent upon its follicle environment during development, but it is unclear whether PCOS or polycystic ovarian (PCO) morphology alone affects oocyte metabolism and energy-demanding processes such as meiosis. Oocytes have a large quantity of mitochondria, which play a crucial role in egg maturation and fertilizing potential[84,85] as well as embryonic development.[86] The main role of mitochondria is the production of ATP. Mitochondrial DNA is also associated with epigenetic alterations which can cause altered gene expression and function.[87,88] Alterations in mitochondrial DNA methylation have recently been associated with metabolic disorders.[89-91] It has been reported that mitochondrial distribution is affected in PCO oocytes and the mitochondrial potential is also reduced.[92,93] The copy number of mitochondrial DNA and its expression is also significantly reduced.[93] This may be associated with high homocysteine levels in follicular fluid in PCOS patients. Abnormal carbon metabolism and methylation of mitochondrial DNA has also been related to mitochondrial dysfunction in PCO oocytes.[93]

EMBRYO IN POLYCYSTIC OVARY

PCOS patients usually suffer from poor outcomes and, most of the times, it is attributed to poor egg quality. Research is now showing us that there are a lot more intricate details involved. Morphokinetic studies have shown that PCOS women had slower embryo development from ICSI till 2 pronuclei (PN), the first cleavage and second cleavage were also affected when compared to a cohort of non-PCOS embryos. When cultured to blastocyst, the observed delay started to recover and there was no difference after 7th cell stage and the embryo kinetics were also similar. There were a few confounding factors in the one of being poorer sperm quality in the PCOS group, which can be one of the reasons for slower embryo development. However, even with lower sperm quality, morphokinetic changes were still observed between control embryos and embryos PCOS women, indicating that the delayed embryo development in embryos derived from hyperandrogenic PCOS women was probably oocyte related.[94] The cleavage time can be used to assess the embryo quality in PCOS patients[95] and a time lapse evaluation of 459 zygotes did show that embryos with a faster cleavage in the first 3 divisions had a higher chance of blastulation and had higher implantation rates.[96,97] Bellver et al. 2013[98] assessed embryos from obese patients (patients $n = 13$, of whom four had PCOS) and found a significant delay at *t2 and t3 division* when compared with embryos from fertile non-obese oocyte donors. The development delay was similar to the one shown in hyperandrogenic PCOS patients and thus it supports the evidence that maternal metabolic status and hormonal disturbances do alter embryonic development *in vitro*.[98] However in both studies, the pattern of embryonic development had no direct effect on implantation and pregnancy rates so it is hard to conclude whether these patterns have a clinical significance or not. The maternal effect on embryo morphokinetics may be because of the dependence on RNA transcription until the embryonic genome takes over.[100] This is a possible explanation for the initial delayed cleavage but a subsequent restoration of normality once the 8 cell stage is complete. To further support this notion sibling embryo studies have shown the same pattern of embryo development in different culture medias.[99]

Murine models have shown that diabetes and obesity, associated with insulin resistance, have a direct effect on oocyte quality and embryonic development. It has also shown that such eggs and embryos have ultrastructural mitochondrial abnormalities and metabolic irregularities.[101] Insulin resistance and obesity also had a direct correlation with the amount of oxidative stress generated in mice eggs and had a significant effect on the mitochondrial abnormalities in them.[102]

We know that mitochondrial inheritance is solely by the mother and paternal mitochondria cannot survive in the oocyte.[103] Thus slow embryonic development can also be because of the mitochondrial dysfunction in the oocytes, an entity which is already well established in PCOS women.

STRATEGIES FOR MANAGING PCOS IN THE LAB

In Vitro Fertilization vs Intracytoplasmic Sperm Injection

Sibling oocyte studies in PCOS patients in which the husband semen samples were normal according to the World Health Organization (WHO) and strict Kruger's criteria have shown that, the percentage of MII oocytes in cases of complete fertilization failure were not different in patients who underwent IVF, but the eggs that were inseminated using ICSI had a better fertilization rate when compared to conventional IVF. Complete fertilization failure was as high as 15% in conventional IVF compared to none in the ICSI group: Other than fertilization rates there was no difference in cleavage rates, morphology and rate of development in both groups. Similar observations have been made in other studies as well[104-106] retrospectively.

Sibling oocytes which underwent ICSI did have a higher fertilization rate, thus suggest that ICSI can overcome low fertilization and high incidence of fertilization failure in PCOS patients. It might be due to the fact that PCOS patients might have some underlying abnormality in the zona pellucida (ZP), and because ICSI bypasses this ZP-sperm binding reaction, the rates with ICSI are much higher, but again more evidence is required to come to a conclusion on the same. Stadtmauer et al.[107] did ICSI in patients with PCOS and previous poor fertilization with IVF and the RCT concluded that ICSI should be performed in all or at least a portion of eggs in PCOS patients **(Fig. 9.5)**.

Fresh Transfer vs Freeze All

Polycystic ovarian syndrome is one of the most common anovulatory disorders in infertility. We may have a high incidence of getting more eggs from PCOS but pregnancy rates have been reported to be similar when compared with controls. New data suggests that women with PCOS tend to have a higher incidence of miscarriages and meta-analysis have shown that such patients have a higher risk of maternal and neonatal complications.[110] Many observational studies have reported to have better outcomes when frozen-thawed embryos were transferred in PCOS patients when compared to a fresh transfer.[108] Some have reported significant correlations between elevated peak serum estradiol and risks of SGA (small for gestation age) as well as preeclampsia in singleton conceived pregnancies.[109]

Elective cryopreservation and transfer reduces the chances of SGA and preeclampsia when compared with fresh transfers in patients with high E2 (>3450 pg/mL). Sadly most of the data is based on retrospective analysis and most studies were uncontrolled, thus better evidence is required to come to a definitive conclusion.[110] In patients, who have a higher risk of OHSS delaying transfer does reduce the maternal complications associated with the same.

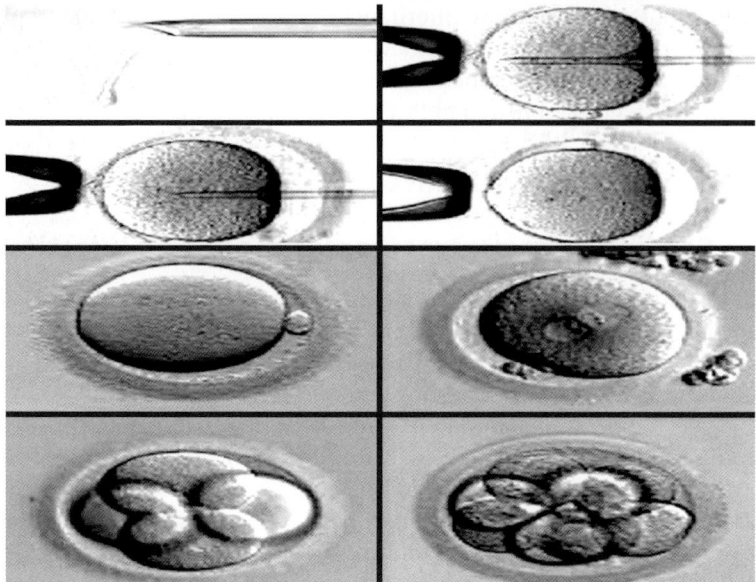

Fig. 9.5 Normal embryo development seen in PCO oocytes

IN VITRO MATURATION

In vitro maturation is a process where oocytes are taken out from ovaries while immature and cultured in vitro to achieve maturity before being fertilized. We have already discussed how the ovarian environment is altered in PCOS and there is an increased risk of getting poor quality eggs due to the various intra- as well as extraovarian factors that influence oogenesis. Thus it was hypothesized that when eggs are matured in the laboratory, they would have a more controlled and predictable environment thus leading to better oocyte quality[111-113] than what would have been recovered with a gonadotropin stimulation.[112,113] In vitro maturation of oocytes of PCOS patients can be a very attractive option as it eliminates the problem of immature oocyte recovery after pick up. In this method, eggs are retrieved from cycles which are almost similar to natural cycles and are matured in vitro utilizing special media and then fertilized using ICSI.[114-116] As of now reported pregnancies and implantation rates are lower but the cost as well as complications of stimulations are significantly reduced.[115]

As IVM has the best results with patients with a higher astral follicle count in minimally stimulated ovaries it is all the more beneficial in PCOS, also women who have had poor outcomes with stimulated cycles may benefit from IVM (**Fig. 9.6**).[117]

The most important parameter in controlling IVM outcomes is the culturing environment. Composition of most IVM media is based on mammalian research models.[118] TCM-199 with serum FSH, pyruvate, penicillin, streptomycin and hCG has shown the best maturation rates,[118] but the implantation rates have

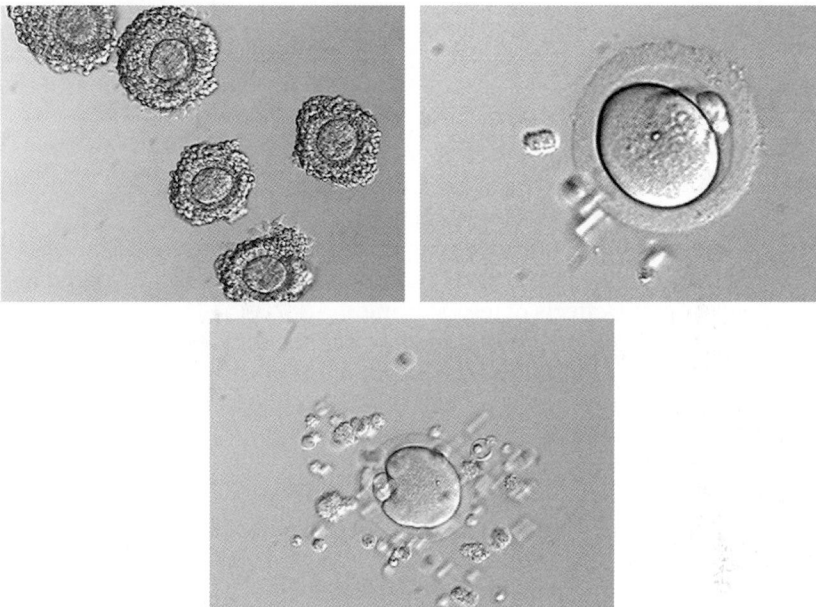

Fig. 9.6 Mature oocyte obtained after in vitro maturation (IVM) of immature comulative oocyte complexes (COCs) obtained from spiny mice. (*Courtesy: Student Research Project Sng Danielle, Arturo Macotella. Monash University. MCE 2014*)

been reported as 8% and clinical pregnancy rates have been reported to be 25% thus, more studies are required to determine how to optimize IVM and how we can improve the culture conditions to make it more successful. We must also take into consideration that this is still an experimental procedure and the efficacy and safety of the technique still needs to be addressed. Only around 400 births have been reported with this method and these children are still quite young if we must look at long-term implications.

Two studies,[119] which have been included in the American Society for Reproductive Medicine (ASRM) opinions on IVM reported 78.8% maturation in 3,079 oocytes collected from PCOS women after priming. Out of these, 69.2% fertilized. In another larger study where 6,860 were matured using IVM and maturation rate of 73% was reported and a fertilization of 79% seen. These meta-analysis reported pregnancy rates ranging from 24 to 34% and implantation ranged from 5 to 21%.[119]

The ASRM committee opinion clearly suggests that this is an experimental procedure which should be performed only at specialized centers after carefully selecting the right candidates for the same. Candidates for this technology include PCOS, PCO-like ovaries and women with estrogen sensitive cancers. ICSI is not necessary to achieve fertilization in such cases and initial results suggest that implantation and pregnancy rates are significantly lower with IVM, a detail which must be mentioned to the patients before starting the treatment.[120]

KEY POINTS

- To understand the pathophysiology of PCOS, both the nature of the dysfunction within the ovary and the external influences that modify ovarian behavior, are considered.
- Women with PCOS have a generalized overactive steroidogenesis.
- LH and insulin stimulate TC androgen production and insulin also amplifies the effects of testosterone.
- Serum LH concentrations may be significantly elevated due to an increased amplitude and frequency of LH pulses.
- Hyperinsulinemia is a key component in the pathogenesis of PCOS, although it is not ubiquitous.
- Poorer oocyte quality is due to effect on internal biology of the oocyte.
- The embryo quality is also affected.
- ICSI tends to have a higher fertilization when compared to conventional IVF.
- Frozen cycles tend to have better outcome but more studies needed
- IVM is a great new frontier for such patients but is still considered experimental.
- Patient undergoing IVM must be counseled for poorer implantation and pregnancy rates.

REFERENCES

1. Moran L, Teede H. Metabolic features of the reproductive phenotypes of polycystic ovary syndrome. Human Reproduction Update. 2009;15(4):477-88.
2. Toulis KA, Goulis DG, Farmakiotis D, Georgopoulos NA, Katsikis I, Tarlatzis BC, et al. Adiponectin levels in women with polycystic ovary syndrome: a systematic review and a meta-analysis. Human Reproduction Update. 2009;15(3):297-307.
3. Cadagan D, Khan R, Amer S. Thecal cell sensitivity to luteinizing hormone and insulin in polycystic ovarian syndrome. Reproductive Biology. 2016;16(1):53-60.
4. Ludwig M, Finas DF, al-Hasani S, Diedrich K, Ortmann O. Oocyte quality and treatment outcome in intracytoplasmic sperm injection cycles of polycystic ovarian syndrome patients. Human reproduction (Oxford, England). 1999;14(2):354-8.
5. Mulders AG, Laven JS, Imani B, Eijkemans MJ, Fauser BC. IVF outcome in anovulatory infertility (WHO group 2)--including polycystic ovary syndrome–following previous unsuccessful ovulation induction. Reproductive biomedicine online. 2003;7(1):50-8.
6. Weghofer A, Munne S, Chen S, Barad D, Gleicher N. Lack of association between polycystic ovary syndrome and embryonic aneuploidy. Fertility and Sterility. 2007;88 (4):900-5.
7. Sahu B, Ozturk O, Ranierri M, Serhal P. Comparison of oocyte quality and intracytoplasmic sperm injection outcome in women with isolated polycystic ovaries or polycystic ovarian syndrome. Archives of Gynecology and obstetrics. 2008;277(3): 239-44.
8. Gianaroli L, Magli MC, Ferraretti AP, Fortini D, Grieco N. Pronuclear morphology and chromosomal abnormalities as scoring criteria for embryo selection. Fertility and Sterility. 2003;80(2):341-9.
9. Gianaroli L, Magli MC, Ferraretti AP, Lappi M, Borghi E, Ermini B. Oocyte euploidy, pronuclear zygote morphology and embryo chromosomal complement. Human Reproduction (Oxford, England). 2007;22(1):241-9.

10. Wang Q, Luo L, Lei Q, Lin MM, Huang X, Chen MH, et al. Low aneuploidy rate in early pregnancy loss abortuses from patients with polycystic ovary syndrome. Reproductive biomedicine online. 2016.
11. Franks S, Roberts R, Hardy K. Gonadotrophin regimens and oocyte quality in women with polycystic ovaries. Reproductive biomedicine online. 2003;6(2):181-4.
12. Dumesic DA, Padmanabhan V, Abbott DH. Polycystic ovary syndrome and oocyte developmental competence. Obstetrical and Gynecological Survey. 2008;63(1):39-48.
13. Wood JR, Dumesic DA, Abbott DH, Strauss JF, 3rd. Molecular abnormalities in oocytes from womene with polycystic ovary syndrome revealed by microarray analysis. Journal of Clinical Endocrinology and Metabolism. 2007;92(2):705-13.
14. Dumesic DA, Richards JS. Ontogeny of the ovary in polycystic ovary syndrome. Fertility and Sterility. 2013;100(1):23-38.
15. Huang X, Hao C, Shen X, Liu X, Shan Y, Zhang Y, et al. Differences in the transcriptional profiles of human cumulus cells isolated from MI and MII oocytes of patients with polycystic ovary syndrome. Reproduction (Cambridge, England). 2013;145(6):597-608.
16. van der Spuy ZM, Dyer SJ. The pathogenesis of infertility and early pregnancy loss in polycystic ovary syndrome. Best Practice and Research Clinical Bbstetrics and Gynaecology. 2004;18(5):755-71.
17. Dumesic DA, Abbott DH, Padmanabhan V. Polycystic ovary syndrome and its developmental origins. Reviews in Endocrine and Metabolic Disorders. 2007;8(2):127-41.
18. Boomsma CM, Fauser BCJM, Macklon NS. Pregnancy complications in women with polycystic ovary syndrome. Semin Reprod Med. 2008;26(1):72-84.
19. Erickson GF, Shimasaki S. The physiology of folliculogenesis: the role of novel growth factors. Fertility and sterility. 2001;76(5):943-9.
20. Padhy N, Latha M, Sathya B, Varma TR. Antral follicle size in the downregulated cycle and its relation to in vitro fertilization outcome. Journal of Human Reproductive sciences. 2009;2(2):68-71.
21. Hillier SG. Current concepts of the roles of follicle stimulating hormone and luteinizing hormone in folliculogenesis. Human Reproduction (Oxford, England). 1994;9(2):188-91.
22. Franks S. Polycystic ovary syndrome in adolescents. International Journal of Obesity. 2008;32(7):1035-41.
23. Cano F, Garcia-Velasco JA, Millet A, Remohi J, Simon C, Pellicer A. Oocyte quality in polycystic ovaries revisited: identification of a particular subgroup of women. Journal of Assisted Reproduction and Genetics. 1997;14(5):254-61.
24. Urman B, Tiras B, Yakin K. Assisted reproduction in the treatment of polycystic ovarian syndrome. Reproductive biomedicine online. 2004;8(4):419-30.
25. Hardy K, Robinson FM, Paraschos T, Wicks R, Franks S, Winston RM. Normal development and metabolic activity of preimplantation embryos in vitro from patients with polycystic ovaries. Human Reproduction (Oxford, England). 1995;10(8):2125-35.
26. Balen AH, Conway GS, Kaltsas G, Techatrasak K, Manning PJ, West C, et al. Polycystic ovary syndrome: the spectrum of the disorder in 1741 patients. Human Reproduction (Oxford, England). 1995;10(8):2107-11.
27. Adams J, Franks S, Polson DW, Mason HD, Abdulwahid N, Tucker M, et al. Multi-follicular ovaries: clinical and endocrine features and response to pulsatile gonado-tropin releasing hormone. The Lancet (London, England). 1985;2(8469-70):1375-9.
28. Homburg R, Jacobs HS. Etiology of miscarriage in polycystic ovary syndrome. Fertility and Sterility. 1989;51(1):196-7.
29. Regan L, Owen EJ, Jacobs HS. Originally published as Hypersecretion of luteinizing hormone, infertility, and miscarriage. The Lancet. 1990;336(8724):1141-4.
30. Sengoku K, Tamate K, Takuma N, Yoshida T, Goishi K, Ishikawa M. The chromosomal normality of unfertilized oocytes from patients with polycystic ovarian syndrome. Human reproduction (Oxford, England). 1997;12(3):474-7.

31. Jabara S, Coutifaris C. In vitro fertilization in the PCOS patient: clinical considerations. Semin Reprod Med. 2003;21(3):317-24.
32. Santos MA, Kuijk EW, Macklon NS. The impact of ovarian stimulation for IVF on the developing embryo. Reproduction (Cambridge, England). 2010;139(1):23-34.
33. Dumesic DA, Schramm RD, Peterson E, Paprocki AM, Zhou R, Abbott DH. Impaired developmental competence of oocytes in adult prenatally androgenized female rhesus monkeys undergoing gonadotropin stimulation for in vitro fertilization. The Journal of Clinical Endocrinology and Metabolism. 2002;87(3):1111-9.
34. Kurzawa R, Ciepiela P, Baczkowski T, Safranow K, Brelik P. Comparison of embryological and clinical outcome in GnRH antagonist vs. GnRH agonist protocols for in vitro fertilization in PCOS non-obese patients. A prospective randomized study. Journal of Assisted Reproduction and Genetics. 2008;25(8):365-74.
35. Ben-Shlomo I. The polycystic ovary syndrome: what does insulin resistance have to do with it? Reproductive biomedicine online. 2003;6(1):36-42.
36. Jamnongjit M, Hammes SR. Ovarian steroids: the good, the bad, and the signals that raise them. Cell cycle (Georgetown, Tex). 2006;5(11):1178-83.
37. Stoklosowa S, Bahr J, Gregoraszczuk E. Some morphological and functional characteristics of cells of the porcine theca interna in tissue culture. Advances in Experimental Medicine and Biology. 1979;112:145-8.
38. Teissier MP, Chable H, Paulhac S, Aubard Y. Comparison of follicle steroidogenesis from normal and polycystic ovaries in women undergoing IVF: relationship between steroid concentrations, follicle size, oocyte quality and fecundability. Human Reproduction (Oxford, England). 2000;15(12):2471-7.
39. Tesarik J, Mendoza C. Nongenomic effects of 17 beta-estradiol on maturing human oocytes: relationship to oocyte developmental potential. The Journal of Clinical Endocrinology and Metabolism. 1995;80(4):1438-43.
40. Okon MA, Laird SM, Tuckerman EM, Li TC. Serum androgen levels in women who have recurrent miscarriages and their correlation with markers of endometrial function. Fertility and Sterility. 1998;69(4):682-90.
41. Tuckerman EM, Okon MA, Li T, Laird SM. Do androgens have a direct effect on endometrial function? An in vitro study. Fertility and Sterility. 2000;74(4):771-9.
42. Craig LB, Ke RW, Kutteh WH. Increased prevalence of insulin resistance in women with a history of recurrent pregnancy loss. Fertility and Sterility. 2002;78(3):487-90.
43. Kezele PR, Nilsson EE, Skinner MK. Insulin but not insulin-like growth factor-1 promotes the primordial to primary follicle transition. Molecular and Cellular Endocrinology. 2002;192(1–2):37-43.
44. Wijeyaratne CN, Balen AH, Barth JH, Belchetz PE. Clinical manifestations and insulin resistance (IR) in polycystic ovary syndrome (PCOS) among South Asians and Caucasians: is there a difference? Clinical Endocrinology. 2002;57(3):343-50.
45. Hsieh YY, Chang CC, Tsai HD, Lin CS. Leukemia inhibitory factor in follicular fluid is not related to the number and quality of embryos as well as implantation and pregnancy rates. Biochemical Genetics. 2005;43(9-10):501-6.
46. Artini PG, Battaglia C, D'Ambrogio G, Barreca A, Droghini F, Volpe A, et al. Relationship between human oocyte maturity, fertilization and follicular fluid growth factors. Human Reproduction (Oxford, England). 1994;9(5):902-6.
47. Franks S, Mason H, Willis D. Follicular dynamics in the polycystic ovary syndrome. Mol Cell Endocrinol. 2000;163(1-2):49-52.
48. Baskind NE, Balen AH. Hypothalamic-pituitary, ovarian and adrenal contributions to polycystic ovary syndrome. Best Practice and Research Clinical Obstetrics and Gynaecology. 2016.
49. Weenen C, Laven JS, Von Bergh AR, Cranfield M, Groome NP, Visser JA, et al. Anti-Müllerian hormone expression pattern in the human ovary: potential implications for initial and cyclic follicle recruitment. Molecular Human Reproduction. 2004;10(2): 77-83.

50. Sadeu JC, Smitz J. Growth differentiation factor-9 and anti-Müllerian hormone expression in cultured human follicles from frozen-thawed ovarian tissue. Reproductive biomedicine online. 2008;17(4):537-48.
51. Stubbs SA, Hardy K, Da Silva-Buttkus P, Stark J, Webber LJ, Flanagan AM, et al. Anti-Müllerian hormone protein expression is reduced during the initial stages of follicle development in human polycystic ovaries. The Journal of Clinical Endocrinology and Metabolism. 2005;90(10):5536-43.
52. Pellatt L, Hanna L, Brincat M, Galea R, Brain H, Whitehead S, et al. Granulosa cell production of anti-Müllerian hormone is increased in polycystic ovaries. The Journal of Clinical Endocrinology and Metabolism. 2007;92(1):240-5.
53. Pellatt L, Rice S, Dilaver N, Heshri A, Galea R, Brincat M, et al. Anti-Müllerian hormone reduces follicle sensitivity to follicle-stimulating hormone in human granulosa cells. Fertility and Sterility. 2011;96(5):1246-51.e1.
54. Wei LN, Huang R, Li LL, Fang C, Li Y, Liang XY. Reduced and delayed expression of GDF9 and BMP15 in ovarian tissues from women with polycystic ovary syndrome. Journal of Assisted Reproduction and Genetics. 2014;31(11):1483-90.
55. Knight PG, Glister C. TGF-beta superfamily members and ovarian follicle development. Reproduction (Cambridge, England). 2006;132(2):191-206.
56. Artini PG, Monti M, Matteucci C, Valentino V, Cristello F, Genazzani AR. Vascular endothelial growth factor and basic fibroblast growth factor in polycystic ovary syndrome during controlled ovarian hyperstimulation. Gynecological endocrinology: the official Journal of the International Society of Gynecological Endocrinology. 2006;22(8):465-70.
57. Hammadeh ME, Fischer-Hammadeh C, Hoffmeister H, Huebner U, Georg T, Rosenbaum P, et al. Fibroblast growth factor (FGF), intracellular adhesion molecule (sICAM-1) level in serum and follicular fluid of infertile women with polycystic ovarian syndrome, endometriosis and tubal damage, and their effect on ICSI outcome. American Journal of Reproductive Immunology (New York, NY: 1989). 2003;50(2):124-30.
58. Goodarzi, Mark O, et al. Polycystic ovary syndrome: etiology, pathogenesis and diagnosis. Nature Review Endocrinology. 2011;7(4):219-31.
59. Westergaard LG, Andersen CY. Epidermal growth factor (EGF) in human preovulatory follicles. Human Reproduction (Oxford, England). 1989;4(3):257-60.
60. Jamnongjit M, Gill A, Hammes SR. Epidermal growth factor receptor signaling is required for normal ovarian steroidogenesis and oocyte maturation. Proceedings of the National Academy of Sciences of the United States of America. 2005;102(45):16257-62.
61. Hsieh M, Zamah AM, Conti M. Epidermal growth factor-like growth factors in the follicular fluid: role in oocyte development and maturation. Semin Reprod Med. 2009;27(1):52-61.
62. Cohen Y, Malcov M, Schwartz T, Mey-Raz N, Carmon A, Cohen T, Lessing JB, Amit A, Azem F. Spindle imaging: a new marker for optimal timing of ICSI? Human Reproduction. 2004(1);19(3):649-54.
63. Dumesic DA, Padmanabhan V, Abbott DH. Polycystic ovary syndrome and oocyte developmental competence. Obstetrical and gynecological survey. 2008;63(1):39.
64. Rajani S, Chattopadhyay R, Goswami SK, Ghosh S, Sharma S, Chakravarty B. Assessment of oocyte quality in polycystic ovarian syndrome and endometriosis by spindle imaging and reactive oxygen species levels in follicular fluid and its relationship with IVF-ET outcome. Journal of human reproductive sciences. 2012;5(2):187.
65. Franks S, Hardy K. Aberrant follicle development and anovulation in polycystic ovary syndrome. In: Annalesd'endocrinologie. Elsevier Masson. 2010;71(3)228-30.
66. Rienzi L, Ubaldi F, Iacobelli M, Minasi MG, Romano S, Greco E. Meiotic spindle visualization in living human oocytes. Reproductive biomedicine online. 2005;10(2):192-8.

67. Eiben B, Borgmann S, Schübbe I, Hansmann I. A cytogenetic study directly from chorionic villi of 140 spontaneous abortions. Human Genetics. 1987;77(2):137-41.
68. Plachot M. Chromosomal abnormalities in oocytes. Molecular and cellular endocrinology. 2001;183:S59-63.
69. Angell RR, Ledger W, Yong EL, Harkness L, Baird DT. Cytogenetic analysis of unfertilized human oocytes. Human Reproduction. 1991;6(4):568-73.
70. De Santis L, Cino I, Rabellotti E, Calzi F, Persico P, Borini A, Coticchio G. Polar body morphology and spindle imaging as predictors of oocyte quality. Reproductive biomedicine online. 2005;11(1):36-42.
71. Wang WH, Meng L, Hackett RJ, Keefe DL. Developmental ability of human oocytes with or without birefringent spindles imaged by polscope before insemination. Human Reproduction. 2001;16(7):1464-8.
72. Inoué S. Polarization optical studies of the mitotic spindle. Chromosoma. 1953;5(1):487-500.
73. Liu L, Oldenbourg R, Trimarchi JR, Keefe DL. A reliable, noninvasive technique for spindle imaging and enucleation of mammalian oocytes. Nature biotechnology. 2000;18(2):223-5.
74. Heijnen EM, Eijkemans MJ, Hughes EG, Laven JS, Macklon N3, Fauser BC. A meta-analysis of outcomes of conventional IVF in women with polycystic ovary syndrome. Human reproduction update. 2006;12(1):13-21.
75. Fernandez H. Oocyte and embryo quality in polycystic ovary syndrome. Gynecol Obstet Fertil. 2003;31:350-4.
76. Tarin JJ, Vendrell FJ, Ten J, Cano A. Antioxidant therapy counteracts the disturbing effects of diamide and maternal ageing on meiotic division and chromosomal segregation in mouse oocytes. Molecular Human Reproduction. 1998;4(3):281-8.
77. Yildirim B, Demir S, Temur I, Erdemir R, Kaleli B. Lipid peroxidation in follicular fluid of women with polycystic ovary syndrome during assisted reproduction cycles. The Journal of Reproductive Medicine. 2007;52(8):722-6.
78. Agarwal A, Gupta S, Sharma R. Oxidative stress and its implications in female infertility-a clinician's perspective. Reproductive biomedicine online. 2005;11(5):641-50.
79. Oyawoye O, Gadir AA, Garner A, Constantinovici N, Perrett C, Hardiman P. Antioxidants and reactive oxygen species in follicular fluid of women undergoing IVF: relationship to outcome. Human Reproduction. 2003;18(11):2270-4.
80. Das S, Chattopadhyay R, Ghosh S, Goswami SK, Chakravarty BN, Chaudhury K. Reactive oxygen species level in follicular fluid—embryo quality marker in IVF?. Human Reproduction. 2006;21(9):2403-7.
81. Zuelke KA, Jones DP, Perreault SD. Glutathione oxidation is associated with altered microtubule function and disrupted fertilization in mature hamster oocytes. Biology of reproduction. 1997;57(6):1413-9.
82. Bedaiwy MA, Falcone T. Peritoneal fluid environment in endometriosis. Minerva Cineol. 2003;55(4):333-45.
83. Rajani S, Chattopadhyay R, Goswami SK, Ghosh S, Sharma S, Chakravarty B. Assessment of oocyte quality in polycystic ovarian syndrome and endometriosis by spindle imaging and reactive oxygen species levels in follicular fluid and its relationship with IVF-ET outcome. Journal of Human Reproductive Sciences. 2012;5(2):187.
84. May-Panloup P, Chretien MF, Jacques C, Vasseur C, Malthiery Y, Reynier P. Low oocyte mitochondrial DNA content in ovarian insufficiency. Human Reproduction. 2005;20(3):593-7.
85. Cummins JM. The role of mitochondria in the establishment of oocyte functional competence. European Journal of Obstetrics and Gynecology and Reproductive Biology. 2004;115:S23-9.

86. Dumollard R, Duchen M, Carroll J. The role of mitochondrial function in the oocyte and embryo. Current topics in Developmental biology. 2007;77:21-49.
87. Rebelo AP, Williams SL, Moraes CT. In vivo methylation of mtDNA reveals the dynamics of protein–mtDNA interactions. Nucleic acids research. 2009;37(20):6701-15.
88. Metodiev MD, Lesko N, Park CB, Cámara Y, Shi Y, Wibom R, Hultenby K, Gustafsson CM, Larsson NG. Methylation of 12S rRNA is necessary for in vivo stability of the small subunit of the mammalian mitochondrial ribosome. Cell Metabolism. 2009;8;9(4): 386-97.
89. Iacobazzi V, Castegna A, Infantino V, Andria G. Mitochondrial DNA methylation as a next-generation biomarker and diagnostic tool. Molecular genetics and metabolism. 2013;110(1):25-34.
90. Feng S, Xiong L, Ji Z, Cheng W, Yang H. Correlation between increased ND2 expression and demethylated displacement loop of mtDNA in colorectal cancer. Mol Med Rep. 2012;6(1):125-30.
91. Janssen BG, Byun HM, Gyselaers W, Lefebvre W, Baccarelli AA, Nawrot TS. Placental mitochondrial methylation and exposure to airborne particulate matter in the early life environment: An ENVIR ON AGE birth cohort study. Epigenetics. 2015;3;10(6): 536-44.
92. Crider KS, Yang TP, Berry RJ, Bailey LB. Folate and DNA methylation: a review of molecular mechanisms and the evidence for folate's role. Advances in Nutrition: An International Review Journal. 2012;3(1):21-38.
93. Jia L, Li J, He B, Jia Y, Niu Y, Wang C, Zhao R. Abnormally activated one-carbon metabolic pathway is associated with mtDNA hypermethylation and mitochondrial malfunction in the oocytes of polycystic gilt ovaries. Scientific reports. 2016;6.
94. Azzarello A, Hoest T, Mikkelsen AL. The impact of pronuclei morphology and dynamicity on live birth outcome after time-lapse culture. Human Reproduction. 2012;27(9):2649-57.
95. Dal Canto M, Coticchio G, Renzini MM, De Ponti E, Novara PV, Brambillasca F, Comi R, Fadini R. Cleavage kinetics analysis of human embryos predicts development to blastocyst and implantation. Reproductive biomedicine online. 2012;25(5):474-80.
96. Meseguer M, Herrero J, Tejera A, Hilligsøe KM, Ramsing NB, RemohíJ. The use of morphokinetics as a predictor of embryo implantation. Human reproduction. 2011;26(10):2658-71.
97. Lemmen JG, Agerholm I, Ziebe S. Kinetic markers of human embryo quality using time-lapse recordings of IVF/ICSI-fertilized oocytes. Reproductive biomedicine online. 2008;17(3):385-91.
98. Bellver J, Pellicer A, García-Velasco JA, Ballesteros A, Remohí J, Meseguer M. Obesity reduces uterine receptivity: clinical experience from 9,587 first cycles of ovum donation with normal weight donors. Fertility and Sterility. 2013;100(4):1050-8.
99. Basile N, Morbeck D, García-Velasco J, Bronet F, Meseguer M. Type of culture media does not affect embryo kinetics: a time-lapse analysis of sibling oocytes. Human Reproduction. 2013;28(3):634-41.
100. Braude P, Bolton V, Moore S. Human gene expression first occurs between the four- and eight-cell stages of preimplantation development. Nature. 1988;332(6163): 459-61.
101. Jungheim ES, Schoeller EL, Marquard KL, Louden ED, Schaffer JE, Moley KH. Diet-induced obesity model: abnormal oocytes and persistent growth abnormalities in the offspring. Endocrinology. 2010;151(8):4039-46.
102. Igosheva N, Abramov AY, Poston L, Eckert JJ, Fleming TP, Duchen MR, McConnell J. Maternal diet-induced obesity alters mitochondrial activity and redox status in mouse oocytes and zygotes. PloS one. 2010;5(4):e10074.
103. Craigen WJ. Mitochondrial DNA mutations: an overview of clinical and molecular aspects. Mitochondrial Disorders: Biochemical and Molecular Analysis. 2012:3-15.

104. Hwang JL, Seow KM, Lin YH, Hsieh BC, Huang LW, Chen HJ, Huang SC, Chen CY, Chen PH, Tzeng CR. IVF versus ICSI in sibling oocytes from patients with polycystic ovarian syndrome: a randomized controlled trial. Human Reproduction. 2005;20(5):1261-5.
105. Sengoku K, Tamate K, Takuma N, Yoshida T, Goishi K, Ishikawa M. The chromosomal normality of unfertilized oocytes from patients with polycystic ovarian syndrome. Human Reproduction. 1997;12(3):474-7.
106. Ludwig M, Finas DF, Al-Hasani S, Diedrich K, Ortmann O. Oocyte quality and treatment outcome in intracytoplasmic sperm injection cycles of polycystic ovarian syndrome patients. Human Reproduction. 1999;14(2):354-8.
107. Stadtmauer LA, Toma SK, Riehl RM, Talbert LM. Metformin treatment of patients with polycystic ovary syndrome undergoing in vitro fertilization improves outcomes and is associated with modulation of the insulin-like growth factors. Fertility and Sterility. 2001;75(3):505-9.
108. Imbar T, Kol S, Lossos F, Bdolah Y, Hurwitz A, Haimov-Kochman R. Reproductive outcome of fresh or frozen-thawed embryo transfer is similar in high-risk patients for ovarian hyperstimulation syndrome using GnRH agonist for final oocyte maturation and intensive luteal support. Human Reproduction. 2012;27(3):753-9.
109. Hu XL, Feng C, Lin XH, Zhong ZX, Zhu YM, Lv PP, Lv M, Meng Y, Zhang D, Lu XE, Jin F. High maternal serum estradiol environment in the first trimester is associated with the increased risk of small-for-gestational-age birth. The Journal of Clinical Endocrinology and Metabolism. 2014;99(6):2217-24.
110. Imbar T, Kol S, Lossos F, Bdolah Y, Hurwitz A, Haimov-Kochman R. Reproductive outcome of fresh or frozen-thawed embryo transfer is similar in high-risk patients for ovarian hyperstimulation syndrome using GnRH agonist for final oocyte maturation and intensive luteal support. Human Reproduction. 2012;27(3):753-9.
111. Almahbobi G, Trounson AO. The role of intraovarian regulators in the aetiology of polycystic ovarian syndrome. Reproductive Medicine Review. 1996;5(03):151-68.
112. Baker SJ, Spears N. The role of intraovarian interactions in the regulation of follicle dominance. Human Reproduction Update. 1999;5(2):153-65.
113. Cha KY, Koo JJ, Ko JJ, Choi DH, Han SY, Yoon TK. Pregnancy after in vitro fertilization of human follicular oocytes collected from nonstimulated cycles, their culture in vitro and their transfer in a donor oocyte program. Fertility and Sterility. 1991;55(1):109-13.
114. Borghol N, Lornage J, Blachère T, Garret AS, Lefèvre A. Epigenetic status of the H19 locus in human oocytes following in vitro maturation. Genomics. 2006;87(3):417-26.
115. Cha KY, Han SY, Chung HM, Choi DH, Lim JM, Lee WS, Ko JJ, Yoon TK. Pregnancies and deliveries after in vitro maturation culture followed by in vitro fertilization and embryo transfer without stimulation in women with polycystic ovary syndrome. Fertility and sterility. 2000;31;73(5):978-83.
116. Cha KY, Chung HM, Lee DR, Kwon H, Chung MK, Park LS, Choi DH, Yoon TK. Obstetric outcome of patients with polycystic ovary syndrome treated by in vitro maturation and in vitro fertilization–embryo transfer. Fertility and sterility. 2005;31;83(5):1461-5.
117. Child TJ, Abdul-Jalil AK, Gulekli B, Tan SL. In vitro maturation and fertilization of oocytes from unstimulated normal ovaries, polycystic ovaries, and women with polycystic ovary syndrome. Fertility and Sterility. 2001;76(5):936-42.
118. Lin YH, Hwang JL, Huang LW, Mu SC, Seow KM, Chung J, Hsieh BC, Huang SC, Chen CY, Chen PH. Combination of FSH priming and hCG priming for invitro maturation of human oocytes. Human Reproduction. 2003;18(8):1632-6.
119. Chian RC, Buckett WM, Tan SL. In-vitro maturation of human oocytes. Reproductive biomedicine online. 2004;31;8(2):148-66.
120. American Society for Reproductive Medicine. In vitro maturation: a committee opinion. Fertility and Sterility. 2013;99(3):663-6.

SECTION 4

AREAS OF CONCERN

10. Polycystic Ovarian Syndrome in Lean and Obese Women
11. Polycystic Ovarian Syndrome in Adolescents
12. Implications of Polycystic Ovarian Syndrome on Pregnancy
13. Psychological and Cognitive Problems in Polycystic Ovarian Syndrome
14. Long-term Sequel of Polycystic Ovarian Syndrome
15. Medicolegal Aspects of Polycystic Ovarian Disease

CHAPTER 10

Polycystic Ovarian Syndrome in Lean and Obese Women

Kundan Vasant Ingale

INTRODUCTION

Polycystic ovarian syndrome (PCOS) is a frequent endocrine-metabolic dysfunction, characterized by chronic anovulation and hyperandrogenism affecting the reproductive function of young women and that is closely associated with insulin resistance (IR) which plays preponderant role in chronic anovulation and long-term metabolic consequences of the syndrome. The clinical manifestations of PCOS are heterogeneous and vary according to the patient's age. In general, they begin during perimenarche with menstrual alterations, mainly oligomenorrhea, hyperandrogenism and android obesity. Hyperinsulinemia and insulin resistance are characteristic features of obese and nonobese women with PCOS. In the original description of Stein and Leventhal, obesity was one of the main characteristics of PCOS, besides infertility and hirsutism. Since the first description of the syndrome, numerous studies focused on the role of obesity in the pathogenetic process of PCOS. It is known that nearly half of the women with PCOS are either overweight or obese[1] and when present, obesity worsens the clinical presentation of PCOS.[2] Overweight and obesity contribute to a significant proportion of menstrual disorders in women with PCOS. Mechanisms by which obesity interferes with the pathophysiology and clinical expressions of PCOS are complex and not completely understood. There is enough evidence to show that obesity does paly a role in the clinical appearance in PCOS women, however, the exact pathogenetic pathways in this process remain to be elucidated. There are endocrine and metabolic differences between lean and obese women with PCOS. One of the aim of this chapter is to reveal the facts and theories on the role of obesity in PCOS and to elucidate the probable pathophysiological mechanisms (**Fig. 10.1**).

CHANGES IN BODY WEIGHT AND MENSTRUATION

Changes in body weight are a critical factor in regulating menstrual cycles and reproduction. Apparently, there are significant associations between obesity and pubertal development,[3] irregular menstrual cycles, reduced spontaneous and induced fertility. Generally, changes in circulating sex hormones involving androgens, estrogens and those in sex hormone binding globulin (SHBG) levels, appear to underline the obesity related menstrual and reproductive disorders. Though the exact etiology of PCOS is unclear, the facts that the history of weight gain frequently precedes the onset of clinical manifestations, obese women have more severe hyperandrogenism,[4] and the presence of anovulatory cycles, oligomenorrhea and/or hirsutism are significantly higher in obese than in normal-weight women,[5] suggest a pathogenetic role of obesity in the development of PCOS and related infertility. Obesity in women with PCOS is also associated with adverse effects on the outcome of assisted reproductive technology (ART) treatments and an increased risk of miscarriage.[6]

It has been proposed that the pathogenesis of PCOS is different in obese and nonobese women, with insulin resistance and hyperinsulinemia playing a central role in obese women.[7]

NEUROENDOCRINE ABNORMALITIES IN POLYCYSTIC OVARIAN SYNDROME

In PCOS, LH levels are disproportionately elevated in comparison to follicular stimulating hormone (FSH), resulting in 94% of women with irregular cycles having an elevated LH/FSH ratio.[8] The LH amplitude response to exogenous GnRH is exaggerated in women with PCOS. Furthermore, the GnRH pulse frequency in increased in PCOS to approximately one pulse per 50–60 minutes, similar to the menopausal pulse frequency, and there is an increase in the overall amount of GnRH secreted that is similar in magnitude to the increase in pulse frequency.[9] This pattern of GnRH secretion favors the synthesis and secretion of LH over FSH. Altogether, the increase in GnRH pulse frequency and the increased pituitary responsiveness to GnRH suggest that neuroendocrine dysfunction may be a primary event in the pathogenesis of PCOS.

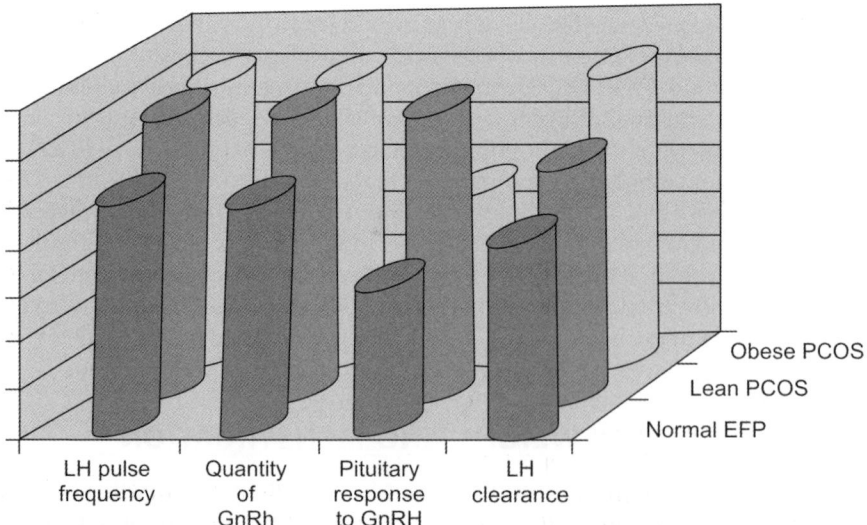

Fig. 10.1 Neuroendocrine features of lean and obese PCOS women relative to normal women in the early follicular phase (EFP)

Hypothalamic function, indicated by LH (GnRH) pulse frequency and overall quantity of GnRH, is increased in PCOS, but not affected by obesity, while the pituitary response to GnRH is increased in PCOS but attenuated by obesity. The effect of obesity on pituitary responsiveness and the increased clearance of LH that occurs in obese PCOS both contribute to the relative normalization of both LH levels and the LH/FSH ratio in obese PCOS. Thus, in setting PCO morphology, an abnormal gonadotropin environment is required for development of menstrual dysfunction.

While a high LH/FSH ratio is common in PCOS, in very obese women with PCOS, this ratio may be relatively normal. Although there is an increase in both GnRH pulse frequency and overall amount in PCOS, there is no effect of BMI on either of these markers of hypothalamic activity,[9] indicating that obesity does not exert its effect on LH secretion at the hypothalamic level and provides evidence that the effect of obesity on gonadotropin secretion is exerted at the pituitary. Both insulin and leptin have been considered as pituitary mediators of the effects of obesity on gonadotropin secretion.

IMPACT OF OBESITY ON POLYCYSTIC OVARIAN SYNDROME

Polycystic Ovarian Syndrome with Superimposed Obesity

The prevalence of obesity in PCOS (42–74%) is much higher than in the general population (~25%).[10-12] Obese individuals, regardless of whether they have PCOS, are more insulin-resistant than normal-weight women with PCOS. When obesity is superimposed on PCOS, the more profound hyperinsulinemia promotes androgen production from ovarian theca cells, inhibits hepatic sex hormone-binding globulin (SHBG) synthesis, enhances pituitary LH secretion, and increases the ovarian androgenic response to LH. The superimposed obesity is also associated with hyperactivity of the hypothalamic–pituitary-adrenal axis, leading to increased adrenal androgens and worsening of the hyperandrogenic state.

Obesity has profound effects on the clinical, hormonal and metabolic features of PCOS, which largely depends on the degree of excess fat and on the pattern of fat distribution.

- *Clinical hyperandrogenism and androgen blood levels*: It has been demonstrated that obese PCOS women are characterized by significantly lower SHBG plasma levels and worsened hyperandrogenemia (particularly total and free testosterone and androstenedione) in comparison with their normal-weight counterparts.[12] A higher proportion of obese PCOS women complain of hirsutism and other androgen-dependent disorders, such as acne and androgenic alopecia, in comparison with normal-weight women.[12] The androgen profile can be further negatively affected in PCOS women by the presence of the abdominal body fat distribution with respect to those with the peripheral phenotype, regardless of BMI values.[12]
- *Hormonal abnormalities*: Several studies have clearly demonstrated that menstrual abnormalities are more frequent in obese than in normal-weight PCOS women.[12] Moreover, there is an evidence of a reduced incidence of pregnancy and blunted responsiveness to pharmacological treatments to

induce ovulation in obese PCOS women.[13,14] In a prospective study carried out in 158 anovulatory women, the dose of clomiphene required to achieve ovulation was in fact positively correlated, whereas ovulatory outcome negatively correlated with body weight.[15] The pregnancy rate after low dose human menopausal gonadotropin (HMG) or pure FSH administration has been found to be significantly lower in obese PCOS women than in normal-weight counterpart.[16] It was also observed that those with obesity had higher gonadotropin requirements during stimulation, fewer oocytes, a higher abortion rate, and a lower live-birth rate than their nonobese counterpart.[17]

- *Metabolic abnormalities*: In 1980, the association between hyperinsulinemia and PCOS was first noted by Burghen, et al. who found a significant positive correlation between insulin, androstenedione and testosterone levels among PCOS women.[18] In fact, recent studies show that hyperinsulinemia is present in 85% of patients with PCOS, including 95% of obese and 65% of lean affected women.[19-21] Many other studies have in fact reported that insulin resistance is very common in the presence of obesity, particularly the abdominal phenotype,[12,22,23] although it may be present even in those with normal weight. It was found that visceral adiposity index (VAI) levels were higher in overweight and/or obese PCOS patients compared to peer controls and non-obese PCOS patients, and associated with some metabolic and inflammatory parameters.[26] Six months of lifestyle modifications enhanced insulin sensitivity by 70% and significantly reduced anovulation in affected obese women.[24-26]

Different studies in American, Asian and Italian cohorts have shown that women with PCOS have a tendency to early development of Type 2 Diabetes Mellitus (T2DM) and that its prevalence was higher when compared with the general population, regardless of ethnicity and geographical area. It was also found that this occurred almost always in those women who were obese and very rarely in their nonobese counterparts. Therefore, obesity seems to represent a condition for the development of T2DM in PCOS women.

Cheal et al found that, although insulin resistance and the presence of the metabolic syndrome were significantly associated ($p<0.001$), the sensitivity and positive predictive values equaled 46 and 76%, the presence of overweight with high triglycerides, low HDL-cholesterol or elevated blood pressure being the most common factors included in the diagnosis of the metabolic syndrome itself.[27] It therefore appears that obesity plays a major role in distinguishing those with and without the metabolic syndrome.

The metabolic syndrome (at least three should be present)
- Abdominal obesity > 88 cm - Triglycerides ≥ 150 mg/dL - High density lipoprotein (HDL)-C <50 mg/dL - Blood pressure ≥ 130/85 mm Hg - Abnormal oral glucose tolerance test

Abha Mujumdar et al. showed in her study that the prevalence of menstrual irregularities [79.2% vs. 44%, P=0.000, 95% confidence interval (CI) = 0.26–0.44)] and clinical hyperandrogenism (74.2% vs. 50.6%, P=0.000, 95% CI=0.14–0.32) was

TABLE 10.1 Comparative data of various clinical features in lean vs obese women with polycystic ovarian syndrome

	Group A Obese n = 300 (%)	Group B Lean n = 150 (%)	P-value Odds ratio 95%CI
Mean age in years	29.1	28.4	
Waist to hip ratio:			P–0.056 (OR–1.486, 0.99–2.21)
>0.85	143 (47.7)	57 (38)	(Power 88%)
≤0.85	157 (52.3)	93 (62)	
Menstrual cycles:			P–0.000 (OR–4.88, 3.18-7.48)
Abnormal	238 (79.2)	66 (44)	(Power 100%)
Withdrawal bleed	126 (42)	14 (9.4)	
Delayed	78 (26)	21 (14)	
Early	23 (7.6)	27 (18)	
Variable	11 (3.6)	04 (2.6)	
Normal	62 (20.8)	84 (56)	
Oligo-ovulation	18 (6)	22 (14.6)	
Normal ovulation	44 (14.8)	62 (41.4)	
Clinical hyperandrogenism:			P–0.000 (OR–2.82, 1.86–4.25)
Clinical hyperandrogenism present	223 (74.2)	76 (50.6)	(Power 100%)
Hirsutism	101 (33.6)	42 (28)	
Acne and oily skin	122 (40.6)	34 (22.6)	
Hirsutism acne and oily skin	56 (18.6)	25 (16.6)	
Clinical hyperandrogenism absent	77 (25.8)	74 (49.4)	

Abbreviation: OR = Odds ratio

significantly higher in the obese group, whereas android central obesity (waist to hip ratio >0.85) was similar in both groups, irrespective of body weight (47.7% vs. 38%, P=0.056, 95% CI –0.06 to + 0.18) **(Table 10.1)**.[28]

Similar prevalence of prehypertension in obese and lean PCOS women (23% vs. 29.2%, RR 0.8) and higher prevalence of frank hypertension in obese women (18% vs. 6%, RR 3). Her study also revealed an increase in prevalence of endometrial hyperplasia in obese compared with lean PCOS patients (P = 0.055, RR 2.8). Atypical endometrial hyperplasia in obese group with withdrawal bleeding (four cases) was seen **(Table 10.2)**.[28]

Polycystic ovarian syndrome emerges as a clinically heterogeneous condition with increased prevalence of menstrual irregularities and clinical hyperandrogenism in the obese. Prevalence of hypertension and altered waist to hip ratio is independent of obesity. Impaired glucose tolerance (IGT), diabetes,

TABLE 10.2 Comparative data of various health manifestations in lean vs. obese women with polycystic ovarian syndrome

	Group A Obese n = 300 (%)	Group B Lean n = 150 (%)	P-value Odds ratio 95%CI
Hypertension			P–0.261 (OR–1.27, 0.84–1.91)
Normotensive	177 (59)	97 (64.8)	(Power 58%)
Prehypertensive	69 (23)	44 (29.2)	
Hypertensive	54 (18)	09 (6)	
Stage 1	32 (10.6)	07 (4.6)	
Stage 2	22 (7.4)	02 (1.4)	
PreHT + HT	123 (41)	53 (35.2)	
Diabetes			P–0.000 (OR–3.1, 1.85–4.99)
No diabetes	190 (63.2)	126 (84)	(Power 100%)
IGT	75 (25)	15 (10)	
Diabetes	35 (11.8)	09 (6)	
IGT + diabetes	110 (36.8)	24 (16)	
Endometrium			
Day 2 ET < 4 mm on USG	226 (75.4)	134 (89.2)	
Day 2 ET > 4 mm on USG	74 (24.6)	16 (10.6)	
No endometrial hyperplasia	57 (19)	13 (8.6)	

Abbreviations: IGT, impaired glucose tolerance; HT, hypertension; ET, endometrium.

and endometrial hyperplasia appear to be more prevalent in the obese, putting them at a greater risk of having morbid problems at a much younger age than the lean ones and, therefore, needing more rigorous management.[28]

Treatment of Obese Polycystic Ovarian by Insulin-sensitizing Drugs

Sparse to nonexistent data supporting a role of insulin-sensitizing drugs (ISDs) for prevention of T2DM, cardiovascular disease, hypertension or endometrial cancer for women with PCOS.

For the management of ovulatory infertility in the nonobese PCOS population (BMI<30 kg/m^2), there is moderate quality evidence demonstrating that metformin monotherapy improves the odds of ovulation and chance of achieving clinical pregnancy.

In the nonobese population of women with PCOS-related subfertility, there is moderate quality evidence demonstrating the absence of reproductive benefit when metformin is combined with clomiphene citrate (CC) therapy. CC alone remains the mainstay pharmacological therapy for this group.

For obese women (BMI ≥ 30 kg/m^2) with PCOS associated subfertility, there is low quality evidence showing the failure of metformin monotherapy to improve reproductive endpoints. In view of considerable side effects profile, metformin therapy may not be recommended for fertility management in this group of women. There is moderate quality evidence to support the beneficial effect of metformin in combination with CC therapy in increasing the likelihood of ovulation and clinical pregnancies.

For women with CC resistant subfertility, there is moderate quality evidence to support that metformin co-treatment increases ovulation rates. There is also low-quality evidence demonstrating that metformin/CC combination therapy may be associated with higher live births than laparoscopic ovarian drilling (LOD). Women with CC-resistant PCOS may be given the benefit of a trial of medical ovulation induction using combination therapy prior to committing to the more invasive and expensive alternative of LOD.

For women with PCOS undergoing IVF/ICSI treatments, there is moderate evidence to support the failure of metformin co-administration to improve the Clinical outcomes of live births, clinical pregnancies or miscarriages. There is moderate evidence demonstrating a significant reduction in the risk of OHSS with metformin co-treatment, when human chorionic gonadotropin (hCG) is used to trigger final oocyte maturation.

For women with symptomatic PCOS-related androgen excess, there is limited evidence available to support that metformin monotherapy improves hirsutism and acne, compared with more established antiandrogenic drugs. There is sufficient evidence demonstrating that the addition of metformin to the oral contraceptives piles (OCP) is more effective than OCP alone in improving hirsutism and acne.

The majority of women with PCOS are overweight and therefore likely to benefit from weight-reduction strategies. Successful weight loss can be through combination of dietary modifications and restrictions. Minimizing intake of simple carbohydrates, saturated fats and omega-6-fatty acids, optimizing dietary fiber and omega-3-fatty acid content, ensuring against spells of starvation and encouraging intake of frequent and small meals are strategies that will facilitate improvements in metabolic as well as phenotypic burden of PCOS. Regular physical activity of moderate intensity in conjunction with the specified dietary modification is sure to further enhance the overall health benefit.

The selection of therapy for PCOS generally depends on the physical symptoms and patients' desire for childbearing. For obese women with PCOS, weight loss should be considered as a first option. For infertile patients, clomiphene citrate is the first line option. If clomiphene fails to induce ovulation and pregnancy, treatment with metformin alone, or in combination with clomiphene can be the second resort. In resistant women, other treatment modalities such as laparoscopic ovarian drilling or ovulation induction with gonadotropins have been proposed as alternative therapies. IVF should be considered as a last option.

SUMMARY

Women with PCOS, though a complex pathophysiology, show different etiopathogenesis, clinical manifestation and treatment response when it comes to phenotypic difference (Lean and Obese women). In lean PCOS women, increased hypothalamic function in form of increased LH pulse frequency and increased GnRH levels is a primary event while in obese women, increased pituitary responsiveness in the form of increased LH clearance is a primary event.

Obese women have more profound hyperandrogenemia with hirsutism, menstrual irregularities and higher risk for metabolic syndrome. Obese women with PCOS will have lower pregnancy rates, low response to gonadotropins, less oocytes, higher miscarriage rates in comparison with counterparts. Insulin sensitizers like metformin can increase ovulation and clinical pregnancy rates without much effect on live birth rate, mainly in obese PCOS women while not beneficial in lean PCOS women.

KEY POINTS

- Change in body weight is a critical factor in regulating menstrual cycle and reproduction.
- Pathogenesis of PCOS is different in obese and nonobese women, with insulin resistance and hyperinsulinemia playing a central role in obese women.
- While a high LH/FSH ratio is common in PCOS, in every obese woman with PCOS, this ratio may be relatively normal.
- Impaired glucose tolerance (IGT), diabetes, and endometrial hyperplasia are more prevalent in the obese, putting them at a greater risk of having morbid problems at a much younger age than that of the lean ones.
- During the management of ovulatory infertility in the nonobese PCOS, metformin monotherapy improves the odds of ovulation and chance of achieving clinical pregnancy.
- For obese PCOS women associated with subfertility, metformin is administered as monotherapy to improve reproductive endpoint.

REFERENCES

1. Rogers J, Mitchell GW. The relation of obesity to menstrual disturbances. N Engl J Med. 1952;247:53-6.
2. EK I, Arner P, Bergqvist A, Carlstrom K, Wahrenberg H. Impaired adipocyte lipolysis in nonobese women with the polycystic ovarian syndrome: a possible link to insulin resistance? J Clin Endocrinol Metab. 1997;82(4):1147-53.
3. Frisch RE. Pubertal adipose tissue: is it necessary for normal sexual maturation? Evidence from the rat and human female. Fed Proc. 1980;39:2395-400.
4. Pasquali R, Casimirri F. The impact of obesity on hyperandrogenism and polycystic ovarian syndrome in premenopausal women. Clin Endocrinol (Oxford). 1993;39:1-16.
5. Hartz AZ, Barboriak PN, Wong A, Katayama KP, Rimm AA. The association of obesity with infertility and related menstrual abnormalities in women. Int J Obes. 1979;3(!):57-73.
6. Hamilton-Fairly, Kiddy D, Watson H, Paterson C, Franks S. Association of moderate obesity with a poor pregnancy outcome in women with polycystic ovarian syndrome treated with low dose gonadotropin. Br J ObstetGynecol. 1992;99(2):128-31.
7. Poretsky L, Cataldo NA, Rosenwaks Z, Guidice LC. The insulin-related ovarian regulatory system in health and disease. Endocr Rev. 1999;20:535-82.

8. Taylor AE, McCourt B, Martin MA, Anderson EJ, Adams JM, Schoenfeld D, Hall JE. Determinants of abnormal gonadotropin secretion in clinically defined women with polycystic ovarian syndrome. J Clin Endocrinol Metab. 1997;82:2248-56.
9. Pagan YL, Srouji SS, Jimenz Y, Emerson A, Gill S, Hall JE. Inverse relationship between LH and BMI in PCOS: investigation of hypothalamic and pituitary contributions. J Clin Endocrinol Metab. 2006;91:1309-16.
10. Nestler JE. Metformin for the treatment of the PCOS. N Engl J Med. 2008;358:47-54.
11. Azziz R, Woods KS, Reyna R, Key TJ, Knochenhauer ES, Yildiz BO. The prevalence and features of the PCOS in an unselected population. Clin Endcrinol Metab. 2004;89:2745-9.
12. Gambineri A, Pelusi C, Vicennati V, Pagotta U, Pascquali R. Obesity and the polycystic ovarian syndrome. Int J Obes Relat Metab Dis. 2002;26:883-96.
13. Lobo RA, Gysler M, March CM, Goebeleman U, Mischell DR Jr. Clinical and laboratory predictors of clomiphene response. Fertil Steril. 1982;37:168-74.
14. Nestler JE, Jakubowicz DJ, Evans WS, Pasquali R. Effects of metformin on spontaneous and clomiphene-induced ovulation in the polycystic ovarian syndrome. N Engl J Med. 1998;25:1876-80.
15. De Leo V, La Marca A, Petraglia F. Insulin-lowering agents in the management of polycystic ovarian syndrome. Endocr Rev. 2003;24:633-7.
16. White DM, Polson DW, Kiddy D, Sagle P, Watson H, Gilling-smith C, Hamilton-fairly D, Franks S. Induction of ovulation with low-dose gonadotropins in polycystic ovarian syndrome: an analysis on 109 pregnancies in 225 women. J Clin Endocrino Metab. 1996;81:3821-4.
17. Fedorcsak P, Dale PO, Storeng R, Tanbo T, abyholm T. The impact of obesity and insulin resistance on the outcome of IVF or ICSI in women with polycystiuc ovary syndrome. Hum Reprod. 2001;16:1086-91.
18. Burghen GA, Givens JR, Kitabchi AE. Correlation of hyperandrogenism with hyper-insulinism in polycystic ovarian disease. J Clin Endocrinol Metab. 1980;50(1):113-6.
19. Teede H, Deeks A, Moran L. Polycystic ovary syndrome: a complex condition with psychological, reproductive and metabolic manifestations that impacts on health across the lifespan. BMC Med. 2010;8:41.
20. Teede HJ, Misso ML, Deeks AA, Moran LJ, Stuckey BG, Wong JL, et al. Assessment and management of polycystic ovarian syndrome: summary of an evidence-based guideline. Med J Aust. 2011;195,S65–S112. 10.5694/mja11.10915.
21. Stepto NK, Cassar S, Joham AE, Hutchison SK, Harrison CL, Goldstein RF, et al. Women with polycystic ovarian syndrome have intrinsic insulin resistance on euglycaemic-hyperinsulaemic clamp. Hum. Reprod. 2013;28:777-84. 10.1093/humrep/des463.
22. Dunaif A. Insulin resistance and polycystic ovarian syndrome: mechanism and implications for pathogenesis. Endocr Rev. 1997;18:774-800.
23. PoretsktL, Cataldo NA, Rosenwaks Z, Guidice LC. The insulin related ovarian regulatory system in health and disease. Endocr Rev. 1999;20:535-82.
24. Baillargeon JP, Iuorno MJ, Nestler JE. Insulin sensitizers for polycystic ovarian syndrome. Clin Obstet Gynecol. 2003;46:325-40. 10.1097/00003081-200306000-00011.
25. Diamanti-Kandarakis E, Dunaif A. Insulin resistance and the polycystic ovary syndrome revisited: an update on mechanisms and implications. Endocr Rev. 2012;33:981-1030.
26. Durmus U, Duarn C, Ecirli S Visceral adiposity index levels in overweight and/or obese, and non-obese patients with polycystic ovarian syndrome and its relationship with metabolic and inflammatory parameters J Endocrinol Invest. 2016;12.
27. Cheal KL, Abbasi F, Lamendola C, Mclaughlin T, Reaven GM, Ford ES. Relationship to insulin resistance of the Adult treatment Panel III Diagnostic Criteria for Identification of the Metabolic Syndrome. Diabetes. 2004;53:1195-2000.
28. Abha Majumdar, Tejashree A Singh. Comparison of clinical features and health manifestations in lean vs. obese Indian women with polycystic ovarian syndrome. J Hum Reprod Sci. 2009;2(1):12-7.

CHAPTER 11

Polycystic Ovarian Syndrome in Adolescents

Sanjeev Khurd, Sadhana Khurd, Aditya Khurd

INTRODUCTION

Polycystic ovarian syndrome (PCOS), previously called as polycystic ovarian disease (PCOD), which in a sense is a misnomer, is the most common endocrine disorder that occurs in women of reproductive age. About 6–12% of women in this age group in the general population worldwide, are affected with PCOS[1] and present with symptoms of menstrual irregularity, hirsuitism, acne, alopecia and obesity, either singular or in a cluster, with their ovaries revealing a polycystic morphology on sonography scan. PCOS women may have difficulty in conceiving naturally and therefore, may confront the problem of infertility. Although the exact etiology and pathophysiology of PCOS remains still unknown, it is now becoming apparent that the syndrome may have a genetic background,[2] familial occurrence and a multifactorial etiology. The endocrinopathy is driven by metabolic aberrations which results in multisystemic manifestations. This means that the women destined to have PCOS are born with a genetic predisposition, clinical features of which may be brought forth following environmental stimulus.[3] The earliest that this is likely to happen is during the period of adolescence. The environmental stimuli are likely to be triggered by enormous and abrupt endocrine and metabolic changes which occur during adolescence in these predisposed girls. The adolescent age therefore, offers an opportunity to make an early clinical diagnosis of PCOS.

An early diagnosis becomes important since, the alarm bells about PCOS have already started ringing, not only because its incidence has increased considerably in the last three decades, especially in south Asia, but more so because of the realization of the lifelong health implications of the syndrome, such as infertility, metabolic syndrome/type 2 diabetes mellitus and endometrial cancer. The good news is that majority of these complications may be preventable, provided we make an early diagnosis and start interventions early, and then continue them over the years to give multiple health benefits to the woman. The adolescent age seems to be the right time to initiate these, however, the diagnosis of PCOS, and more so in the adolescent girl, remains a big challenge. Although we continue to treat these adolescent girls with lifestyle modifications and pharmacotherapy, from our experience borrowed from treating adult PCOS, to date, there are no published guidelines for treating adolescents with PCOS.

HISTORY AND PATHOGENESIS (FIG. 11.1)

The PCOS has existed for ages, and finds relevant references at different periods, since the time of Aristotle (384-322 BC), in whose work we find the following description, "discharge from the uterus occurs in some women but not in others. It is found in those who are fair skinned and feminine type generally, but not in those who are fat, dark and masculine in appearance." In 1721, A Valliserni in Italy, referred to "young married peasant woman, moderately obese and infertile, with two larger than normal ovaries, bumpy, shiny and whitish just like pigeon eggs", while Chereau in 1844, describes "sclerocystic changes in the ovaries".

True scientific study however, commenced only 80 years ago, when two American doctors Irwing F Stein and Micheal L Leventhal from Chicago, described the syndrome for the first time in 1935. They published their findings in the same year in their landmark paper titled "Amenorrhea associated with bilateral polycystic ovaries", in the American Journal of Obstetrics and Gynecology. As a part of their study, they performed wedge biopsies of the bulky, polycystic ovaries at laparotomy, in 7 amenorrheic, hirsuitism, infertile women. They observed that all seven of them resumed menstruation and two subsequently conceived as well. Since then, for the next four decades, surgical wedge resection of the ovaries, by laparotomy, became a standard treatment for women who presented with symptoms of PCOS, only to be replaced in the eighties by laparoscopic 'ovarian drilling', which was equally effective, minimally invasive and most importantly, minimized the complications of postoperative adhesions, which may follow a laparotomy.

The sixties saw the introduction of medical management, which indeed was a welcome break from the earlier established invasive surgical treatment. The sixties have been a landmark decade for both fertility prevention, with introduction of the oral contraceptive pill (OCP), and for fertility promotion, with clomiphene

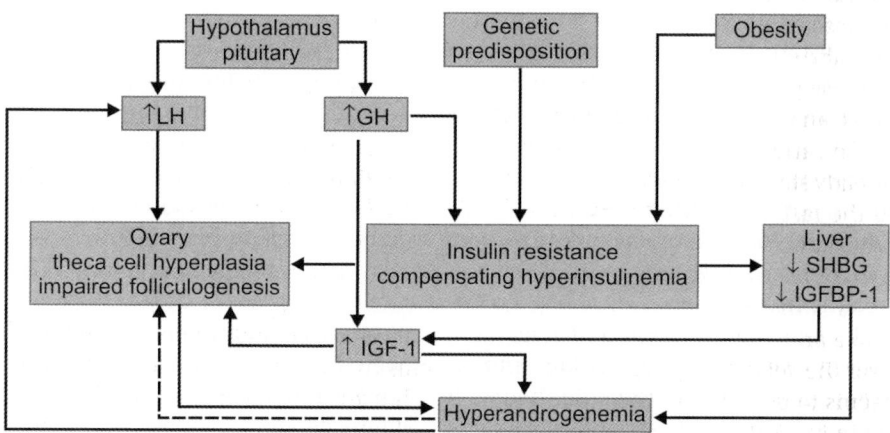

Fig. 11.1 Pathogenesis of polycystic ovarian syndrome

citrate and gonadotropins being introduced for treating anovulatory infertile women. Besides their contraceptive action, OCP have also proved effective as cycle regulators and for the treatments of acne and hirsuitism in PCOS women.

The eighties gave physicians a better insight into the pathophysiology of PCOS and the understanding that increased insulin resistance and compensatory hyperinsulinemia, and its consequences, including procoagulant[4,5] and proinflammatory states[6-8] and endothelial dysfunction[9-11] is one of the key feature of the syndrome. Compensatory hyperinsulinemia, which occurs in response to insulin resistance, causes hyperandrogenemia by promoting excess androgen production from ovarian theca cells, by enhancing pituitary LH secretion and increasing the ovarian androgenic response to LH. Hyperinsulinemia also inhibits hepatic sex hormone–binding globulin (SHBG) synthesis,[12-14] with less androgen now being bound to globulin results in increased bioavailability of free androgens for the target tissues. The resulting hyperandrogenemia is the cause of chronic anovulation, reflected as menstrual irregularity, and symptoms of androgen excess viz. hirsuitism, acne and alopecia. This led to the introduction of insulin sensitizer metformin in the management of PCOS to counter the effects of insulin resistance. Similar insulin sensitizers like pioglitazone, inositols, berberin have also been added subsequently to counter the effects of increased insulin resistance.

PATHOGENESIS OF POLYCYSTIC OVARIAN SYNDROME

The effects of excess weight gain due to excess adiposity in PCOS women were also being realized. The prevalence of obesity in PCOS (42–74%) is much higher than in the general population (~25%).[15-17] Adipose tissue serves multiple functions and is involved in normal metabolism and maintenance of normal endocrine and immune status. Accumulation of excess adiposity that accumulates in obesity causes dysfunction of the adipose tissue compartment, which ultimately leads to immune alteration characterized by chronic low grade inflammation, which causes metabolic derangements and endocrine imbalance in the form of increased insulin resistance and compensatory hyperinsulinemia. This consequently worsens the already existing chronic low grade inflammation and insulin resistance caused due to the PCOS pathology, causing profound hyperinsulinemia in these obese women and magnifies the manifestations of the syndrome. Thus, when obesity, and more so, central obesity gets superimposed on underlying PCOS, overweight and obese women are seen to have more severe symptoms and more severe complications of the syndrome. In the PCOS management therefore, much, stress has been laid on undertaking changes in 'life-style' to reduce and optimize body weight through proper diet, nutrition and exercise programs to compliment various forms of medical and surgical treatments.

Over all these years, the management of PCOS has largely remained symptom oriented and presently multidisciplinary as well, since the manifestations of the syndrome are multi-systemic. Today, besides gynecologists and pediatricians, endocrinologists and physicians, nutritionists and exercise trainers, dermatologists and cosmetologists, infertility specialists and at times bariatric surgeons and oncosurgeons, all team up in the management of PCOS women.

POLYCYSTIC OVARIAN SYNDROME DIAGNOSIS IN ADULTS

In general, PCOS is a diagnosis of exclusion and is defined by a cluster of signs and symptoms, after other causes like thyroid disorder, hyperprolactinemia, primary or secondary ovarian insufficiency, late onset congenital adrenal hyperplasia and androgen producing tumors have been excluded.

The diagnosis of PCOS has always remained a matter of debate and controversy, since PCOS women are a heterogenous group, with the classical cases at one end of the PCOS spectrum, presenting with all the classical features, while some at the other end of the spectrum have very few of these manifestations, with the majority falling in between. The signs and symptoms of PCOS also vary with age, race, weight and medications, adding to the challenges of accurate diagnosis.

The first unifying approach to adult PCOS was proposed during a 1990 consensus meeting at the National Institute of Health (NIH) in the USA. The so-called NIH criteria require presence of chronic anovulation and clinical and/or biochemical hyperandrogensim. In 2003, another consensus workshop at Rotterdam in the Netherlands, held by the European Society of Human Reproduction and Embryology (ESHRE) and American Society of Reproductive Medicine (ASRM) broadened the definition to allow ultrasound evidence of polycystic ovaries (PCO) to substitute for either anovulation or hyperandrogenism. Therefore, presence of any two out of the three criteria qualified for the diagnosis of PCOS.[18] Appreciating the need for clarification, the Androgen Excess Society (AES) convened in 2006 to define PCOS by the presence of hyperandrogenism plus one of the two signs, either ovulatory dysfunction-chronic anovulation (reflected in irregular menstrual cycles or amenorrhea) or ultrasound evidence of the typical PCO morphology (12 or more small follicles 2–9 mm and/or enlarged ovarian volume greater than 10 cms^3, with unilateral manifestation sufficient for PCO diagnosis).

ADOLESCENCE

Adolescence is a transitional stage of physical and psychological human development that generally occurs during the period from puberty to customarily defined adulthood.[19-21] Major pubertal and biological changes occur in the sex organs, height, weight and muscle mass, as well as significant changes occur in brain structure and organization. Menarche, the beginning of menstruation, is a relatively late development which follows a long series of hormonal changes.[22] It is usually associated with irregular menstrual cycles and generally, regular ovulation and regular menstrual cycles follow menarche by about two years.[23]

ADOLESCENTS AND POLYCYSTIC OVARIAN SYNDROME

PCOS is characterized by menstrual irregularities in 80–90% cases. 70% of these have hirsuitism, 30–40% has acne, less than 5% have alopesia, while more than 50% are overweight and obese. The symptomatology of PCOS poses concerns not only to the adolescent girls but also to their families. The menstrual irregularities and symptoms of androgen excess viz. hirsuitism, acne and alopecia are problems of much concern to the adolescent girls in terms of negative self-esteem. Also, the excess adiposity that occurs in the obese PCOS girls may add to their psychological depression, since adolescence is characterized by consciousness and enhanced sensitivity about their body image. The parents of the adolescent PCOS girls on the other hand are worried about their marriage and future fertility. The long- term metabolic complications of PCOS viz. diabetes, hypertension, dyslipidemia, coronary artery disease and endometrial cancer are not of immediate concern to the adolescent girls or their parents. However, it is important to make them aware about the future course of the syndrome as these complications are largely preventable, provided these adolescent girls adopt a healthy life-style, consume balanced, nutritious diet and exercise regularly to keep their weight to the optimum and continue following this regimen over the subsequent years.

Diagnosis of Polycystic Ovarian Syndrome in Adolescents

Premature adrenarche is recognized as heralding PCOS and 20% of affected girls develop clinically significant hyperandrogenism as adults. However, when it comes to laying down diagnostic criteria for PCOS in adolescence, there is no consensus. Transferring adult diagnostic criteria for PCOS to adolescent girls has proven to be confusing, mainly due to overlapping symptoms of normal puberty and limitations in the application of the technological investigative tools in the adolescent population.

In puberty, central axis immaturity and physiologic insulin resistance are often coupled with ovarian anovulation (leading to menstrual irregularity) and mild acne/hirsuitism, mimicking PCOS phenotype. In many cases, the differentiation to bona fide PCOS lies merely in the degree of clinical and biochemical expression. Genetically predisposed adolescents may exhibit an exaggerated ovarian response to physiologic and non-physiologic (e.g. obesity) stimuli at puberty, with an ensuing hormonal cascade that is well recognized in the context of PCOS. Girls with PCOS, therefore, tend to continue having menstrual irregularity well beyond two years, by which time it regularizes in a majority of non-PCOS girls and may therefore suggest the presence of the syndrome.

Presence of biochemical hyperandrogenemia (despite the absence of clinical hyperandrogenism) is the singular finding that crystallizes PCOS from other pubertal 'noise' of adolescence.[24] The most sensitive indicator of biochemical hyperandrogenemia is the determination of free testosterone through equilibrium dialysis.[25] However, this method is not widely available and technically complex and expensive. Since laboratory assays vary widely between laboratories, the actual comparable cut-offs for free testosterone remains elusive. Also, the normative data for testosterone levels in adolescents is lacking.[26] Alternative, the free androgen index (FAI) correlates well with free testosterone measured through equilibrium analysis. It is calculated from measures of total testosterone and sex hormone-binding globulin (SHBG).[27] However, in general, adolescent normative data for total testosterone and FAI are lacking.

Abdominal sonography, as opposed to transvaginal sonography in adults, limits the assessment of ovarian morphology in adolescents girls. Also, reference data regarding normal ovarian size in adolescence have not been identified.

Currently, expert panels or societies in the field have not endorsed any criteria for diagnosis of adolescent PCOS. However, some workers have made suggestions for diagnosis of PCOS in adolescent girls.

Sultan and Paris recommended that the adolescent girl meet four of the five following criteria: oligo – or amenorrhea for >2 years after menarche, clinical hyperandrogenism, biochemical hyperandrogenism, insulin resistance or hyperinsulinemia and polycystic ovaries on ultrasound.[28]

Carmina et al. have suggested that for adolescents, the diagnosis of PCOS can be securely made only when all the three Rotterdam criteria are met, viz. hyperandrogenemia along with chronic anovulation and classic ovarian PCO morphology. The authors suggest that adolescents who exhibit only two out of

TABLE 11.1 Differential diagnosis of PCOS

Assessment considerations		Implications
Supporting PCOS		
Clinical	• Premature adrenarche • Menstrual disturbance of oligomenorrhea, primary or secondary amenorrhea • Physical examination of facial hair/hirsuitism, acne, alopecia, central weight distribution, acanthosis nigricans • Family history of PCOS, infertility, gestational diabetes, type 2 diabetes	
Laboratory	Elevation of morning, free testosterone (low sex-hormone binding globulin), total testosterone and free androgen index (FAI)	>200 ng/dL suggestive of ovarian androgen secreting tumor
Imaging	Transabdominal ultrasound with findings of spherical enlarged ovary(ies) where mostly the central stroma is increased—peripheral arrangement of small follicles (necklace of pearls)	
Ruling out other conditions		
Laboratory	Thyroid stimulating hormone	Thyroid disorder
	Prolactin	Prolactinoma or drug induced cause for elevated prolactin
	Follicle-stimulating hormone (FSH), luteinizing hormone (LH), estradiol (E2)	Elevated FSH/LH and low E2 suggest primary ovarian insufficiency. Normal to low FSH, LH and low E2 suggest hypothalamo—pituitary dysfunction
	Morning 17-hydroxyprogesterone	>200 ng/dL suggestive of late—onset congenital adrenal hyperplasia

Contd...

Contd...

Assessment considerations		Implications
	Dehydroepiandrosterone-sulfate	Adrenal hyperandrogenism/ >800 ug/dL suggestive of adrenal tumor
	Urinary cortisol assessment/ dexamethasone suppression test	Rare conditions such as Cushing's syndrome are not routinely ruled out but should be considered if clinical suspicion arises (e.g. adolescent with elevated blood pressure)
	Urine/serum human chorionic gonadotropin	Rule out pregnancy

the three criteria may probably have PCOS and they should be followed up and their symptoms re-evaluated **(Table 11.1)**.[30]

Treatment of Adolescent Polycystic Ovarian Syndrome

Although several avenues of therapy have been suggested, there are no published guidelines for treating adolescents with PCOS. Similar to adult therapy, treatment in adolescence focuses on the dual approach of (1) symptomatic relief and (2) preventative strategy. The three interrelated targets of therapy are anovulation, hyperandrogenemia and insulin resistance. To date, Ibanez et al have contributed the majority of systematic studies examining therapeutic modalities in lean adolescents with PCOS;[30-32] these authors have moved the field forward in terms of therapeutic options for young girls diagnosed with PCOS. Given the narrow ethnic and clinical PCOS spectrum of the Ibanez and Zegher cohorts, the transferability of the data to obese adolescents of other ethnic backgrounds still needs to be examined.

PRINCIPLES OF MANAGEMENT

The principles are:
- To establish menstrual cyclicity
- To treat clinical (hirsuitism, acne, alopecia) and biochemical (testosterone and DHEASO4) hyperandrogenicity
- To counteract immediate and long-term sequel of hyperinsulinemia.

ACTUAL MANAGEMENT PROTOCOLS

Management of adolescent PCOS includes:
- Lifestyle modifications and weight loss in obese
- Insulin sensitizing agents (metformin, pioglitazone, inositol, beberin)
- Combined ethinyl estradiol and progestin/oral contraceptive pill
- Antiandrogens (cyproterone acetate, flutamide, spironolactone, fenestride)

- Combined ethinyl estradiol and cyproterone acetate
- Cosmetic treatment (epilation, waxing, electrolysis, laser).

Lifestyle Modification and Weight Loss

Intensive lifestyle modifications, even with only a modest change in body mass index (BMI) have shown to improve menstrual cycle irregularity and normalize serum androgens in the adolescents with PCOS.[33,34]

This acts by lowering circulating free androgen and insulin levels. These beneficial effects occur because; weight loss increases sex hormone-binding globulin (SHBG). This reduces the level of circulating free testosterone, as SHBG is the carrier of two sex steroid hormones, namely estrogen and testosterone. Even 7% weight reduction may lead to spontaneous resumption of menses and improvement in hirsuitism in adolescent PCOS girls.[35] However, maintaining life style changes becomes challenging and therefore, pharmacotherapy often becomes necessary.

Insulin-sensitizing Agents

The commonly used drug is metformin and is a good choice for both lean and overweight adolescents. Pioglitazone, inositols, berberine are less commonly used insulin sensitizing agents.

Metformin has an excellent safety profile in patients with healthy kidney and liver function and can be used in patients with concern of thromboembolic risk.

Metformin was the first antidiabetic drug to be examined in the context of treating PCOS condition in adult PCOS in the eighties and nineties.[36] In 2001, the first studies emerged examining the effect of metformin in adolescent PCOS. For a group of 18 non-obese girls with PCOS and a history of premature adrenarche, Ibanez et al. found that 14 (78%) had restored menstrual cycle regularity by 6 months of metformin therapy. Six months of metformin restored normal menstrual cycles in 10/11 obese PCOS[37] and improved both ovarian an adrenal hyperandrogenemia in another group of obese subjects.[38] A double-blind placebo controlled study in obese girls with PCOS found that metformin/lifestyle versus placebo/lifestyle were more effective in reducing testosterone levels and menstrual cycle regularity than lifestyle alone.[39]

The mode of action of these drugs is through two ways:
1. They regulate hyperinsulinemia.
2. They also regulate reproductive endocrine axis.

Regulation of hyperinsulinemia is brought about in three ways:
1. By directly sensitizing insulin receptors (postreceptor translation mechanism—by correcting serine tyrosine phosphorylation).
2. By preventing neoglucogenesis.
3. By reducing absorption of glucose from intestine.

Regulation of endocrine reproductive axis is achieved by:
- Increasing the level of SHBG and thereby decreasing the level of bioactive free testosterone
- Because the level of insulin is reduced, there is no LH mediated activity of theca cells for excess testosterone production
- Metformin also reduces the level of leptin production.

Dose, Duration and Schedule of Metformin Treatment

Dose of metformin is slowly and incrementally increased to 1500–2000 mg, divided twice or thrice daily and taken with food. Sustained release preparations are now also available. They can be taken once a day and they therefore have better patient compliance and also have lesser gastrointestinal side effects. The period of treatment should be for a minimum of 6 months to maximum 2 years. The schedule of treatment should be either alone or in combination with estrogen-progestin pill/oral contraceptive pill, along with weight reduction in obese PCOS, through diet modifications and regular exercise.

Side Effects

The side effects consist of gastrointestinal symptoms like nausea and diarrhea. Long-term effect may be hyperhomocystinemia and supplementation by daily Vitamin B_{12} can prevent this long-term use effect. Hepatic dysfunction is another significant complication. Therefore, after 6 months to 1 year treatment, alternate therapy with N-acetylcystene, twice daily may be continued as a substitute for metformin.

Combined Estrogen and Progestin Pills/Oral Contraceptive Pills

Combined estrogen-progestin (EP) pills/oral contraceptive pills (OCPs) containing both an estrogen and progesterone component, not only regularize the menstrual cycle but also alleviate clinical features such as hirsuitism and acne.[40] It may take 6–12 months of this treatment for these symptoms to show amelioration.

The mechanisms of action of these drugs are as follows:
- Estrogen component of the combined pill specifically, increases hepatic production of sex hormone-binding globulin (SHBG), which leads to reduction in circulating free and bioavailable androgens. Also, estrogen competes with testosterone for receptors, thereby prevents conversion of testosterone to more potent androgens, i.e. dihydrotestosterone (DTH).
- The progestin component of the combined pill ensures endometrial decidualization and thus protects against proliferative endometrial pathologies, including endometrial hyperplasia. Therefore, potential risk of endometrial cancer resulting from prolonged periods of anovulation is reduced.
- The combined EP pill/OCP also suppress bioactivity of follicular stimulating hormone (FSH) and leutinizing hormone (LH) through negative feed-back on gonadotropin releasing hormone (GnRH) secretion from pituitary and may regularize FSH : LH ratio, thereby lowering LH driven ovarian androgen production.
- Progestins in the combined EP pill/OCP can also contribute to the improving hyperandrogenemia. Progestational anti-androgen like cyproterone acetate and 4th generation progestins such as drospirenone have an added anti-androgenic effect, and therefore have been deemed more effective in improving PCOS symptoms.[41]

Composition of Oral Contraceptive Pills with Drospirenone

Ethinylestradiol 30 ug + drospirenone 3 mg.

What is Drosperinine?

It is a 4th generation progestin. The molecule is a synthetic progestin, analog to spironolactone, chemically and structurally similar to spironolactone. It is closer to natural progesterone and is a progestin with some differences.
The pharmacological properties are:
- Antimineralocorticoid effect.
- Counteracts estrogen stimulated activity of the rennin-angiotensin-aldosterone system, thereby influences regulation of water and electrolytes. There is less water retention; therefore there is no breast tenderness.
- It also has mild anti-androgenic effect, thereby improving skin condition (hirsuitism, acne alopecia).
- Acts as potassium sparing diuretic.

Currently Available Progestins and their Androgenic Effects

The following **Table 11.2** illustrates that, of all the available progestins, drospirenone is the only progestin which has a positive antiandrogenic effect.

Advantages of Drospirenone

- Exhibits both progestogenic and anti-androgenic effect
- Inhibits LH therefore, less availability of androgens
- More hepatic clearance of androgens
- Direct inhibition of androgen action at receptor site
- One study was even able to demonstrate that switching to the antiandrogenic 4th generation progestin OCP from a 3rd generation progestin OCP improves adiposity in adolescents.[42]

TABLE 11.2 Different types of progestine and their androgenic effects

Progestin	Androgenic effect
Levonorgestrel	High
Norgestrel	High
Norethindrone	Medium
Norethindrone acetate	Medium
Ethynodiol diacetate	Low
Norgestimate	None
Desogestrel	None
Drospirenone	Anti-androgenic

Contraindications

- Hepatic dysfunctions
- Renal insufficiency
- Adrenal insufficiency
- Previous history of deep venous thrombosis (DVT), stroke or thrombosis
- Factor V Leiden mutation, greatly enhance risk of thromboembolism.

Drospirenone is also contraindicated in association with:

- ACE inhibitors
- Angiotension-II receptors agonists
- Potassium sparing diuretics
- Potassium supplementation
- Heparin
- Aldosterone antagonists
- NSAID
- Smokers

Concerns about drospirenone:

Somewhat higher thromboembolic risk compared to older third-generation formulations.[43-45] There are concerns like increasing insulin resistance and elevated lipid profile with use of drospirenone; but these have not been substantiated. Rather, unlike other OC pills, drospirenone reduces metabolic abnormalities.

Combined Estrogen and Progestin Pill/OCP and Metformin

Metformin combination with EP pill/OCP has additional beneficial effects, in improving body composition and dispilidemia. A recent double blind placebo—controlled study in obese adolescents confirmed this beneficial effective of this combination therapy.[35] Adding metformin to EP pill/OCP and lifestyle improved total testosterone and HDL and waist circumference. It appears that adding metformin to EP pill/OCP ameliorates some of the negative effects of EP pill/OCP with its contraceptive benefits. Therefore, in sexually active, overweight adolescent PCOS with cardiometabolic risk, combination of OCP and metformin may be the best choice rather than monotherapy.

Antiandrogens

Hyperandrogenemia is not only closely tied to the pathogenesis of the condition but also responsible for the metabolic complications. Hyperandrogenemic obese adolescents have greater risks of metabolic syndrome and inflammatory state than nonhyperandrogenemic, similar obese counterparts.[46,47] Therefore, antiandrogen therapy may be indicated not only to benefit cosmetic manifestations such as hirsuitism, acne and alopecia, but also as a metabolic management strategy.

In young women at risk for pregnancy, antiandrogens must only be used with secure contraceptives due to the potential effect of undervirilization of a male conceptus.

The following antiandrogens are used:
1. *Cyproterone acetate:* Administered in a small dose of 2.5 mg. The only disadvantage is mild antiglucocorticoid effect, which is more apparent at a higher dose.
It was first used in 1964 and has been the first antiandrogen in clinical use. It is a synthetic steroidal antiandrogen, progestin and antigonadotropin. It acts by preventing endogenous androgens from interacting with androgen receptor and also by suppressing androgen biosynthesis. Cyproterone acetate in the dose of 2.5 mg is combined with ethinyl estradiol and causes overall improvement in the symptoms of acne in 75–90% cases, besides acting as a cycle regulator. In severe hirsuitism daily dose of 50–100 mg is recommended. Its mild antiglucocortecoid effect is a disadvantage, which is more apparent at a higher dose. Cyproterone acetate is presently not approved by US FDA due to concerns of hepatotoxicity.
2. *Flutamide:* A nonsteroidal drug with a potent androgen receptor blocker has been very effective in both cosmetic and metabolic effects when added to EP pill/OCP and metformin in PCOS treatment regimen.[42,48,49] There have been concerns about its hepatoxic effect. However, this effect is dose dependant and in low dose of 62.5 mg/day it was shown to be safe in a meta-analysis of 12 prospective studies.[50] Ibanez and Zegher confirmed the efficacy and safety of flutamide for young women with hirsuitism in combination therapy.[51]
3. *Spironolactone:* An aldesterone antagonist has been used for decades as potassium sparing diuretic and was found to have antiandrogen effects in 1970s.[52] Its antiandrogenic effect is carried out through a dual mechanism of androgen receptor blockade, and via spironlactone's inhibition of 5 alpha reductase, thus reducing the conversion of testosterone to its biologically more potent metabolite, di-hydrotestosterone. Studies in adult women have shown higher doses of 100 mg daily to be safe and effective in improving hirsuitism scores over time. Spironolactone, while more commonly used to help women with hirsuitism, has the unnerving side effect of irregularizing menses. Therefore, it is often used in combination with EP pill/OCPs in patients with PCOS.
4. *Finasteride* is predominantly a type 2, 5 alpha-reductase inhibitor, an enzyme that converts testosterone to dihydrotesterone, thereby inhibits the production of dihydrotestosterone. Used in the treatment of hirsuitism as has efficacy similar to spironolactone. It has to be given orally, in the daily dose of 5 mg for 3–6 months. It is combined with EP pill/OCP to increase its efficacy. It has renal and hepatic toxicity.

Ethinylestradiol with Cyproterone Acetate[53-55] with or without Metformin

This schedule of treatment is specifically indicated in obese PCOS girls with symptoms of hirsuitism and acne. Dual therapy is better than monotherapy. Metformin is an insulin sensitizing agent, thereby reduces the level of insulin. It also reduces the level of androgens.

TABLE 11.3 Therapeutic regimens for management of polycystic ovarian syndrome

Treatment	Menstrual dysfunction	Hyperandrogenism	Metabolic benefit
Insulin sensitizer metformin	+/−	+/−	+
Oral contraceptive pill (OCP)	+	+	−
Cyclic progesterone	+	−	−
OCP + metformin	+	+	+
Antiandrogen	+/−	+	+/−
Estrogen + antiandrogen	+	+	+/−

Ethinyloestradiol increases hepatic synthesis of SHBG and there by reduces the level of free testosterone. Cyproterone acetate.[56,57] is antiandrogenic drug and is administered in a small dose (2.5 mg).

The **Table 11.3** identifies efficacy of the commonly utilized therapeutic regimens against the common symptoms of PCOS.

SUMMARY

The incidence of PCOS has shown a remarkable increase both in adult and adolescent population in the last three decades. A timely diagnosis of PCOS in the afflicted adolescent allows an opportunity of not only successfully addressing the burdensome symptoms but also initiating preventative strategies aimed at mitigating long-term sequelae of this chronic disorder. While the manifestations of PCOS during adolescence may be similar to those seen in the adults, diagnostic dilemmas abound and diagnostic criteria are less studied compared to the adults. Hyperandrogenemia is the most reliable finding in the adolescent PCOS, however the laboratory assays and cut offs for free testosterone widely vary between laboratories. There is presently no consensus on the diagnostic criteria and there are no published guidelines for treating adolescent PCOS. Presently, life-style modifications and weight loss in obese, along with insulin sensitizers, antiandrogenic progestational agents like cyproterone acetate and drospirenone containing estrogen progestin pills and antandrogens form the core of management in adolescent girls with PCOS for symptomatic relief and prevention of long-term complications of the syndrome.

KEY POINTS

- Adolescence is a transitional stage of physical and psychological human development which occurs during the period from puberty to customarily defined adulthood.

- Treating adolescent girls with life style modifications and pharmacotherapy, to date, there are no published guidelines for treating adolescents with PCOS.
- PCOS is characterized by menstrual l irregularities in 80–90% cases. 70% of these have hirsuitism, 30–40% has acne, less than 5% have alopesia, while more than 50% are overweight and obese.
- In the obese PCOS girls, the excess adiposity, add to their psychological depression.
- It is important to make them aware about the future course of the syndrome so that these adolescent girls adopt a healthy lifestyle, consume balanced, nutritious diet and exercise regularly to keep their weight to the optimum and maintain.
- Diagnosis of PCOS in adolescent can be securely made only when all the three Rotterdam criteria are met.
- Management is aimed to establish menstrual cyclicity, to treat clinical and biochemical hyperandrogenicity and to counteract immediate and long-term sequel of hyperinsulinemia.

REFERENCES

1. Yildiz BO, Bozdag G, Yapici Z, et al. Prevalence, phenotype and cardiometabolic risk of polycystic ovary syndrome under different diagnostic criteria. Hum Reprod. 2012;27(10):3067-73.
2. Carmina E, Oberfield SE, Lobo RA. The diagnosis of polycystic ovary syndrome in adolescents. Am J obstet Gynecol. 2010;203:201.e1-5.
3. Shayya R, RJ Chang. Reproductive endocrinology of adolescent polycystic ovary syndrome. Br Jr Obstetrics & Gynaecology. 2010;117(2)150-5.
4. Velazquez EM, Mendoza SG, Wang P, Glueck CJ. Metformin therapy is associated with a decrease in plasma plasminogen activator inhibitor-1, lipoprotein (a), and immunoreactive insulin levels in patients with the polycystic ovary syndrome. Metabolism. 1997;46(4):454-7.
5. Kelly CJG, Lyall H, Petrie JR, Gould GW, Connel JMC, Rumley A, et al. A specific elevation in tissue plasminogen activator antigen in women with polycystic ovarian syndrome. J Clin Endocrinol Metab. 2002;87(7):3287-90.
6. Sampson M, Kong C, Patel A, Unwin R, Jacobs HS. Ambulatory blood pressure profiles and plasminogen activator inhibitor (PAI-1) activity in lean women with and without the polycystic ovary syndrome. Clin Endocrinol (Oxf). 1996;45(5):623-9.
7. Bahceci M, Tuzcu A, Canoruc N, Tuzun Y, Kidir V, Aslan C. Serunm C-reactive protein (CRP) levels and insulin resistance in non-obese women with polycystic ovarian syndrome, and effect of bicalutamide on hirsuitism, CRP levels and insulin resistance. Horm Res. 2004;62(6):283-7.
8. Talbott EO, Zborowski JV, Boudreaux MY, McHugh-Pemu KP, Sutton Tyrell K, Guzick DS. The relationship between C-reactive protein and carotid intima-media wall thickness in middle-aged women with polycystic ovary syndrome. J Clin Enocrinol Metab. 2004;89(12):6061-7.
9. Boulman N, levy Y, Leiba R, Sachar S, Linn R, Zinder O, et al. Increased C-reactive protein levels in the polycystic ovary syndrome: a marker of cardiovascular disease. J Clin Endocrinol Metab. 2004;89(5):2160-5.

10. Tarkun I, Arslan BC, Canturk Z, Turemen E, Sahin T, Duman C. Endothelial dysfunction in young women with polycystic ovary syndrome : relationship with insulin resistance and low-grade chronic inflammation. J Clin Endocrinol Metab. 2004;89(11):5592-6.
11. Orio F. Palomba S, Cascella T, De Simone B, Di Biase S, Russo T, et al. Early impairment of endothelial structure and function in young normal-weight women with polycystic ovary syndrome. J Clin Endocrinol Metab. 2004;89(9):4588-93.
12. Paradisi G, Steinburg HO, Hempfling A, Cronin J, Hook G, Shepard MK, et al. Polycystic ovary syndrome is associated with endothelial dysfunction. Circulation. 2001;103(10):1410-5.
13. Morales AJ, Laughlin GA, Butzow T, Maheshwari H, Baumann G. Yen SS. Insulin, somatotropic and luteinizing hormone axes in lean and obese women with polycystic ovary syndrome: common and distinct features. J Clin Endocrinol Metab. 1996;81:2854-64.
14. Ford ES, Li C. Metabolic syndrome and health related quality of life among U.S. adults. Ann Epidemiol. 2008;18:165-71.
15. Boutzios G, Karalaki M, Zapanti E. Common pathophysiological mechanisms involved in luteal phase deficiency and polycystic ovary syndrome impact on fertility. Endocrine. 2012.Doi:10.1007/s12020-012-9778-9.
16. Nestler JE. Metformin for treatment of polycystic ovary syndrome. N Engl J Med 2008;358:47-54.
17. Azziz R, Woods KS, Reyna R, Key TJ, Knochenhauer ES, Yildiz BO. The prevalence and features of the polycystic ovary syndrome in unselected population. Clin Endorinol Metab. 2004;89:2745-9.
18. Azziz R, Sanchez LA, Knochenhauer ES, Moran C, Lazenby J, Stephens KC, et al. Androgen excess in women: experience with over 1000 consecutive patients. Clin Endorinol Metab. 2004;89:453-62.
19. Rotterdam ESHRE/ASRM – Sponsored PCOS Consensus criteria and long term health risks related to polycystic ovary syndrome society. Fertil Steril. 2004;81:19-25.
20. Macmillan Dictionary for Students Macmillan, Pan Ltd. 1981;14:456. Retrieved 2010-7-15.
21. "Adolescence". Merriam-Webster. Retrieved May 9, 2012.
22. "Puberty and adolescence". Medline Plus. Archived from the original on 23 July 2010. Retrieved. 2010-07-30.
23. Dorn LD, Nottelmann ED, Sussman EJ, Inoff-Germain G, Dr, Chrousos GP. "Variability in hormone concentrations and self-reported menstrual histories in young adolescents: Menarche as an Integral part of a developmental process." Journal of Youth and Adolescence. 1999;28(3):283-304. Doi: 10.1023? A:1021680726753
24. Hafetz E. Parameters of sexual maturity in man. In: E. Hafetz (Ed.). Perspectives in human reproduction, Vol. 3: Sexual maturity: Physiological and clinical parameters. Ann Arbor, MI: Ann Arbor Science Publishers; 1999.
25. Fauser BC, Tarlatiz BC, Rebar RW, Legro RS, Balen AH, Lobo R, et al. Consensus on women's health aspects of polycystic ovary syndrome (PCOS): the Amsterdam ESHRE/ASRM – Sponsored 3rd PCOS Cosensus Workshop Group. Fertil Steril. 2012; 97(1):28-38.e25. PubMed PMID: 22153789.
26. Azziz R, Carmina E, Dewailly D, Diamanti-Kandarkis E, Escobar-Moreale HF, Futterweit W, et al. The Androgen Excess and PCOS criteria for polycystic ovary syndrome: the task force report. Fertil Steril. 2009;91(2):456-88. PubMed PMID: 18950759.
27. Rosner W, Vesper H. Towards excellence in testosterone testing: a consensus statement. J Clin Enocrinol Metab. 2010;95(10):4542-8. PubMed PMID: 20926540. eng
28. Hahn S, Kuehnel W, Tan S, Kramer K, Schmidt M, Roesler S, et al. Diagnostic value of calculated testosterone. Indices in the assessment of polycystic ovary syndrome. Clin Chem Lab Med. 2007;45(2):202-7. PubMed PMID: 17311509.

29. Sultan C, Paris F. Clinical expression of polycystic ovary syndrome in adolescent girls. Fertil Steril. 2006;86(Suppl 1):S6.
30. Carmina E, Oberfield SE, Lobo RA. The diagnosis of polycystic ovary syndrome in adolescents. Am J Obstet Gynecol. 2010;203:201.el-201.e5
31. Ibanez L, de Zegher F. Flutamide-metformin plus ethinyl estradiol-drospirenone for lipolysis and antiatherogenesis in young women and ovarian hyperandrogenesim: the key role of metformin at the start and after more than one year of therapy. J Clin Endocrinol Meetab. 2005;90(1):39-43. PubMed PMID: 15483105
32. Ibanez L, Valls C, Ferrer A, Marcos MV, Rodriguez–Hierro F, de Zegher F. Sensitization to insulin induces ovulation in nonobese adolescents with anovulatory hyperandrogenism. J Clin Endocrinol Metab. 2001:86(8):3595-8. PubMEd PMID: 11502783
33. Ibanez L, Diaz M, Sebastini G, Sanchez-Infantes D, Salvador C, Lopez-Bermelo A, et al. Treatment of androgen excess in adolescent girls: ethinyl estradiol-cyproterone acetate versus low-dose pioglitazone-flutamide-metformin. J Clin Endocrinol Metab. 2001;96(11):3361-6. PubMed PMID: 21865363
34. Lass N, Kleber M, Winkel K, Wunsch R, Reinehr T. Effect of lifestyle intervention on features of polycystic ovarian syndrome, metabolic syndrome, and intima-media thickness in obese adolescent girls. J Clin Endocrinol Metab. 2011;96(11):3533-40. PubMed PMID 21880803.
35. Hoeger K, Davidson K, Kochman L, Cherry T, Kopin L, Guzick DS. The impact of metformin, oral contraceptives, and lifestyle modification on polycystic ovary syndrome in obese adolescent women in two randomized, placebo-controlled clinical trials. J Clin Endocrinol Metab. 2008;93(11):4299-306. PubMed PMID; 18728175, Pubmed Central PMCID: 2582568.
36. Pasquali R, Antenucci D, Casmirri F, Venturoli S, Paradisi R, Fabbri R, Balestra V, Melchionda N, Barbara L. Clinical and hormonal characteristics of obese amenorrheic hyperandrogenic women before and after weight loss. J Clin Endocrinol Metab. 1989; 68:173-9.
37. Velazquez EM, Mendoza S, Hamer T, Sosa F, Glueck CJ. Metformin therapy in polycystic ovary syndrome reduces hyperinsulinemia, insulin resistance, hyperandrogenemia, and systolic blood pressure, while facilitating normal menses and pregnancy. Metabolism. 1994;43(5):647-54. PubMed PMID: 8177055.
38. Glueck CJ, Wang P, Fontaine R, Tracy T, Sieve-Smith L. Metformin to restore normal Menses in oligo – amenorrheic teenage girls with polycystic ovary syndrome (PCOS). J Adolesc Health. 2001;29(3):160-9. PubMed PID: 11524214.
39. Arslanian SA, Lewy V, Danadian KK, Saad R. Metformin therapy in obese adolescents With polycystic ovary syndrome and impaired glucose tolerance: amelioration of exaggerated adrenal response to adrenocorticotropin with reduction of insulinemia/ insulin resistance. J Clin Endocrinol Metab. 2002;87(4):1555-9. PubMed PMID: 11932281.
40. Bridger T, MacDonald S, Baltzer F, Rodd C. Randomized placebo-controlled trial of metformin for adolescents with polycystic ovary syndrome. Arch Pediatr Adoles Med. 2006;160(3):241-6. pubMed PMID: 16520442.
41. Geller DH, Pacaud D, Gordon CM, Misra M. The Therapeutics Committee of the Pediatric Endocrine. State of the art review: emerging therapies; the use of insulin sensitizers in the treatment of adolescents with polycystic ovary syndrome (PCOS). Int J Pediatr Endocrinol. 2011:9. PubMed PMID: 21899727, Pubmed Central PMCID: 3180691.
42. Kriplani A, Periyasamy AJ, Agarwal N, Kulshretha V, Kumar A, Ammini AC. Effect of oral contraceptive containing ethinyl estradiol combined with drospirenone vs. deogestrel on clinical and biochemical parameters in patients with polycystic ovary syndrome. Contraception. 2010;82(2):139-46. PubMed PMID: 2065754.

43. Ibanez L, de Zegher F. Flutamide-metformin plus an oral contraceptive (OC) for young women with polycystic ovary syndrome: switch from third-to-fourth-generation OC reduces body adiposity. Hum Reprod. 2004;19(8):1725-7. PubMed PMID: 15229206.
44. Dunn N. The risk of deep venous thrombosis with oral contraceptives containing drospirenone. BMJ. 2011;342:d2519. PubMed PMID: 21511807.
45. Jick SS, Hernandez RK. Risk of non-fatal venous thromboembolism in women using oral contraceptives containing drospirenone compared with women using oral contraceptives containing levonorgestrel: case-control study using United States claims data. BMJ. 2011;342:d2151. PubMed PMID: 21511805, Pubmed Central PMCID: 3081040.
46. Parkin L, Sharples K, Hernadez RK. Kick SS. Risk of venous thromboembolism in women using oral contraceptives containing drospirenone or levonorgestrel: nested case-control study based on UK General Practice Research Database BMJ. 2011;342: d:2139. PubMed PMID: 21511804, Pubmed Central PMCIS: 3081041.
47. Rosner W, Auchus RJ, Azziz R, Sluss PM, Raff H. Position statement: utility, limitations and pitfalls in measuring testosterone: and Endocrine Society position statement. J Clin Endocrinol Metab. 2007;92(2):405-13. Pub Med PMID: 17090633.
48. Alemzadeh R, Kichler J, Calhoun M. Spectrum of metabolic dysfunction in relationship with hyperandrogenemia in obese adolescent girls with polycystic ovary syndrome. Kur J Endocrinol. 2010;162(6):1093-9. PubMed PMID: 20371657.
49. Ibanez L, Valls C, Cabre S, De Zegher F. Flutamide-metformin plus ethinylestradiol-drospirenone for lipolysis and antiatherogenesis in young women with ovarian hyperandrogenism: the key role of early, low-dose flutamide. J Clin Endocrinol Metab. 2004;89(9):4716-20. PubMed PMID: 15356085.
50. Ibanez L, de Zegher F. Low-dose flutamide-metformin therapy for hyperinsulinemic hyperandrogenism in nonobese adolescents and women. Fertile Steril. 2006;86(Suppl 1:S)24-5. PubMed PMID: 16798281.
51. de Zegher F, Ibanez L. Low-dose flutamide for women with androgen excess: anti-androgenic efficacy and hepatic safety. J Endocrinol Invests. 2009;32(1):83-4. PubMed PMID: 19337022.
52. Paradisi R, Fabbri R, Porcu E, Battaglia C, Seracchioli R. Venturoli S. Retrospective observational study on the effects and tolerability of flutamide in a large population of patients with acne and seborrhea over a 15 year period, Gynecol Endocrinol. 2011;27(10):823-9. PubMed PMID: 21117864.
53. Stipp B, Taylor AA, Bartter FC, Gillette JR, Loriaux DL, Easley R, et al. Effect of spironolactone on sex hormones in man. J Clin Endocrinol Metab. 1975;41(4):777-81. PubMed PMID: 1176584.
54. Golland IM, Elstein ME. Results of an open one-year study with diane-35 in women with polycystic ovarian syndrome. Ann NY Acad Sci. 1993;687:263-8.
55. Sarih Y, Diber S, Kelestimur F. Comparison of Diane 35 and Diane 35 plus nasteride in the treatment of hirsuitism. Fertile Steril. 2001;75:496-500.
56. van Wayhen RG, van den Ende A. Experience in the long term treatment of hirsuitism and/or acne with cyproterone acetate–containing preparations. Efcacy, metabolic and endocrine effects. ExpCLin Endocrinol Diabetes. 1995;103:241-51.
57. Harborne L, Fleming R, Lyall H, Sattar N, Norman J. Metformin orantoandrogen in the treatment of hirsuitism in polycystic ovary syndrome. J Clin Endocrinol Metab. 2003;88:4116-23.

CHAPTER **12**

Implications of Polycystic Ovarian Syndrome on Pregnancy

Milind R Shah, Nirmal N Gujarathi

INTRODUCTION

Polycystic ovarian syndrome is a very common metabolic and reproductive disorder of reproductive age associated with obesity, hyperandrogenemia, and insulin resistance **(Fig. 12.1)**. It is always discussed as one of the major hurdle of pregnancy. But with advances in understanding this disease over years, we also understood the battle is not over once we achieve pregnancy in case of PCOS. There are so many issues we need to tackle when woman gets pregnant if she is known case of PCOS. PCOS affects pregnancy and also long-term health of a woman. Nowadays a growing body of evidence points to a high prevalence of pregnancy complications in PCOS women. As a result, PCOS is not only related to metabolic abnormalities, menstrual irregularity or infertility as previously reported, but becoming increasingly recognized and related to the problems of gestational diabetes mellitus (GDM), pre-eclampsia, premature delivery rate, neonatal birth weight, cesarean section rate, and admission to an neonatal intensive care unit

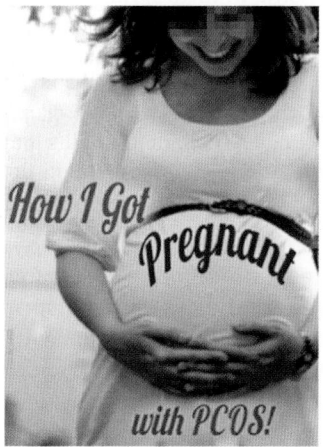

Fig. 12.1 Pregnancy with PCOS

(NICU), which are all considered to be adverse pregnancy outcomes of PCOS during pregnancy. The elevated risk for adverse obstetric complications that was observed in women presenting PCOS varied widely depending on the different phenotypes and features of PCOS.[1] However, it was not possible to account for how the prevalence of pregnancy and neonatal complications changes follow the phenotypic variants of PCOS, as the research literature lacked of the stratification of different PCOS phenotype.

Women with PCOS can conceive spontaneously but with a delayed fertile window since there is a tendency of irregular menstrual cycles with advancing age. Women with PCOS are slightly older than women without PCOS. So we need to consider that advanced maternal age is also strongly correlated with many of the adverse pregnancy outcomes.

Women with PCOS tend to require ovulation induction or assisted reproductive technology (ART) in order to become pregnant due to oligo-ovulation or anovulation. This treatment for infertility often results in an evaluated rate of multiple births. In order to explore the relationship between PCOS and pregnancy outcomes completely, the use of metformin, ovulation induction or ART must be taken into account. However many studies including Norwegian study, which reported that adverse outcomes are attributable to the factors leading to infertility rather than to factors related to reproductive technology.[2] It is said that irrespective of the use of assisted reproduction, PCOS is associated with preterm birth, gestational diabetes, and pre-eclampsia.

Polycystic ovarian syndrome (PCOS) is one of the most common endocrine disorders in women of reproductive age. The prevalence of PCOS is approximately 5-20% in general population.[3] It all depends on diagnostic criteria applied. Out of all women suffering from normogonadotropic anovulation, 70% presents with endocrine or ultrasound features of PCOS.[4] The Rotterdam ESHRE/ASRM criteria for PCOS include, oligo-ovulation or anovulation, biochemical or clinical hyperandrogenism and polycystic ovaries on ultrasound examination.[5] In 50% cases obesity has been found associated with PCOS.[6] PCOS coincides with the metabolic syndrome which is associated with increased chances for cardiovascular disease later in life.[7] Considering current lifestyle and food habits, incidence of PCOS will be rising in future, rather seen to be very much increased in our day to day practice.

PCOS shows many negative effects on pregnancy and evidences are increasing. Pregnancy itself is insulin resistance state, which may manifest as impaired glucose tolerance or gestational diabetes. PCOS women are at an increased risk of developing gestational diabetes as incidence of insulin resistance in PCOS ranges from 25-70%.

Moreover, the 'Barker hypothesis' of fetal programming *in utero* suggests that the fetal nutrition and endocrine environment (e.g. hyperinsulinemia) may effect neuroendocrine systems regulating body weight, food intake and metabolism, with consequences for long-term health in the offspring.[8]

Considering subfertility issue, many women with PCOS undergo ovulation induction or assisted reproductive techniques, which increases chance of multifetal gestation.[9]

PATHOPHYSIOLOGY OF POLYCYSTIC OVARIAN SYNDROME

The pathophysiological mechanisms behind the increased risk of adverse pregnancy outcomes among women with polycystic ovarian syndrome (PCOS) are not fully known. Disordered endocrine milieu, resulted from chronic anovulation, morphologically represents as polycystic ovaries. Polycystic ovaries and clinical features of PCOS show a functional derangement in follicular development, resulting in chronic anovulation **(Fig. 12.2)**.

Woman with PCOS exhibits increased LH levels and low-normal FSH levels and increased LH:FSH ratios. Because of pulsatile pattern of GnRH secretion, LH secretory dynamics changes. Decrease in FSH levels are seen because of increased GnRH pulse frequency and elevated estrone levels derived from

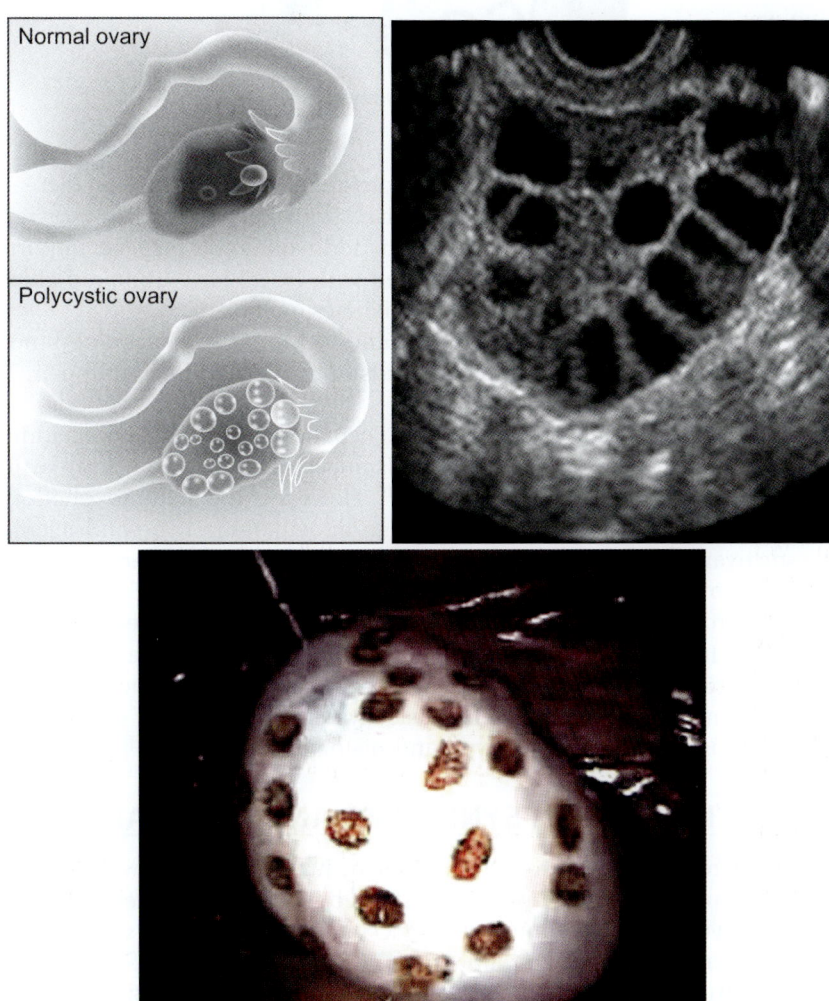

Fig. 12.2 Normal and polycystic ovaries

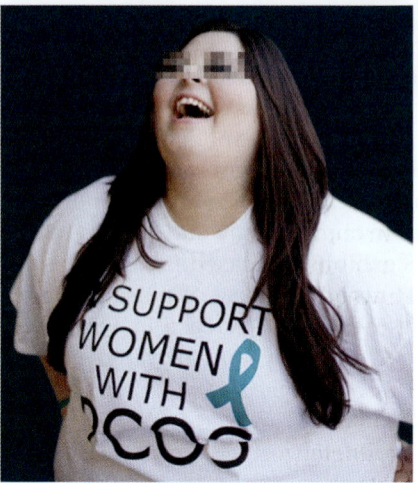
Fig. 12.3 Obesity and PCOS

peripheral aromatization of increased androstenedione. Normal or increased levels of inhibin B are noted, which are derived from small follicles.

Insulin resistance and compensatory hyperinsulinemia play an important role in pathophysiology. About 35% women with PCOS have impaired glucose tolerance and 10% fits in criteria of type 2 diabetes mellitus.

Increased androgens and insulin combine to inhibit sex hormone-binding globulin (SHBG) production from liver, leads to increase in free androgen. This aggravates insulin resistance.

Obesity, a characteristic of 60–80% of PCOS patients, has a malignant additive effect on features of PCOS such as insulin resistance, hyperandrogenism, infertility, hirsutism and pregnancy complications.[10] However, the definite phenotype of PCOS (different combinations of oligo/anovulation, hyperandrogenism, polycystic ovaries), as well as the extent of obesity in PCOS patients influences the variation of insulin resistance level **(Fig. 12.3)**.[11]

Hyperandrogenism is a major feature due to excess androgen production from ovaries. Increased LH and insulin stimulation leads to increased androgen production from ovary. Stromal expansion in PCOS women becomes more sensitive to insulin and LH and intrinsic dysregulation of key steroidogenic enzymes, helps in aggravation of hyperandrogenism.[12]

POLYCYSTIC OVARIAN SYNDROME AND PREGNANCY

In a systemic review and meta-analysis done by Jun Z Qin et al, it was found that PCOS affects pregnancy negatively and affects both mother and fetus. A total of 27 studies, involving 4982 women with PCOS and 119692 controls were eligible for the meta-analysis. Women with PCOS demonstrated a significantly higher risk of developing GDM (OR 3.43; 95% CI: 2.49–4.74), PIH (OR 3.43; 95% CI: 2.49–4.74), pre-eclampsia (OR 2.17; 95% CI: 1.91–2.46), preterm birth (OR 1.93; 95% CI: 1.45–2.57), cesarean section (OR 1.74; 95% CI: 1.38–2.11) compared to controls. Their babies had a marginally significant lower birth weight (WMD –0.11 g; 95%

CI: –0.19 – –0.03), and higher risk of admission to NICU (OR 2.32; 95% CI: 1.40–3.85) compared to controls.[13]

This meta-analysis shows insignificance between-study heterogeneity detected, women with PCOS demonstrated significantly elevated risk of gestational diabetes mellitus, pregnancy-induced hypertension, pre-eclampsia, premature delivery, preterm, cesarean section rate, and admission to an NICU pregnancy compared with controls, and marginally significant lower birth weight in PCOS group is found out. However, the results of previous meta-analytic data showed that no increased risk of cesarean section rate in women with PCOS compared with controls, and birth weight was almost the same in the both groups. Other findings of the present meta-analysis were similar with the results of previous meta-analytic data.

Implications of PCOS on pregnancy are as follows:
1. Maternal
    - Subfertility and multifetal gestation
    - Spontaneous abortions
    - Gestational diabetes mellitus
    - Gestational hypertension
    - Higher cesarean section rate.

2. Fetal
    - Premature births
    - Neonatal weight issues
    - Perinatal mortality and morbidity
    - Admission to neonatal intensive care unit
    - Lactation issues.

MATERNAL COMPLICATIONS

Subfertility

In PCOS women chronic anovulation is most common cause of subfertility. Along with this, poor oocyte quality, endometrial factors and implantation abnormalities also contribute to it. These subfertility women are candidates for ovulation induction. Ovulation induction should be done with clomiphene citrate as a first choice and in resistant cases metformin and other insulin sensitizers should be used. If this does not work then ovarian drilling or treatment with gonadotropin should be considered. Insulin sensitizers such as metformin, thiazolidinediones and D-chiro-inositol can be used to increase ovulation success.[14,15] Risk of multifetal gestation increases in PCOS patients as most of them require ovulation induction or assisted reproductive techniques for conception.

Spontaneous Abortions

The PCOS is associated with increased risk of first trimester spontaneous abortion. According to the PCOS consensus of 2012, miscarriage rates are suggested to be comparable, although available data show conflicting results (Amsterdam ESHRE/ASRM-Sponsored 3rd PCOS Consensus Workshop Group, 2012). Previous studies have shown 30–50% spontaneous abortion rate compared to normal women.

Wang et al showed that women with PCOS have significantly high risk of spontaneous abortion than non-PCOS women.[11] As per Glueck, metformin therapy throughout pregnancy in women with PCOS reduces the otherwise high rate of first-trimester spontaneous abortion seen among women not receiving metformin. Metformin does not appear to be teratogenic.[16,17] Australian study demonstrated that the miscarriage rate was more frequent in women with PCOS than in controls, although PCOS was not an independent risk factor for pregnancy loss but the miscarriage rate was strongly influenced by BMI.[18]

Gestational Diabetes Mellitus

Insulin resistance due to PCOS and pregnancy being insulin resistant condition, adds together to increase risk of gestational diabetes mellitus. Its early diagnosis is crucial and its careful treatment significantly reduces the incidence of related maternal and neonatal complications.[19,20] Xiao et al showed that risk of gestational diabetes mellitus is 1.5 times more in PCOS women than non-PCOS women.[21] As per Ashrafi and coworkers incidence of GDM in patients undergoing assisted reproduction techniques for PCOS is 44%. They said that it is recommended to do screening test for GDM in PCOS women with ART treatment, irregular menses and high serum triglycerides level in the early stage of pregnancy. Pregestational use of metformin can be effective in reducing the occurrence of GDM.[22] Four small randomized trials have demonstrated that myoinositol supplementation can lead to more than a 50% rate reduction in GDM compared with placebo.[23] There is very limited knowledge about predictive factors to know which of the PCOS women will have GDM for sure. However, Veltman-Verhulst has found that low plasma sex hormone-binding globulin (SHBG) levels may be a better predictor for GDM in women presenting with PCOS.[24]

Preeclampsia

Risk of developing pregnancy-induced hypertension and preeclampsia is more in PCOS women. As per meta-analysis risk of developing pre-eclapmsia is three to four times more in PCOS women.[25] As per study done by Fridstrom et al, incidence of gestational hypertension was more in third trimester in PCOS women.[26] It is well stated that women undergoing assisted reproductive technology are at increased risk of hypertensive disease during pregnancy, which has been attributed to the underlying cause of infertility.[27] One of the reasons quoted is women with PCOS have significantly different microscopic placental characteristics compared with non pcos women, independently from pregnancy complications.[28]

FETAL COMPLICATIONS

Data regarding incidence of adverse fetal outcomes in PCOS pregnancies are controversial. Boomsma et al and Kjerulff et al demonstrated that risk of preterm delivery is 2 times more than non PCOS patient. But recent studies did not find any such increase in risk.[29]

In a large cohort study done by Roos et al, showed infants born to PCOS patients were frequently delivered prematurely and had an increased risk of meconium aspiration.[30]

In nonobese PCOS patients, risk of SGA is more and in obese PCOS patient's risk of LGA is more.[30, 31]

Neonates born to PCOS mothers have two fold increased risk of NICU admission compared to non-PCOS mothers. Low Apgar score at 5 minutes were noted in babies born to PCOS patients. Increased perinatal mortality in babies of PCOS patients was noted in study done by Boomsma et al.

Infants born to mothers with PCOS are more likely to have a low Apgar score at five minutes, have meconium aspiration, and be large for gestational age. Higher proportion of macrosomia and being large for gestational age among infants of mothers with PCOS is controversial since the available studies have not established this association. It is well founded that maternal obesity is associated with increased birth weight in offspring as well as glucose intolerance and gestational diabetes. Women with PCOS are in general more overweight than women without the condition. Looking into body mass index suggests that PCOS may increase the rate of fetal growth independently. Women with PCOS are, regardless of body mass index, at increased risk of developing gestational diabetes. Infants born to mothers with PCOS were more likely to have low Apgar scores at five minutes and to experience meconium aspiration. These infants may be more susceptible to fetal distress during labour. However, there was no association with stillbirth, and the increased risk for neonatal death.

Lactation Issues

Women with PCOS are considered to have a reduced breastfeeding rate that resulted significantly related to midpregnancy androgen levels **(Fig. 12.4)**.[32] Because of this and many hormonal imbalances associated with PCOS, researchers have speculated that some women may have difficulty breastfeeding and producing

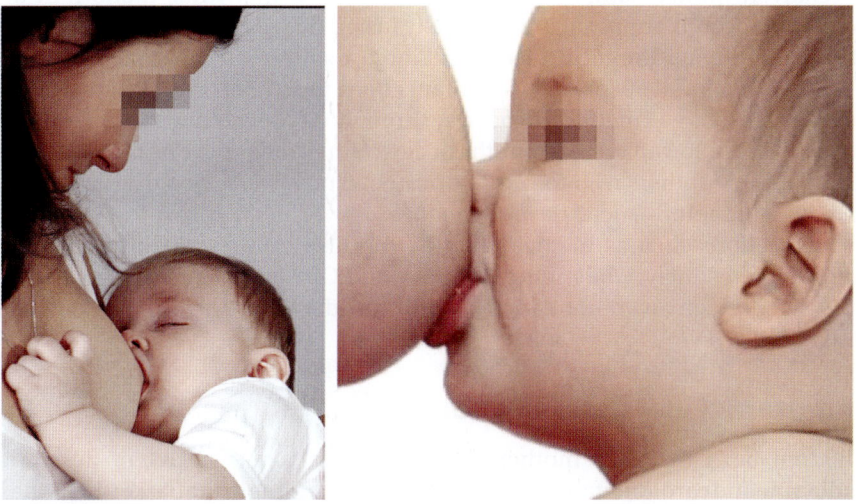

Fig. 12.4 PCOS and lactation

an adequate milk supply for their infants. The hormonal aberrations in PCOS involve insulin, progesterone, and estrogen, all of which are important to breast development and milk-secreting ability. According to Marasco, some women with PCOS may have more difficulty producing adequate milk because the breast tissue fails to undergo the normal physiological changes during pregnancy needed to prepare for lactation or perhaps because not enough breast tissue existed prior to pregnancy.[33] Women with PCOS have low levels of progesterone, which is needed for alveolar growth and breast tissue development. Insulin also plays a role in milk production, and having insulin resistance may contribute to lactation problems in women with PCOS, according to Marasco's research. As a precaution, lactation consultants recommend that all women with PCOS pump after feedings for at least 10–15 minutes on each breast to help establish an adequate milk supply in the first two weeks of initiating nursing. Frequent feedings with full drainage can also help maximize milk production, as can consuming an adequate amount of food and fluid each day. For mothers with a low milk supply, extra breast stimulation via frequent nursing or pumping sessions is crucial. Skin-to-skin contact is also encouraged to boost milk production. Milk supply problems may be prevented or ameliorated by establishing early intervention strategies during pregnancy. This may include obtaining resources for local breastfeeding support groups and preparing to work with a board-certified lactation consultant soon after giving birth. Good breastfeeding management, including proper latch and positioning, are imperative to successful milk production and proper infant growth and development. Using progesterone supplements and metformin during pregnancy may also help support an adequate milk supply in women with PCOS and possibly support breast development during pregnancy. Since many women choose to take metformin during pregnancy for the obvious benefits, they may be inclined to continue taking metformin while they breastfeed to prevent a rebounding of PCOS symptoms after birth, control insulin levels, and possibly help produce an adequate milk supply. However, the use of metformin during lactation is controversial. The few studies that are available have consisted of relatively limited sample sizes, and results show that while metformin does cross into the milk supply, it is in clinically insignificant amounts with no adverse effects on infants. The most recent and largest study was conducted among 61 nursing infants and 50 formula-fed infants born to mothers with PCOS who took an average of 2.5 g of metformin per day throughout pregnancy and lactation. The infants were followed up to 6 months of age, with results showing that the breast-fed infants of mothers who took metformin had no adverse health risks in regard to growth or motor—social development.[34]

Medications such as metoclopramide can also be prescribed to boost milk supply. Interestingly, while some women with PCOS experience low milk supply, others report an overabundance of milk production. This area needs more research.

Long-term Fetal Complications

Children born to PCOS mothers have lifetime increased risk of developing endocrine and cardiometabolic dysfunction.[35] According to the Barker-hypothesis, lifetime health can be strongly related to the intrauterine environment, i.e. being born to a mother who has suffered pregnancy complications may increase the risk of metabolic abnormalities, such as obesity and early IR, in PCOS offspring. The increased incidence of GDM observed in women with PCOS could influence negatively the cardiovascular risk factors of their offspring.

DIET AND MEDICATION CONCERNS IN PCOS PREGNANCY

The PCOS women face particular challenges as far pregnancy and its complications one help them to achieve healthy pregnancies by addressing their special emotional, health, and dietary needs **(Fig. 12.5)**. Proper medical management and medical nutrition therapy are imperative to prevent the onset of these complications and optimize fetal growth and development. Many women with PCOS who are able to conceive may have misconceptions about eating healthfully during pregnancy. Popular diet guidelines for PCOS recommend a very low-carbohydrate diet, but current evidence does not support it. Women who follow

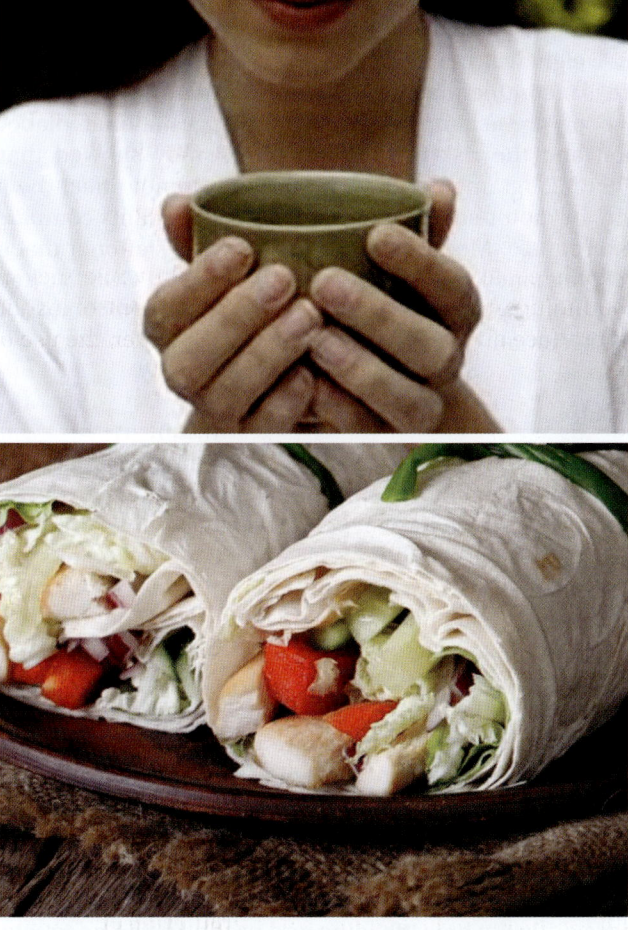

Fig. 12.5 Diet and medication in PCOS

these recommendations may feel apprehensive about eating foods containing carbohydrates during pregnancy, including fruits, vegetables, legumes, and grains all of which provide important vitamins, minerals, and fiber and are essential for fetal growth and development. Women may also be inclined to limit carbohydrates out of fear of gaining too much weight or to prevent gestational diabetes mellitus. Currently, no evidence supports limiting carbohydrates during pregnancy to prevent gestational diabetes mellitus. Dieticians should screen patients with PCOS for negative attitudes toward food and weight and convey the importance of consuming whole grain and whole food carbohydrates in sufficient amounts.

On the other hand, some women may think pregnancy gives them license to eat anything they want. This could lead to binging during pregnancy, resulting in excessive weight gain. Additionally, women who already struggle with anxiety and depression may feel that these conditions are exacerbated during pregnancy and may turn to food for emotional support. A study published in the Journal of American Dietic Association in 2005 found that pregnant women who reported high stress, anxiety, and fatigue consumed more carbohydrates, fats, and protein and less vitamin C and folate. Body image issues can also be of concern during pregnancy, as those who have struggled with their weight most of their lives may fear that their weight will spiral out of control.

Metformin is recommended for pregnant women with PCOS, as it can reduce the incidence of pre-eclampsia, macrosomia, gestational diabetes mellitus, preterm labor, and the risk of miscarriage. A study showed that at dosages between 1.5 and 2.5 grams per day, metformin did not affect the birth weight, length, growth, or motor-social development of 126 infants compared with their control counterparts.[36] Metformin helps prevent gestational diabetes mellitus and improve pregnancy outcomes in women with PCOS by helping reduce preconception and pregnancy weight gain, hyperinsulinemia, and insulin resistance and secretion.

CONCLUSION

In PCOS patients, insulin resistance and hyperandrogenism are main causative factors, leading to different complications in pregnancy. Furthermore, the interaction of insulin resistance, hyperandrogenism and obesity results in an increased risk of diabetes mellitus type 2 (DM2), metabolic syndrome (MS), cardiovascular diseases (CVD), pregnancy loss and late pregnancy complications (pre-eclampsia, gestational diabetes). This indicates that PCOS is a chronic disease that impacts women across the lifespan.[37]

This information may be vital in clinical practice for the management of pregnancy in women with PCOS. These women should be given notice of the additional risks their pregnancies may have, stronger surveillance and attention should be provided, as well as screening for these complications during pregnancy and parturition. However, in order to manage pregnancy in woman with PCOS more effectively, further investigation into the importance of glucose control, hormonal status regulation, lifestyle modification and medical therapy among women with PCOS during pregnancy should be done. Some women with PCOS may have difficulty breastfeeding and producing an adequate milk supply for their infants due to hormonal imbalances. Dieticians can play an integral part in the health of women with PCOS during pregnancy and throughout the lactation period.

It is necessary to establish guidelines for supervision during pregnancy and parturition to prevent these complications.

KEY POINTS

- The pregnancy can pose additional concerns to women with PCOS, as they are at a higher risk for miscarriage and obstetrical complications such as gestational diabetes mellitus, preterm labor, pregnancy-induced hypertension, higher cesarean rates, more NICU admissions and macrosomia.
- Some women may be resistant to eating carbohydrate foods while others may consume too many of them, posing additional risks to mother and fetus. Dieticians must educate patients about the benefits of a good diet and lifestyle to sustain a healthy pregnancy.
- In general, PCOS in pregnancy should be considered a state of pre-gestational diabetes mellitus and dietary guidelines should resemble those for gestational diabetes mellitus.
- In addition, some women with PCOS may have difficulty breast-feeding and producing an adequate milk supply for their infants due to hormonal imbalances.
- Metformin or myoinositol used throughout period of pregnancy is beneficial to reduce these complications, however their use during lactation is controversial.

REFERENCES

1. Carmina E, Azziz R. Diagnosis, phenotype, and prevalence of polycystic ovarian syndrome. Fertil Steril. 2006;86(Suppl 1):S7-S8.
2. Romundstad LB, Romundstad PR, Sunde A, von During V, Skjaerven R, Gunnell D, et al. Effects of technology or maternal factors on perinatal outcome after assisted fertilisation: a population-based cohort study. Lancet. 2008;372:737-43.
3. Archer JS, Chang RJ. Hirsutism and acne in polycystic ovarian syndrome. Best Pract Res Clin Obstet Gynaecol. 2004;18(5):737-54.
4. Laven JSE, Imani B, Eijkemans MJC, Fauser BCJM. New approach to polycystic ovarian syndrome and other forms of anovulatory infertility. Obstet Gynecol Surv. 2002; 57(11):755-67.
5. The Rotterdam ESHRE/ASRM-sponsored PCOS consensus workshop group. Revised 2003 consensus on diagnostic criteria and long-term health risks related to polycystic ovarian syndrome (PCOS). Hum Reprod. 2004;19(1):41-7.
6. Norman RJ. Improving reproductive performance in overweight/obese women with effective weight management. Hum Reprod Update. 2004;10(3):267-80.
7. Wild RA. Long-term health consequences of PCOS. Hum Reprod Update. 2002; 8(3):231-41.

8. Barker DJP. Fetal programming of coronary heart disease. Trends Endocrinol Metab. 2002;13(9):364-8.
9. Fauser BCJM, Devroey P, Macklon NS. Multiple births resulting from ovarian stimulation for subfertility treatment. Lancet. 2005;365(9473):1807-16.
10. Galtier-Dereure F, Boegner C, Bringer J. Obesity and pregnancy complications and cost. Am J Clin Nutr. 2000;71:1242S-8S.
11. Chang WY, Knochenhauer ES, Bartolucci AA, Azziz R. Phenotypic spectrum of polycystic ovarian syndrome: clinical and biochemical characterization of the three major clinical subgroups. Fertil Steril. 2005;83:1717-23. 10.1016/j.fertnstert.2005.01.096.
12. Fritz MA, Speroff L. Clinical Gynecologic Endocrinology and Infertility. Lippincott Williams and Wilkins; 2011. p. 1439.
13. Obstetric complications in women with polycystic ovarian syndrome: a systematic review and meta-analysis by Jun Z Qin, et al. Reproductive Biology and Endocrinology. 2013;11:56.
14. Boomsma CM, Eijkemans MJC, Hughes EG, Visser GHA, Fauser BCJM, Macklon NS. A meta-analysis of pregnancy outcomes in women with polycystic ovarian syndrome. Hum Reprod Update. 2006;12(6):673-83.
15. Metformin increases ovulation and pregnancy rates in anovulatory women with PCOS - meta-analysis. Evidence-based Obstetrics and Gynecology. 2004;6(3):129-30.
16. Wang JX. Polycystic ovarian syndrome and the risk of spontaneous abortion following assisted reproductive technology treatment. Hum Reprod. 2001;16(12):2606-9.
17. Glueck CJ, Phillips H, Cameron D, Sieve-Smith L, Wang P. Continuing metformin throughout pregnancy in women with polycystic ovarian syndrome appears to safely reduce first-trimester spontaneous abortion: a pilot study. Fertil Steril. 2001;75(1):46-52.
18. Joham AE, Ranasinha S, Zoungas S, Moran L, Teede HJ. Gestational diabetes and type 2 diabetes in reproductive-aged women with polycystic ovarian syndrome. J Clin Endocrinol Metab. 2014;99(3):E447-52.
19. Ngai I, Govindappagari S, Neto N, Marji M, Landsberger E, Garry DJ. Outcome of Pregnancy When Gestational Diabetes Mellitus Is Diagnosed Before or After 24 Weeks of Gestation. Obstetrics and Gynecology. 2014;123:162S-3S.
20. Poolsup N, Suksomboon N, Amin M. Effect of treatment of gestational diabetes mellitus: a systematic review and meta-analysis. PLoS One. 2014;9(3):e92485.
21. Xiao Q, Cui Y-Y, Lu J, Zhang G-Z, Zeng F-L. Risk for Gestational Diabetes Mellitus and Adverse Birth Outcomes in Chinese Women with Polycystic ovarian syndrome. Int J Endocrinol. 2016:5787104.
22. Ashrafi M, Sheikhan F, Arabipoor A, Hosseini R, Nourbakhsh F, Zolfaghari Z. Gestational diabetes mellitus risk factors in women with polycystic ovarian syndrome (PCOS). Eur J Obstet Gynecol Reprod Biol. 2014;181:195-9.
23. Froehlich R, Werner E. The Potential Role for Myoinositol in the Prevention of Gestational Diabetes Mellitus. Am J Perinatol. 2016;33(13):1236-41.
24. Veltman-Verhulst SM, van Haeften TW, Eijkemans MJ, de Valk HW, Fauser BC, Goverde AJ: Sex hormone-binding globulin concentrations before conception as a predictor for gestational diabetes in women with polycystic ovarian syndrome. Hum Reprod. 2010;25(12):3123-8. 10.1093/humrep/deq272.
25. Palomba S, de Wilde MA, Falbo A, Koster MPH, La Sala GB, Fauser BCJM. Pregnancy complications in women with polycystic ovarian syndrome. Hum Reprod Update. 2015; 21(5):575-92.
26. Fridström M, Nisell H, Sjöblom P, Hillensjo T. Are Women with Polycystic ovarian syndrome at an Increased Risk of Pregnancy-Induced Hypertension and/or Preeclampsia? Hypertens Pregnancy. 1999;18(1):73-80.

27. Kallen B, Finnstrom O, Nygren KG, Olausson PO, Wennerholm U-B. In vitro fertilisation in Sweden: obstetric characteristics, maternal morbidity and mortality. BJOG. 2005;112(11):1529-35.
28. Koster MPH, de Wilde MA, Veltman-Verhulst SM, Houben ML, Nikkels PGJ, van Rijn BB, et al. Placental characteristics in women with polycystic ovarian syndrome. Hum Reprod. 2015;30(12):2829-37.
29. Qin JZ, Pang LH, Li MJ, Fan XJ, Huang RD, Chen HY. Obstetric complications in women with polycystic ovarian syndrome: a systematic review and meta-analysis. Reprod Biol Endocrinol. 2013;11(1):56.
30. Roos N, Kieler H, Sahlin L, Ekman-Ordeberg G, Falconer H, Stephansson O. Risk of adverse pregnancy outcomes in women with polycystic ovarian syndrome: population based cohort study. BMJ. 2011;343(oct13 1):d6309-d6309.
31. Kjerulff LE, Sanchez-Ramos L, Duffy D. Pregnancy outcomes in women with polycystic ovarian syndrome: a metaanalysis. Am J Obstet Gynecol. 2011;204(6):558.e1-6.
32. Vanky E, Isaksen H, Moen MH, Carlsen SM. Breastfeeding in polycystic ovarian syndrome. Acta Obstet Gynecol Scand. 2008;87(5):531-5.
33. Marasco L, Marmet C, Shell E. Polycystic ovarian syndrome: A connection to insufficient milk supply? J Hum Lact. 2000;16(2):143-8.
34. Glueck CJ, Salehi M, Sieve L, Wang P. Growth, motor, and social development in breast-and formula-fed infants of metformin-treated women with polycystic ovarian syndrome. J Pediatr. 2006;148(5):628-32.
35. Kent SC, Gnatuk CL, Kunselman AR, Demers LM, Lee PA, Legro RS. Hyperandrogenism and hyperinsulinism in children of women with polycystic ovarian syndrome: a controlled study. J Clin Endocrinol Metab. 2008;93(5):1662-9.
36. Glueck C, Goldenberg N, Pranikoff J, et al. Height, weight, and motor-social development during the first 18 months of life in 126 infants born to 109 mothers with polycystic ovarian syndrome who conceived on and continued metformin through pregnancy. Hum Reprod. 2004;19(6):1323-30.
37. Wild RA. Long-term health consequences of PCOS. Hum Reprod Update. 2002;8(3):231-41. 10.1093/humupd/8.3.231.

CHAPTER 13

Psychological and Cognitive Problems in Polycystic Ovarian Syndrome

Vidya Pancholia, AK Pancholia

INTRODUCTION

Polycystic ovarian syndrome (PCOS) is a common endocrine disorder affecting an estimated 5–10% of reproductive age group women.[1] The diagnosis of PCOS can be made as early as in adolescent years. The Rotterdam criteria and National Institute of Child Health and Development suggest the following criteria for diagnosis of PCOS: chronic oligoovulation or anovulation, clinical or biochemical evidence of androgen excess, the presence of polycystic ovaries on an ultrasound examination, and the exclusion of other known disorders.

The PCOS encompasses a range of reproductive and metabolic manifestations including infertility, menstrual dysfunction, insulin resistance, acne, hirsutism, and obesity.[2] These symptoms are associated with undesirable mental health outcomes and impairment in quality of life at the emotional, physical, and social levels.[2-6] **(Fig. 13.1)** These undesirable manifestations of PCOS have been

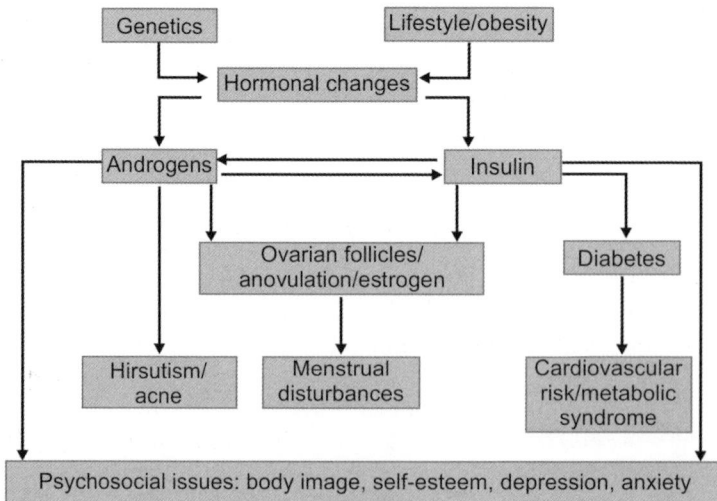

Fig. 13.1 Reproductive, metabolic and psychiatric manifestations of PCOS

TABLE 13.1 Psychiatric disorders in PCOS

Psychiatric disorders	Group		
	PCOS (%)	Control (%)	Total (%)
Present	58 (52.7)	4 (10.0)	62 (41.3)
Absent	52 (47.3)	36 (90.0)	88 (58.7)
Total	110 (100.0)	40 (100.0)	150 (100.0)

$x^2 = 22.084$; df = 1; p < 0.001

Abbreviation: PCOS, Polycystic ovarian syndrome

well studied in adult age groups. For instance, PCOS may induce a feeling of stigmatization in afflicted women due to their inability to conform to the societal norms of appearance and reproductive capabilities.[7-8] No studies have assessed the psychosocial impact of PCOS on adolescent age groups. Not surprisingly, the prevalence of depression and anxiety in women with PCOS is 29–50% and 57%, respectively.[9-10] Moreover, the life-time incidence of depressive episodes is 3.8 times higher in women with PCOS compared to age-matched controls **(Table 13.1)**. The biological causes of depression in women with PCOS have been linked to hyperandrogenism, insulin resistance, and impaired fasting glucose, and can be independent of obesity in some cases.[9-10] The reported high rates of depression and anxiety among women with PCOS highlight the need for increased screening for psychiatric symptoms and incorporating the management of these symptoms, if present, in the treatment plan of women with PCOS.[9]

Regarding cognitive dysfunction in PCOS, It is generally accepted that there are sex difference in cognition.[11-13] However, the nature of the cognitive functions which discriminate between males and females is not entirely clear. There is reasonable evidence that women typically outperform men on tasks requiring verbal memory, perceptual speed, perceptual accuracy and fine motor skills and demonstrate greater bilateral advantage than men, whereas men typically outperform women on tasks of spatial ability and mathematical reasoning.[14] Cognitive functioning may be affected in women with PCOS as a result of both hyperandrogenism and hyperestrogenism. Systematic searches of journal databases failed to find any research assessing cognitive function in PCOS. It was hypothesized that women with PCOS would demonstrate enhanced performance, relative to healthy controls, due to hyperandrogenism and hyperestrogenism on sexually dimorphic cognitive tasks.

REDUCED QUALITY OF LIFE INDICATORS

According to the World Health Organization (WHO) definition of 1948, health is a state of physical, mental and social well-being and not merely the absence of disease. There is also a term 'quality of life', introduced by Schipper, which is related to the above definition of health.[15] Quality of life depending on health, Health Related Quality of Life (HRQOL) enables the assessment of the therapeutic process from the perspective of the patient. The symptoms of polycystic ovarian syndrome, such as hirsutism, acne, menstrual disturbances, infertility and obesity are strong factors that can influence the quality of life. A series of studies, using both questionnaires general and specific for PCOS, has been carried out.

All of these studies, mostly case-controlled, have shown that PCOS significantly reduces quality of life compared to healthy women[16-20] or patients with other mild gynecological problems.[21] Another case-control, the study by Coffey et al., has shown that women with PCOS have a 20% lower quality of life than patients with asthma, diabetes mellitus, epilepsy and chronic back pain. According to most studies, obesity is the most noticeable factor that lowers the quality of life in PCOS patients. On a scale where 1 means the worst quality of life, and 7 the best, obesity reaches an average value of 2.1,[22] 2.33,[23] 2.85,[24] 2.86,[17] and 2.94.[25] Infertility is the second most important factor influencing negatively the quality of life in women with PCOS. Trent et al. studied 97 adolescents with this syndrome and compared them to 186 healthy women matched for age.[21] Patients with PCOS significantly more often (3.4 times) had concerns about their ability to become pregnant in the future, which corresponded to the reduced quality of life indicators. Hirsutism is another symptom of PCOS that plays a significant role in reducing quality of life in women with this syndrome. Lipton et al. studied 88 women with hirsutism localized on the face and found a reduction in quality of life in the field of social life and interpersonal relationships.[26] The studied patients spent an average of 104 minutes a week checking the degree of hair excess: two thirds by looking in the mirror and 76% by touch. Cultural factors have an important influence on the relationship between the individual components or symptoms of PCOS and deterioration in quality of life.

DEPRESSION

Depressive disorders are defined as a deep and persistent lowering of mood. According to DSM-IV (Diagnostic and Statistical Manual of Mental Disorders) major depression, dystymia and unspecified depressive disorders can be distinguished. According to the data from the National Institutes of Health (NIH), depression affects about 5% of the population in a year, and 13% of people during their whole life. Many researchers in longitudinal studies have shown an increased incidence of depression in women with PCOS,[27-28] and some have even reported a seven-fold increase in the incidence of suicide among women with this syndrome. Kerchner et al. found depression in 40% of 60 women diagnosed with PCOS.[27] In this group, ten women met the criteria for the diagnosis of depression, while 14 others had already been receiving antidepressants. After comparing these findings with the results from previous studies in the same group of women, it appeared that within an average of 22 months 19% (11 of 60) of women with PCOS have developed depression. Hollinrake et al. assessed the prevalence of depression among 103 women with PCOS compared to an equally-sized control group.[28] Depression, both previously diagnosed and treated, and newly found during the study, concerned 35% of patients with PCOS, compared to 10.7% of women in the control group. Fatigue (96%) and sleep disturbances (88%) were the most commonly reported symptoms of depression. The risk of depressive disorders in a subgroup of obese women with PCOS was assessed as 44% compared to 14.7% in obese women from the control group. Women with PCOS and depression had higher BMI and lower values of insulin sensitivity indices compared to PCOS patients without depression. Anxiety disorders often coexist with depression. On the basis of a questionnaire study, Benson

Table 13.2 Comparison of various disorders for HR and CI

	HR	95% CI	P value
Schizophrenia	0.83	0.433–1.588	0.573
Bipolar disorder	0.979	0.520–1.840	0.946
Depressive disorder	1.296	1.084–1.550	0.004*
Anxiety disorder	1.392	1.121–1.729	0.003*
Sleep disorder	1.495	1.176–1.899	0.001*

Abbreviations: HR, hazard ratio; CI, confidence interval
*Statistical significance

et al. found anxiety disorders in 34% of 448 women with PCOS. These symptoms were associated mainly with acne and fertility problems.[29] The same disorders found in PCOS that are associated with decreased quality of life contribute to the manifestation of depression. Among them are obesity, infertility, hirsutism and acne. Furthermore, it is believed that increased levels of testosterone, which is one of the key abnormalities in PCOS, is associated with an increased risk of developing depression[30] **(Table 13.2)**.

BIPOLAR DISORDERS

Bipolar disorders are characterized by the alternating occurrence of periods of mania and depression. They are divided into bipolar disorder I (full-blown mania and major depression), bipolar disorder II (hypomania and episodes of major depression) and unspecified bipolar disorder (bipolar symptoms that do not meet criteria I or II). There is little evidence on the relationship of bipolar disorder and PCOS. Opinions of the authors concerning the links between these conditions are divergent. Some of them claim that the development of PCOS is influenced by the valproic acid (VPA) itself, which is used to treat bipolar disorder. Others believe that there is a direct relationship between both these diseases, and they explain it by disturbances that are common to PCOS and bipolar disorder at the hypothalamic-pituitary-ovary level[31] and the similarity of metabolic abnormalities in these diseases.[32] Only a few studies have focused on the impact of the drugs used to treat bipolar disease, especially valproic acid, on the occurrence of menstrual disturbances.[33,34] McIntyre et al. compared 18 women treated with VPA with 20 female patients treated with lithium, and they found a higher incidence of menstrual disturbances in the first group (50% versus 15%).[34] In addition, patients treated with VPA had significantly higher levels of androgens (total testosterone, free testosterone and androstenedione), more atherogenic lipid profile (higher total cholesterol, low-density lipoprotein (LDL) cholesterol and triglycerides, and lower high-density lipoprotein (HDL) cholesterol levels) and higher serum leptin concentrations. In another study concerning 80 women with bipolar disorder, PCOS was diagnosed in 6% of patients treated with VPA and in none treated with other antipsychotic drugs. Klipstein et al. studied the incidence of bipolar disorder in 78 patients previously diagnosed with PCOS: 28% of the women had been diagnosed with bipolar disorder or met the criteria for the diagnosis according to the MDS questionnaire

(Mood Disorders Questionnaire).[31] Ninety seven per cent of patients in whom bipolar disorder was diagnosed before or during the study had not been treated with valproic acid before the time of diagnosis of PCOS. So, valproic acid therapy alone cannot explain the linkage between bipolar disorder and PCOS. Due to the coexistence of metabolic disturbances such as insulin resistance, obesity or hyperglycemia, found in both these diseases, a common pathogenic background seems possible.[31]

EATING DISORDERS

According to DSM-IV, three types of eating disorders are distinguished: anorexia nervosa, bulimia nervosa, and periodic overeating, binge-eating disorder (BED). In addition, subgroups of nonspecific eating disorders, Eating Disorders Not Otherwise Specified (EDNOS) are recognized. McCluskey et al. found that one-third of 153 studied women with PCOS fulfilled the diagnostic criteria for eating disorders, and bulimia was diagnosed in 6% of them.[35] Other studies have shown an increased incidence of polycystic ovaries on ultrasound image in women with bulimia, and even the normalization of these changes after recovery from bulimia.[9] Morgan et al. studied the prevalence of eating disorders in a group of 80 women with hirsutism, including 68 patients with PCOS.[36] In 36.3% of the women, eating disorders were diagnosed (all the women were from the PCOS group): in 22.5% EDNOS was recognized, in 12.6% bulimia nervosa and in 1.3% anorexia nervosa. In contrast to the above mentioned results, Michelmore et al. found no association between PCOS or polycystic ovaries on the ultrasound image and eating disorders.[37] They studied a group of 230 young women. Picture of polycystic ovaries in ultrasound was found in 74 women (33%), and 59 of them were diagnosed with PCOS. Thirty percent of the participants admitted to episodes of binge eating, while 4% had used extreme methods to maintain body weight. No statistically significant differences between the incidence of eating disorders in women with PCOS and women with normal ovaries were found.

ANXIETY AND FEARS

Recently, researchers showed an increased level of anxiety,[38,39] and social anxiety in PCOS women compared to controls. The finding of reduced sleep in women with PCOS might be explained by a higher prevalence of sleep apnea in obese women with PCOS.[40] An interesting issue is determining which characteristics of PCOS are related to anxiety. It has been shown that not only visual features of PCOS such as a higher body weight and an excessive growth of bodily hair were related to an increased experience of fear of what other people thought about their appearance, but also the absence of their cycle (amenorrhea) was negatively associated with fear of appearance evaluation.[41] The association between fear of negative appearance evaluation and nonvisual characteristics might be explained by a reduced feeling of femininity. The experience of women with PCOS feeling less feminine seems to be related to menstrual irregularities and hirsutism.[42] Contrasting findings have been found with respect to the relation between anxiety and hirsutism. Some studies reported women with hirsutism showing greater anxiety levels and social fears.[43] Moreover, one study found that higher anxiety scores were indicated in PCOS women with hirsutism than in women with newly diagnosed gynecological cancer. Furthermore, both acne and an unfulfilled wish to conceive seem to be a risk factor for clinically relevant anxiety in women with PCOS. Livadas et al.[44] studied whether anxiety was associated with hormonal and metabolic profile. PCOS women with higher anxiety scores showed significantly elevated HOMA-IR (insulin resistance) and free androgen index (FAI) values than PCOS women with lower anxiety scores, independently of BMI; however, no relation was found with hormonal values such as testosterone, androstenedione, sex hormone-binding globulin levels, dehydroepiandrosterone sulfate, and estradiol. In the same line, the relation between greater FAI values and greater levels of anxiety was previously reported by Mansson et al.[8] Moreover, Deeks and colleagues[29] indicated in a cross-sectional study in PCOS women and control that poor perception of self-worth and body image as well as health evaluation predicted higher anxiety levels. It has also been found that anxiety in PCOS women is associated with having a passive coping style.

SELF-ESTEEM AND BODY SATISFACTION

A recent study demonstrated a more negative body image in women with PCOS compared to healthy controls.[45] It has been indicated that women with facial hair and decreased self-esteem have higher depression and anxiety scores as well as poorer QoL, although poorer self-esteem compared to the general population was not confirmed, amenorrhea was associated with poorer self-esteem whereas hyperandrogenism and acne were found to be associated with body dissatisfaction. In line with our previous findings, it has been shown that women with PCOS and clinical symptoms of hirsutism and acne have greater body dissatisfaction than healthy controls with regular cycles, even after adjustment for BMI.[46] Furthermore, poorer self-esteem in PCOS women has been linked to higher levels of depression and anxiety.[47]

POTENTIAL MECHANISMS

Both testosterone and estrogen provide potential mechanisms for the alterations in cognitive performance observed in PCOS.[13,48,49] Extrapolating from other areas of research may provide insight into the current findings. In particular, research involving exogenous administration of estrogen and testosterone during gender reassignment provides causal evidence for the activational effects of these hormones.[50,51] A growing body of research has demonstrated that exogenous administration of androgens, both in gender reassignment and in healthy males, directly improves spatial functioning and indirectly improves verbal functioning via aromatization to estradiol.[50,51,52] However, the story is not quite as simple as this. O'Connor et al.[53] demonstrated that exogenous administration of large doses of testosterone impairs spatial performance whilst improving verbal performance in healthy males. O'Connor et al.[53] have proposed that testosterone influences spatial performance in an inverted "U"-shaped pattern with moderate levels associated with optimal performance and excessively low or high levels associated with impaired performance.[53] Conversely, they postulate that estrogen (and estradiol) demonstrates a "U"-shaped curve on verbal performance with excessively low or high levels associated with enhanced verbal functioning. Such a curvilinear relationship cannot explain the current finding because the elevations of estrogen in PCOS are relatively small and equate to those seen in the midfollicular phase, when verbal functioning is at its best. Testosterone is thought to influence cognitive functioning, yet there was no evidence of this in the current research. This implies that the levels of testosterone seen in PCOS might be insufficiently high enough to affect cognitive functioning. PCOS is associated with abnormalities in the levels of other hormones, besides testosterone and estrogen, especially follicle-stimulating hormone (FSH), luteinizing hormone (LH), progesterone and prolactin. Any of these hormonal abnormalities, individually or in combination, could be responsible for the effects of PCOS on cognition. The role of these hormones on cognition in the general population has largely been neglected in favor of studying estrogen and testosterone. No research has been identified assessing the effects of prolactin, FSH or LH on cognition. There is a limited amount of research into the effects of progesterone. In particular, animal models have shown that progesterone may have a neuroprotective effect.[54] However, meta-analyses have failed to find any advantage to estrogen replacement therapy (ERT) supplemented with progesterone compared to ERT without progesterone on cognitive functioning in healthy postmenopausal women or in Alzheimer's disease.[55] Brett and Baxendale[56] review the effects of exogenous progesterone on cognitive functioning. Only two studies were identified. One found evidence for impaired spatial memory in rats and the other found impaired paragraph recall in healthy females. Overall, without further scientific exploration, it is not possible to theorize about the effects of these hormones on cognition in PCOS.

MANAGEMENT

The management of depression and anxiety in patients with PCOS does not differ from the usual management of unipolar depression and anxiety disorders. Stepped care approach recommended by the National Institute for Health and Clinical Excellence is shown in **Table 13.3**.[57]

TABLE 13.3 Stepped care approach recommended by National Institute for Health and Clinical Excellence

Stages of depression	Nature of interventions
Step 1: All known and suspected presentations of depression	Assessment, support, psychoeducation, watchful waiting/active monitoring and referral for further assessment and interventions
Step 2: Persistent sub threshold depressive symptoms; mild to moderate depression	Low-intensity psychological interventions. Medications, and referral for further assessments and interventions
Step 3: Persistent sub threshold depressive symptoms or mild to moderate depression with inadequate response to initial interventions; moderate to severe depression	Medications, high-intensity psychological interventions, combined treatments, collaborative care, and referral for further assessments and interventions
Step 4: Severe and complex depression; risk to life; severe self-neglect	Medications, high-intensity psychological interventions, electroconvulsive therapy, crisis service, combined treatments, multi-professional and inpatient care

Medications usually preferred as first line agents are from group of selective serotonin reuptake inhibitors (SSRIs) like escitalopram (5–20 mg/day), fluoxetine (10–20 mg/day), sertraline (50–100 mg/day) followed by serotonin norepinephrine reuptake inhinitors (SNRIs) like venlafaxine (37.5–75 mg/day) and duloxetine (20–40 mg/day). These drugs are preferred over other classes of drugs like tricyclic antidepressants (TCAs) because of their better safety profile and decreased drug interactions.

Other nonpharmacological modes of treatments are as follows:

Lifestyle modifications: Lifestyle modification is the first form of therapy which combines dietary, behavioral techniques (reduction of psychosocial stressors), and exercises. Studies have shown that combined physical activity and dietary interventions reduced depressive symptoms and elevations in quality of life in patients with PCOS.[58,59]

Psychological treatment: Most women are afraid of infertility, body image, sexuality, loss of femininity and lower self-worth which can contribute to poorer outcomes with respect to the mental health.[59] Psychological features needs to be acknowledged, discussed and if needed counseling to be considered to enable lifestyle change which is unlikely to be successful without first addressing education and psychosocial issues.[60] Use of motivational interviewing (MI) strategies into the counseling sessions have been proven to enhance participant motivation in lifestyle modification programs. MI process activates participants to engage in self-actualization behaviors to improve health.[61] Rofey et al. observed that a manual-based Cognitive Behavioural Training and Primary and Secondary Control Enhancement Training showed promising effects with significant reductions in obesity and depression in adolescents with PCOS. They also observed decreased rates of physiological comorbidities such as menstrual irregularity; high percent of fat mass, sleep-related breathing disorder; blood pressure and mid-region adiposity associated with PCOS.[62] Techniques such as relaxation and cognitive behavioral therapy (CBT) to treat stress can be used to address the cortisol secretion abnormalities often present in PCOS women.

Exercises: Exercises improves strength, endurance, quality of life parameters, it helps to reduce stress, improves mood, health related quality of life and psychosocial factors depression and social support). Even it reduces the symptoms of depression as demonstrated by UPBEAT study.[63]

SUMMARY

The PCOS is the most common endocrine disorder in premenopausal women. More and more is known about the relationship between PCOS and impaired mental health. However, it seems that clinicians still attach too little importance to this aspect of the disease. It should be remembered that significantly reduced quality of life and the more frequent occurrence of depression and eating disorders may be associated with this condition. Gynecologists are the front-line professionals to diagnose and treat PCOS among adolescent girls. To that end, it is necessary to incorporate short self-reported screening tools for general psychological difficulties and mood and anxiety related difficulties. It is judicious to conduct long-term follow-up studies on the same population when clinical symptoms of PCOS are more severe in order to investigate any differences and for earlier intervention before onset of symptoms during adulthood.

KEY POINTS

- PCOS induces a feeling of stigmatization in afflicted women due to their inability to conform to the societal norms of appearance and reproductive capabilities.
- Cognitive functioning is affected in women with PCOS as a result of both hyperandrogenism and hyperestrogenism.
- PCOS significantly reduces quality of life compared to healthy women
- Anxiety disorders often coexist with depression.
- PCOS that are associated with decreased quality of life contribute to the manifestation of depression.
- The linkage between bipolar disorder and PCOS, due to the coexistence of metabolic disturbances, found in both these diseases, a common pathogenic background seems possible.
- PCOS fulfilled the diagnostic criteria for eating disorders, and bulimia was diagnosed in 6% of them.
- Anxiety in PCOS women is associated with having a passive coping style.
- Poorer self-esteem in PCOS women has been linked to higher levels of depression and anxiety.
- Management of depression and anxiety in PCOS does not differ from the usual management of unipolar depression and anxiety disorders.

REFERENCES

1. Arslanian SA, Lewy V, Danadian K, et al. Metformin therapy in obese adolescents with polycystic ovarian syndrome and impaired glucose tolerance: reduction of insulinemia/insulin resistance. J Clin Endocrinol Metab 2002;87:1555.
2. Thomson RL, Buckley JD, Lim SS, et al. Lifestyle management improves quality of life and depression in overweight and obese women with polycystic ovarian syndrome. Fertil Steril. 2010;94:1812.
3. Benson S, Hahn S, Tan S, et al. Maladaptive coping with illness in women with polycystic ovarian syndrome. J Obstet Gynecol Neonatal Nurs. 2010;39:37.
4. Ching HL, Burke V, Stuckey BG. Quality of life and psychological morbidity in women with polycystic ovarian syndrome: body mass index, age and the provision of patient information are significant modifiers. Clin Endocrinol (Oxf). 2007;66:373.
5. Himelein MJ, Thatcher SS. Polycystic ovarian syndrome and mental health: A review. Obstet Gynecol Surv. 2006;61:723.
6. Mansson M, Holte J, Landin-Wilhelmsen K, et al. Women with polycystic ovarian syndrome are often depressed or anxiousea case control study. Psychoneuroendocrinology. 2008;33:1132.
7. Pastore LM, Patrie JT, Morris WL, et al. Depression symptoms and body dissatisfaction association among polycystic ovarian syndrome women. J Psychosom Res. 2011;71:270.

8. Rasgon NL, Rao RC, Hwang S, et al. Depression in women with polycystic ovarian syndrome: clinical and biochemical correlates. J Affect Disord. 2003;74:299.
9. Deeks AA, Gibson-Helm ME, Teede HJ. Anxiety and depression in polycystic ovarian syndrome: a comprehensive investigation. Fertil Steril. 2010;93:2421.
10. Hollinrake E, Abreu A, Maifeld M, et al. Increased risk of depressive disorders in women with polycystic ovarian syndrome. Fertil Steril. 2007;87:1369.
11. Lezak, DM. Neuropsychological Assessment, 3rd edn. Oxford University Press, Oxford; 1995.
12. Halpern DF, LaMay ML. The smarter sex: a critical review of sex differences in intelligence. Educ. Psychol Rev. 2000;12(2):229-46.
13. Sanders G, Sjodin M, de Chastelaine M. On the elusive nature of sex differences in cognition: hormonal influences contributing to within-sex variation. Arch Sex Behav 2002;31(1):145-52.
14. Hampson E, Kimura D. Sex differences and hormonal influences on cognitive function in humans. In: Becker JB, Breedlove SM, Crews D (Eds). Behavioral Endocrinology. Massachusetts Institute of Technology, London. 199.pp.357-98.
15. Schipper H, Clinch J, Powell V. Quality of life studies: definitions and conceptual issues. In: Spilker B (Eds). Quality of life and pharmacoeconomics in clinical trials. Philadelphia, Lippincott-Raven. 1996;1-24.
16. Barnard L, Ferriday D, Guenther N, et al. Quality of life and psychological well being in polycystic ovarian syndrome. Hum Reprod. 2007;22:2279-86.
17. Ching HL, Burke V, Stuckey BGA. Quality of life and psychological morbidity in women with polycystic ovarian syndrome: body mass index, age and the provision of patient information are significant modifiers. Clin Endocrinol (Oxf). 2007;66:373-9.
18. Elsenbruch S, Hahn S, Kowalsky D, et al. Quality of life, psychosocial well-being, and sexual satisfaction in women with polycystic ovarian syndrome. J Clin Endocrinol Metab. 2003;88:5801-7.
19. Guyatt G, Weaver B, Cronin L et al. Health-related quality of life in women with polycystic ovarian syndrome, a self-administered questionnaire, was validated. J Clin Epidemiol. 2004;57:1279-87.
20. Mansson M, Holte J, Landin-Wilhelmsen K, et al. Women with polycystic ovarian syndrome is often depressed or anxious—a case control study. Psychoneuroendocrinology. 2008;33:1132-8.
21. Trent ME, Rich M, Austin SB, et al. Quality of life in adolescent girls with polycystic ovarian syndrome. Arch Pediatr Adolesc Med. 2002;156:556-60.
22. Coffey S, Bano G, Mason HD. Health-related quality of life in women with polycystic ovarian syndrome: a comparison with the general population using the polycystic ovarian syndrome questionnaire (PCOSQ) and the Short Form-36 (SF-36). Gynecol Endocrinol. 2006;22:80-6.
23. McCook JG, Reame NE, Thatcher SS. Health-related quality of life issues in women with polycystic ovarian syndrome. J Obstet Gynecol Neonatal Nurs. 2005;34:12-20.
24. Guyatt G, Weaver B, Cronin L, et al. Health-related quality of life in women with polycystic ovarian syndrome, a self-administered questionnaire, was validated. J Clin Epidemiol. 2004;57:1279-87.
25. Jones GL, Hall JM, Balen AH et al. Health-related quality of life measurement in women with polycystic ovarian syndrome: a systematic review. Hum Reprod Update. 2008;14:15-25.
26. Lipton MG, Sherr L, Elford J et al. Women living with facial hair: the psychological and behavioural burden. J Psychosom Res. 2006;61:161-8
27. Kerchner A, Lester W, Stuart SP, et al. Risk of depression and other mental health disorders in women with polycystic ovarian syndrome: a longitudinal study. Fertil Steril. 2009;91:207-12.22.
28. Hollinrake E, Abreu A, Maifeld M, et al. Increased risk of depressive disorders in women with polycystic ovarian syndrome. Fertil Steril. 2007;87:1369-76.

29. Benson S, Arck PC, Tan S, et al. Disturbed stress responses in women with polycystic ovarian syndrome. Psychoneuroendocrinology. 2009;34:727-35.
30. Rohr UD. The impact of testosterone imbalance on depression and women's health. Maturitas. 2002;15:41(Suppl 1):S25-46.
31. Klipstein KG, Goldberg JF. Screening for bipolar disorder in women with polycystic ovarian syndrome: A pilot study. J Affect Disord. 2006;91:205-9.
32. Freeman MP, Gelenberg AJ. Bipolar disorder in women: reproductive events and treatment considerations. Acta Psychiatr Scand. 2005;112:88-96.
33. Rasgon NL, Altshuler LL, Fairbanks L, et al. Reproductive function and risk for PCOS in women treated for bipolar disorder. Bipolar Disord. 2005;7:246-59.29.
34. McIntyre RS, Mancini DA, McCann S, et al. Valproate, bipolar disorder and polycystic ovarian syndrome. Bipolar Disord. 2003;5:28-5.
35. McCluskey S, Evans C, Lacey JH, et al. Polycystic ovarian syndrome and bulimia. Fertil Steril. 1991;55:287-91.
36. Morgan JF, McCluskey SE, Brunton JN, et al. Polycystic ovarian morphology and bulimia nervosa: a 9-year follow-up study. Fertil Steril. 2002;77:928-31.
37. Michelmore KF, Balen AH, Dunger DB. Polycystic ovaries and eating disorders: Are they related? Hum Reprod. 2001;16:765-9.
38. Benson S, Hahn S, Tan S, Mann K, Janssen OE, Schedlowski M, et al. Prevalence and implications of anxiety in polycystic ovarian syndrome: results of an internet-based survey in Germany. Hum Reprod. 2009;24(6):1446-51.
39. Deeks AA, Gibson-Helm ME, Paul E, Teede HJ. Is having polycystic ovarian syndrome a predictor of poor psychological function including anxiety and depression? Hum Reprod. 2011;26(6):1399-407.
40. Vgontzas AN, Legro RS, Bixler EO, Grayev A, Kales A, Chrousos GP. Polycystic ovarian syndrome is associated with obstructive sleep apnea and daytime sleepiness: role of insulin resistance. J Clin Endocrinol Metab. 2001;86(2):517-20.
41. de Niet JE, de Koning CM, Pastoor H, Duivenvoorden HJ, Valkenburg O, Ramakers MJ, et al. Psychological well-being and sexarche in women with polycystic ovarian syndrome. Hum Reprod. 2010;25(6):1497-503.
42. Kitzinger C, Willmott J. 'The thief of womanhood': women's experience of polycystic ovarian syndrome. Soc Sci Med. 2002;54(3):349-61.
43. Sonino N, Fava GA, Mani E, Belluardo P, Boscaro M. Quality of life of hirsute women. Postgrad Med J. 1993;69(809):186-9.
44. Livadas S, Chaskou S, Kandaraki AA, Skourletos G, Economou F, Christou M, et al. Anxiety is associated with hormonal and metabolic profile in women with polycystic ovarian syndrome. Clin Endocrinol (Oxf). 2011;23.
45. Deeks AA, Gibson-Helm ME, Paul E, Teede HJ. Is having polycystic ovarian syndrome a predictor of poor psychological function including anxiety and depression? Hum Reprod. 2011;26(6):1399-407.
46. Weiner CL, Primeau M, Ehrmann DA. Androgens and mood dysfunction in women: comparison of women with polycystic ovarian syndrome to healthy controls. Psychosom Med. 2004;66(3):356-62.
47. Rofey DL, Szigethy EM, Noll RB, Dahl RE, Lobst E, Arslanian SA. Cognitive-behavioral therapy for physical and emotional disturbances in adolescents with polycystic ovarian syndrome: a pilot study. J Pediatr Psychol. 2009;34(2):156-63.
48. Ditkoff EC, Fruzzetti F, Chang L, Stancyzk FZ, Lobo RA. The impact of estrogen on adrenal androgen sensitivity and secretion in polycystic ovarian syndrome. Clin J. Endocrinol. Metab. 1995;80(2):603-7.
49. Greene RA, Dixon W. The role of reproductive hormones in maintaining cognition. Obstet. Gynecol Clin North Am. 2002;29(3):437-53.
50. Van Goozen SH, Slabbekoorn D, Gooren LJ, Sanders G, Cohen-Kettenis PT. Organizing and activating effects of sex hormones in homosexual transsexuals. Behav Neurosci. 2002;116(6):982-8.

51. Slabbekoorn D, van Goozen SH, Megens J, Gooren LJ, Cohen-Kettenis PT. Activating effects of cross-sex hormones on cognitive functioning: a study of short-term and long-term hormone effects in transsexuals. Psychoneuroendocrinology. 1999;24(4):423-47.
52. Cherrier MM. Androgens and cognitive function J Endocrinol Investig. 2005;28(3):65-75.
53. O'Connor DB, Archer J, Hair WM, Wu FC. Activational effects of testosterone on cognitive function in men. Neuropsychologia. 2001;39(13):1385-94.
54. Schumacher M, Guennoun R, Robert F, Carelli C, Gago N, Ghoumari A, Gonzalez Deniselle MC, Gonzalez S, Ibanez C, Labombarda F, Coirini H, Baulieu EE, De Nicola AF. Local synthesis and dual actions of progesterone in the nervous system: neuroprotection and myelination. Growth Horm. IGF Res. 2004;14(Suppl-1):S18-33.
55. Hogervorst E, Yaffe K, Richards M, Huppert F. Hormone replacement therapy for cognitive function in postmenopausal women. Cochrane Database Syst. Rev. 2006a;2(CD003122).
56. Brett M, Baxendale S. Motherhood and memory: a review. Psychoneuroendocrinology. 2001;26(4):339-62.
57. National Institute for Health and Clinical Excellence. Depression: the treatment and management of depression in adults (update). Clinical Guideline 90. 2009.http://www.nice.org.uk/
58. Sachdev M, Kaur J, Garnawat D, Bhatia MS. Psycho-physiotherapeutic treatment of polycystic ovarian syndrome. Delhi Psychiatry Journal. 2015;18(1):151-4.
59. Banting LK, Gibson-Helm M, Polman R. Physical activity and mental health in women with polycystic ovarian syndrome. BMC Women's Health. 2014;14:51.
60. Teede H, Deeks A, Moran L. Polycystic ovarian syndrome: a complex condition with psychological, reproductive and metabolic manifestations that impacts on health across the lifespan. BMC Med. 2010;8:1-10.
61. Mahoney D. Lifestyle modification intervention among infertile overweight and obese women with polycystic ovarian syndrome. J Am Assoc Nurs Practitioners. 2014; 26:301-8.
62. Rofey DL, Szigethy EM, Noll RB. Cognitive-behavioural therapy for physical and emotional disturbances in adolescents with polycystic ovarian syndrome: a pilot study. J Pediatr Psychol. 2009;34(2):156-63.
63. Blumenthal JA, Sherwood A, Rogers SD, Babyak MA, Doraiswamy PM, Watkins L, et al. Understanding prognostic benefits of exercise and antidepressant therapy for persons with depression and heart disease: the UPBEAT study—rationale, design, and methodological issues. Clin Trials. 2007;4(5):548-59.

CHAPTER **14**

Long-term Sequel of Polycystic Ovarian Syndrome

Anu Agarwal

INTRODUCTION

Polycystic ovarian syndrome (PCOS) is a multifactorial, heterogeneous, complex, genetic, endocrine and metabolic disorder, diagnostically characterized by chronic anovulation, polycystic ovaries and biochemical and clinical manifestation of hyperandrogenism. Despite typically having an early onset, PCOS has varied long-term implications on health and longevity. From the current scenario of ovulatory dysfunction, it may evolve eventually into a metabolic syndrome with insulin resistance, hyper insulinemia, abdominal obesity, hypertension and dyslipidemia, culminating in serious long-term consequences such as type II diabetes mellitus, cardiovascular disease, endometrial hyperplasia.

The need to bring conscious lifestyle changes can only be achieved if both short term and long term health implications are deliberated.

METABOLIC DYSFUNCTION IN POLYCYSTIC OVARIAN SYNDROME

Metabolic Syndrome

The metabolic syndrome (MBS), also called as syndrome x or insulin resistance syndrome consist of a group of risk factors that raises your risk for heart disease and other health problems, such as diabetes and stroke as shown in **Flow chart 14.1**.

The National Cholesterol Education Program Adult Treatment Panel (NCEP-ATP) III criteria for metabolic syndrome in women with PCOS are:
- Abdominal obesity> 88 cm (waist circumference)
- Triglycerides> 150 mg/dL (1.7 mmol/L)
- High-density lipoprotein-cholesterol (HDL-C) <50 mg/dL (1.29 mmol/L)
- A systolic blood pressure > 130 mm Hg or a diastolic blood pressure > 85 mm Hg
- *Fasting glucose:* >100 mg/dL (> 5.6 mmol/L).

Presence of three out of five criteria qualifies for the diagnosis of the syndrome. Participants who reported using antihypertensive or antidiabetic medication (insulin or oral agents) were counted as having high blood pressure or diabetes, respectively.

Up to 43% of nondiabetic PCOS women meet metabolic syndrome criteria before the end of their fourth decade, and most of them before the end of their third decade of life.[1,2]

A significant age related trend (P<0.01) has been reported in the prevalence of MBS, increasing from 23% in PCOS women < 20 years, to 45% in women aged 20-29 years, and then to 53% in PCOS women aged 30-39 years.[3] Insulin resistance (71%) is the most common metabolic abnormality in PCOS patient followed by obesity (52%) and dyslipidemia (46.3%) with an incidence of 31.5% for the metabolic syndrome.

Women with MBS had significantly higher BMI values and tend to present more often with hirsutism and acanthosis nigricans than those lacking this conditions.

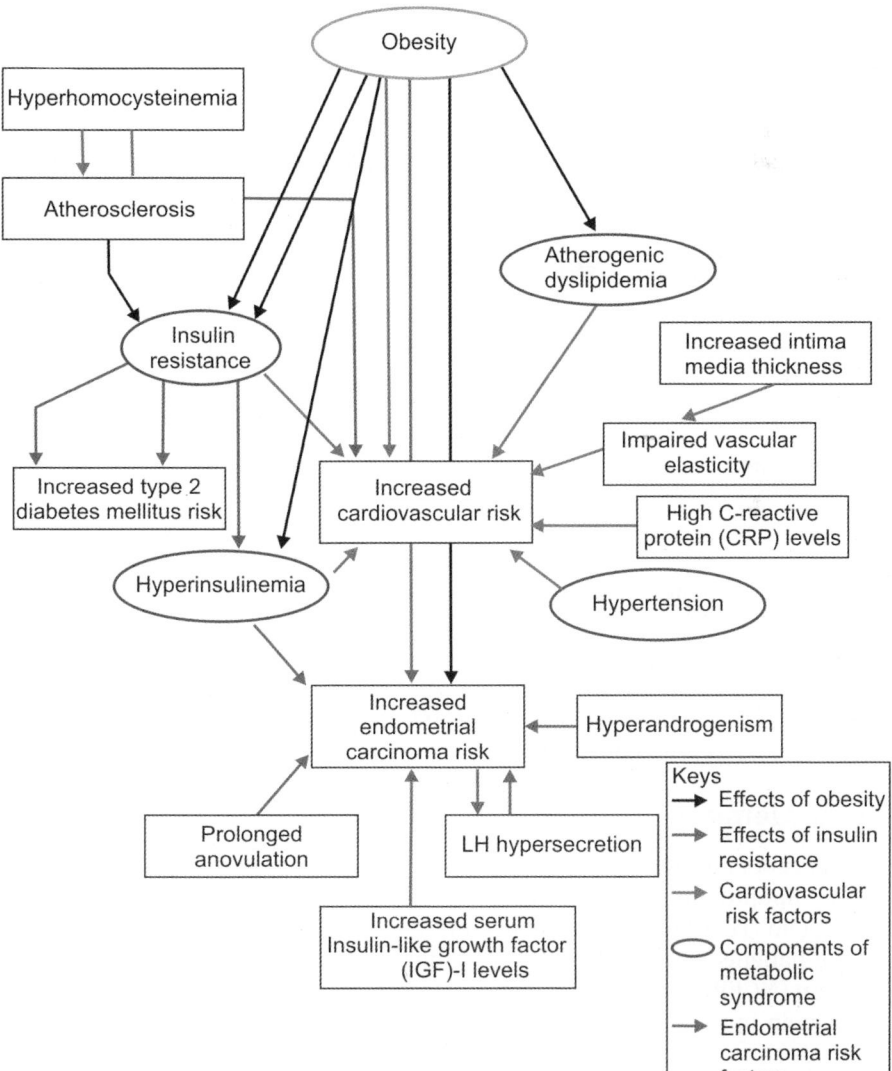

Flow chart 14.1 Metabolic dysfunction in PCOS

Insulin Resistance

"Insulin resistance" is defined as "a decreased ability of insulin to mediate its metabolic actions on glucose uptake, glucose production and lipolysis, requiring increased amounts of insulin to achieve its proper metabolic action."

Insulin resistance occurs in 50 to 80% of women in PCOS[4] and is considered central to the pathogenesis of PCOS. It has a multifactorial pathogenesis, is a precursor of diabetes mellitus (DM), and is additionally associated with components of MBS, such as cardiovascular risk, hypertension and endothelial dysfunction, which are considered the initial step in the process of atherosclerosis and a shorter life span.

Insulin resistance (IR) is one of the important consequences of obesity, the prevalence of which is progressively increasing around the world.

A significantly higher (P < 0.01) prevalence of central obesity, hypertension and high triglycerides and low prevalence of HDL-C has been reported in Asian Indians with the insulin resistance syndrome.[5]

However the risk of developing type II diabetes is also increased in non obese women with PCOS.[6,7]

Anovulatory women with PCOS are relatively hyperinsulinemic and more insulin resistant then weight-matched control subjects[8] and this hormone insensitivity probably contributes to hyperandrogenism.

Etiology of Insulin Resistance

Proposed mechanism for IR is peripheral target tissue resistance, decreased hepatic clearance and increased pancreatic sensitivity. Studies on molecular mechanisms of IR in PCOS suggest that there is dysregulation of insulin receptor phosphorylation.

How to Detect Insulin Resistance?

- A fasting glucose to Insulin ratio < 7— useful index of IR in adolescents[9]
- Oral glucose tolerance test (OGTT) with 75 g of glucose provides information about both insulin resistance and glucose intolerance.

Hyperinsulinemia

Inherent defects in insulin synthesis/secretion, insulin resistance and obesity all contribute to hyperinsulinemia.

Dyslipidemia

Disorders of lipoprotein metabolism associated with increased cholesterol, low-density lipoprotein (LDL) and triglycerides (TG) and decrease in high-density lipoprotein (HDL) cholesterol concentration. Dyslipidemia is reported in up to 70% of patients who have PCOS. According to National Cholesterol Education Program (NCEP) guidelines[10] insulin, estrogen and androgens or known to alter lipoprotein lipid metabolism. Obesity has an important influence on the lipid profile with approximately 50% of patients with PCOS being overweight or obese with abdominal fat. Hyperinsulinemia, due to IR, has been associated with lipid and lipoprotein abnormalities in women with PCOS.

Obesity

More than 50% of PCOS women are overweight (BMI> 25 kg/m^2, or obese BMI> 30 kg/m^2). Obesity contributes significantly to both insulin resistance and hyperandrogenemia in overweight women with or without PCOS. In PCOS there is central or android or visceral obesity. In this there is disproportionate quantity of adipose tissue is distributed in the visceral depots. They have increase waist hip ratio (WHR)> 85, or a waist circumference ≥ 80 cm. → is a marker of metabolic syndrome.

Compared with weight matched controls. Overweight women with PCOS have increase cardiovascular risk factor and evidence of early cardiovascular disease.

Hyperinsulinemia itself contributes to obesity by the anabolic effect on fat metabolism through adipogenesis process—the result is an increase uptake of glucose into adipocytes, the production of triglycerides, and the inhibition of hormone sensitive lipase.[11] Therefore, there is a vicious cycle in which android fat produces android fat and exacerbates the predisposition towards weight gain.

Visceral fat or abdominal fat is metabolically distinct from subcutaneous fat; it is resistant to the antilipolytic action of insulin and releases excessive amounts of free fatty acids, which leads to insulin resistance in the liver and muscle. Excess central adiposity reflects a worsened dyslipidemia profile, with higher triglyceride level and low HDL cholesterol level.

A high prevalence of IR and impaired glucose tolerance among obese women with risk factors, such as obesity (BMI> 30 kg/m^2) or fasting glucose > 100 mg/dL and a relevant family history, makes OGTT and metabolic screen mandatory.

Type II Diabetes Mellitus

PCOS in associated with on approximately 7 fold increased risk of Type II DM.[12]

Insulin resistance and pancreatic β-cell dysfunction are major risk factors for the development of Type II DM.

Women with PCOS also develop abnormal glucose metabolism at a younger age and may demonstrate a more rapid conversion from impaired glucose tolerance to Type to DM.[13]

It is increasingly clear that IGT is also a clinically relevant state where early identification and intervention improve long-term outcome[14] IGT has been found to increase the risk of cardiovascular disease mortality and progression to Type II DM in general population.[15]

Lifestyle interventions, metformin, and glitazones can prevent IGT progression to Type II DM[16] strengthening the argument for early detection of IGT, including in high-risk PCOS women.

Diagnosis

European Society of Human Reproduction and Embryology (ESHRE)/American Society for Reproductive Medicine (ASRM) sponsored PCOS consensus workshop group recommended oral glucose tolerance test (OGTT) in all overweight women with PCOS.[17]

Oral Glucose Tolerance Test

The most accurate method to diagnose insulin resistance is the OGTT after 75 g of glucose challenge. Normal values are as follows:
- Fasting glycemia: 70–100 mg/dL
- 60 minutes after glucose administration < 180 mg/dL
- 120 minutes after glucose administration < 140 mg/dL

Impaired glucose tolerance is defined when glucose level is > 140 mg/dL 2 hours after glucose load, but < 200 mg/dL.

Diabetes is defined when glycemia is > 200 mg/dL 2 hours after glucose load. Emerging data shows increase risk of metabolic complications in first degree family member of women with PCOS.[18,19]

Impaired fasting glucose is a poor predictor of IGT in women in general[20] and in PCOS[21,22]

In PCOS there is 10 fold increased risk of developing gestational diabetes mellitus (GDM) compared to the general population.

Both IGT and Type II DM are significant cardiovascular risk factors in women. Once the diagnosis of diabetes is made the relative risk of cardiovascular disease in women increases four fold to seven fold. Obesity and overweight increase the risk of developing Type II DM in PCOS women, although PCOS represents an independent risk factor for Type II DM.

Obstructive Sleep Apnea

Women diagnosed with PCOS (or their partners) should be asked about snoring and day time fatigue, somnolence and informed of the possible risk of sleep apnoea and offered investigation and treatment when necessary.

Obstructive sleep apnea (OSA) is an independent cardiovascular risk factor and has been found to be more common in PCOS. The difference in prevalence of sleep apnea between PCOS and controls remained significant even when controlled for body mass index (BMI).[23,24]

It has been reported that the strongest predictors for sleep apnea were fasting plasma insulin level and glucose to insulin ratio.[25]

Cardiovascular Risk

Cardiovascular risk factors associated with PCOS include insulin resistance, central obesity, hypertension, dyslipidemia, hyperhomocysteinemia, increased intima media thickness and impaired vascular elasticity.[26] Obesity may contribute to a significant increase in cardiovascular risk either directly, or via its impact on the various components of the metabolic syndrome.

Therefore, it could be assumed that the lifelong metabolic dysfunctions of PCOS are responsible for a worse cardiovascular profile and predispose for CVD with aging.

Both CRP and homocystiene levels have been shown as independent risk factor for CVD[27] CRP is a marker of inflammation, predict the incidence of myocardial infarction, stroke, peripheral arterial disease and sudden death.[28] Elevated CRP level in PCOS group[29] suggest that women with PCOS may indeed be at risk for early onset CVD.

Despite advances in diagnostic techniques and identification of structural markers to address the prevalence of cardiovascular risk factors in PCOS women, owing to limitations, such as poor documentation of clinical cardiovascular events and a relatively young age of women at follow-up in most studies, the incidence of carotid disease in PCOS women has not consistently been demonstrated and no increase association with cardiovascular mortality reported.[30]

Malignancy

Increased risk for endometrial, ovarian and breast cancer in women with PCOS has been suggested. It is important to note that many confounders including obesity, hyperglycemia and anovulation (unopposed estrogen) with resultant infertility make it difficult to define the absolute risk of these neoplasms attributed to PCOS alone. This is especially true in case of ovarian and breast cancer where a paucity of data limits conclusions. However, the link between PCOS and endometrial cancer appears to be supported by both biologic plausibility and the preponderance of evidence suggesting a two to three fold increase risk of endometrial cancer in the setting of anovulation, menstrual irregularity and PCOS.[31,32]

Proper endometrial surveillance (ultrasound and/or sampling) and periodic induction of uterine bleeding with progesterone withdrawal reduce the risk of endometrial cancer. Oral contraceptive also results in a significant reduction in the risk of endometrial and ovarian cancer with no increase in long-term metabolic risk. In those desiring fertility, pregnancy decreases risk of all three cancer types.

Recent evidence supports the use of progesterone releasing progestin intrauterine device (IUD) in the prevention and treatment of uterine hyperplasia and early endometrial cancer, but it use specifically in women with PCOS have not been investigated.

Agents that induce ovulation and improve the chance of pregnancy would also combat the unopposed estrogen and possibly lowers the risk of endometrial hyperplasia and cancer.

It is generally accepted that PCOS women with amenorrhea at greater risk for endometrial hyperplasia and cancer. Therefore ESHRE/ASRM consensus workshop group has established a proper endometrial surveillance with ultrasound and/or biopsy to assess endometrial thickening in women who experience extended period of amenorrhea, based on clinical suspicion and presentation. In these women periodic progestogen withdrawal is recommended, at least four episodes per year.[33]

However, they do not recommended routine surveillance strategy and/or clinical care to detect ovarian and breast cancer in all women with PCOS.

PSYCHOLOGICAL FEATURES OF POLYCYSTIC OVARIAN SYNDROME

Patients with PCOS presents and increased risk for psychological disorder and reduced quality of life (QOL) compared to healthy women. There is increased prevalence of generalized anxiety and increase in mean anxiety scores in women with PCOS compared with control women.[34]

Moreover, the debate remains open about whether the increased prevalence of these psychological disorders is due to the PCOS itself or its features, such as obesity, hirsutism, irregular menses, and infertility.

ESHRE/ASRM consensus group considers offering psychological screening to all women with PCOS.[35]

MANAGEMENT OF LONG-TERM COMPLICATIONS

Metabolic risk- ESHRE/ASRM-Sponsored PCOS consensus workshop group[35] and the Androgen Excess and PCOS (AE-PCOS) Society[36] recommend OGTT as screening test for IGT and Type II DM in PCOS women with classic phenotype (hyperandrogenism and anovulation), obesity (BMI> 30 kg/m^2), acanthosis higricans which represents a pathognomonic sign of IR, and a personal history of gestational diabetes mellitus (GDM) or a family history of Type II DM.

The AE-PCOS Society[37] recommends OGTT also in lean PCOS women with advanced age (> 40 years).

- *Obesity:* It is recommended that BMI and waist circumference should be determined at every visit.[38]
- *Cardiovascular risk*: AE-PCOS Society proposed—To categorize the PCOS related CVD risk as:

"At risk" for PCOS women with any following risk factors:

Obesity, cigarette smoking, hypertension, dyslipidemia, subclinical vascular disease, IGT and/or family history of premature cardiovascular disease (< 55 years of age in male relative, < 65 years of age in female related).

"At high-risk" for PCOS women with metabolic syndrome and/ or T2 DM and/or overt vascular or renal disease.

The all societies[35,39-41] agree to recommended a cardiovascular disease risk assessment at any age,—for BP, complete lipid profile (including total, LDL, HDL cholesterol and triglyceride), waist circumference, BMI, glucose profile, cigarette smoking and a family history of early cardiovascular disease. PCOS patient should also be assed for depression, anxiety and quality of life.

Periodic reassessment for cardiovascular disease risk in suggested but there is no agreement how often the cardiovascular disease risk assessment should be repeated.

Regarding cancers, there is no agreement on the optimal method, whether ultrasound or endometrial biopsy and timing of screening for endometrial cancer. In line with American Cancer Society Guideline[42] the decision to assess for the presence of endometrial cancer should be based especially on the presence of abnormal uterine bleeding or spotting.

Lifestyle changes, including hypocaloric diet and physical exercise, in considered a cornerstone of the management of women with PCOS.

About 5-10% weight loss in considered clinically significant and able to reduce IGT and metabolic syndrome prevalence in general population.

The women with PCOS, both obese and nonobese are characterized by an IR and hyperinsulinemia more relevant compared to that of age and weight-matched control's women, suggesting a tendency towards IR which is independent of obesity. Accordingly, when impaired insulin sensitivity in present, the use of metformin might be suggested.[43,44]

A Cochrane review[45] showed that metformin reduces serum testosterone level and fasting insulin concentrations to a significant extent only among nonobese women.

Metformin is not of benefit in improving weight loss, insulin sensitivity, or lipid profile; hence a long-term prophylactic treatment with metformin is unlikely to prevent progression to diabetes.[45] In line with these considerations, the main societies[35,39,40] agree to consider metformin for prevention of diabetes in women with PCOS and IGT when lifestyle modification is not successful and/or as an adjuvant to general lifestyle modifications that remains the first line therapy for PCOS women at increased metabolic risk.

So overall, woman with PCOS show an increased risk of obstetric, cardiovascular, metabolic and psychological complications compared to non-PCOS women and timely intervention is required.

KEY POINTS

- PCOS may evolve into a metabolic syndrome by its negative impact on physiology and metabolism of body leading to Type II DM, cardiovascular disease, endometrial hyperplasia and quality of life.
- IR has a multifactorial pathogenesis and central to the pathogenesis of PCOS.
- Tests to detect IR:
  a. Fasting glucose to insulin ratio.
  b. OGTT with 75 g of glucose.
- Women with BMI > 30 or a strong family history of Type II DM should have OGTT.
- In PCOS there is central obesity defined as increased waist hip ratio (WHR) > 85 or increased waist circumference > 80 cm.
- Approximately seven fold increase of developing Type II DM in PCOS. There is rapid conversion from IGT to DM II. So early detection and timely intervention is important.
- Obstructive sleep apnea (OSA) is common is PCOS and OSA is an independent cardiovascular risk factor. Strongest predictors for sleep apnea are fasting plasma insulin levels and glucose to insulin ration.
- Despite the increase in cardiovascular risk factor, morbidity and mortality form coronary heart disease among women with PCOS has not been shown to be as high as predicted.
- Amenorrheic or severely amenorrheic women with PCOS should have induced withdrawal bleeding at regular intervals to reduce the risk of developing endometrial hyperplasia.

REFERENCES

1. Ehrmann DA, Liljenquist DR, Kasza K, Azziz R, Legro RS, Ghazzi MN. Prevalence and predictors of metabolic syndrome in women with polycystic ovary syndrome. J Clin Endocrinol Metab. 2006;91(1):48-53.
2. Apridonidze T1, Essah PA, Iuorno MJ, Nestler JE. Prevalence and characteristics of the metabolic syndrome in women with polycystic in ovary syndrome. J Clin Endocrinol Metab. 2005;90(4):1929-35.
3. Zeyneloglu HB, Esinler I. Chronic complications of polycystic ovary syndrome. In: Allahabadia GN, Agarwal R (Eds). Polycystic ovary syndrome. UK: Anshan Publishers.
4. Legro RS, Castracane VD, Kauffman RP. Detecting insulin resistance in polycystic ovary syndrome: purposes and pit falls. Obstet Gynecol Surv. 2004;59:141-54.
5. Dunaif A. Insulin resistance and polycystic ovary syndrome: mechanisms and implication for pathogenesis. Endcr Rev. 1997;18:774-800.
6. Legro RS, Kunselman AR, Dodson WC, Dunaif A. Prevalence and predictors of risk for type 2 diabetes mellitus and impaired glucose tolerance in polycystic ovary syndrome a prospective, controlled study in 254 affected woman. J Clin Endocrinol Metab. 1999;84:165-9.
7. Pierpoint T, McKeigue PM, Isaacs AJ, Wild SH, Jacobs HS. Mortality of women with polycystic ovary syndrome at long term follow-up. J Clin Epidemiol. 1999;51: 779-86.
8. Legro RS, Castracane VD, Kauffman RP. Detecting insulin resistance in polycystic ovary syndrome: purpose and pitfalls. Obstet Gynecol Surv. 2004;59:141-54.
9. Kent SC, Legro RS. Polycystic ovary syndrome in adolescents. Adolesc Med. 2002; 13:73-83.
10. Third report of the national cholesterol education program (NCEP). Expert panel on detection evaluation, and treatment of high blood cholesterol in adults (Adult treatment panel III) final report. Circulation. 2002;106:3143-421.
11. Arner P. Human fat cell lipolysis: biochemistry, regulation and clinical role. Best pract Res Clin Endocrinol Metab. 2005;19:471-82.
12. Jakubowski L. Genetic aspect of polycystic ovary syndrome. EndoKrynol Pol. 2005:56:285-93. (in Polish)
13. Ehrmann DA, Barnes RB, Rosenfield RL, Cavaghan MK, Imperial J. Prevalence of impaired glucose tolerance and diabetes in women with polycystic ovary syndrome. Diabetes Care.1999;22141-146.
14. Knowler WC, Barrett-Connor E, Fowler SE, Hamman RF, Lachin JM, Walker EA, Nathan DM. Reduction in the incidence of type 2 diabetes with lifestyle intervention or metformin. N Engl J Med. 2002;346;393-403 doi:10.1056/NEJMoa012512. (PMC free article) [PubMed (Cross Ref)].
15. Barr ELM, Magliano DJ, Zimmet PZ, Polkinghorne KR, Atkins RC, Dustan DW, Murray SG, Shaw JE. AusDiab 2005: The Australian Diabetes, Obesity and Lifestyle Study. Melbourne, Australia: International Diabetes Institute, 2006.
16. Knowler WC, Barret-Connor E, Flowers SE, Hammn RF, Lachin JM, Walker EA, Nathan DM. Reduction in the incidence of type 2 diabetes with lifestyle intervention or metforim.N Engl J Med. 2002;346:393-403.doi:10.1056/NEJMoa012512.(PMC free article) (PubMed) (Cross Ref).
17. Salley KE, Wickham EP, Cheang KI, Essah PA, Karjane NW, Nestler JE. Glucose intolerance in polycystic ovary syndrome- a position statement of the androgen Excess Society. J Clin Endcrinol Metab. 2007;92:4546-4556 doi:10.1210/jc-2007-1549 [Pubmed (cross Ref)].
18. Sam S, Legro RS, Essah PA, Apridonidze T, Dunaif A. Evidence for metabolic and reproductive phenotypes in mothers of women with polycystic ovary syndrome. Proc Natl Acad Sci USA. 2006:103:7030-35.doi:10.1073/pnas.0602025103. (PMC free article) [PubMed (Cross Ref)].

19. Yilmaz M, Bukan N, Ersoy R, Karakoc A, Yetkin I, Ayvaz G, Cakir N, Arslan M. Glucose intolerance, insulin resistance and cardiovascular risk factors in first degree relative of women with polycystic ovary syndrome. Hum Reprod. 2005;20:2414-2420.doi. 10.1093/humrep/dei070. [PubMed (Cross Ref)].
20. Dunstan D, Zimmet P, Welborne T, Sicree RTA, Atkins R, Cameron A, Shaw J, Chadaban S. Australian Diabetes, Obesity and Lifestyle Report. Melbourne, Australia: the International Diabetes Institute 2001. The Accelerating Epidemic; Diabetes and associated disorders in Australia 2000. pp. 12-5.
21. Legro RS, Kunselman AR, Dodson WC, Dunaif A. Prevalence and predictors of risk for type 2 diabetes mellitus and impaired glucose tolerance in polycystic ovary syndrome a prospective, controlled study in 254 affected woman. J Clin Endocrinol Metab. 1999; 84:165-9 doi:10.1210/jc.84.1.165.[Pub Med] Cross Ref).
22. Ehrmann DA, Barnes RB, Rosenfield RL, Cavaghan MK, Imperial J. prevalence of impaired glucose tolerance and diabetes in women with polycystic ovary syndrome. Diabetes Care.1999:22;141-6doi:
23. Fogel RB, Malhotra A,Pillar G, Pittman SD, Dunaif A, White DP. Increased prevalence of obstructive sleep apnea syndrome in obese women with polycystic ovary syndrome. J Clin Endocrinol. Metab. 2001;86:1175-80.
24. Gopal M, Duntley S, Uhles M, Attarian H. The role of obesity in the increased prevalence of Obstructive sleep apnea syndrome in the patients with polycystic ovarian syndrome. Sleep Med. 2002;3:401-4.
25. Vgontzas AN, Legro RS, Bixler EO, Grayev A, Kales A, Chrousos GP. Polycystic ovary syndrome is associated with obstructive sleep apnea and daytime sleepiness: role of insulin resistance J Clin Endrocrinol Metab. 2001;86:517-20.
26. Ridker PM. Clinical application of C-reactive protein for cardiovascular disease: detection and prevention. Circulation. 2003;107:363-9.
27. Zeyneloglu HB, Esinler I. Chronic complications of polycystic ovary syndrome. UK Anshan Publishers; 2006.pp.102-12.
28. Hahn S, Tan S, Quad beck B, Herrmann BL, Mann K, et al. Clinical and biochemical characterization of women with polycystic ovary syndrome in North Rhine – westphalia. Horm Metab Res. 2005;37:438-44.
29. Zeyneloglu HB, Esinler I. Chronic complications of polycystic ovary syndrome. UK Anshan Publishers; 2006.pp.102-12.
30. Ridker PM. Clinical application of C-reactive protein for cardiovascular disease: detection and prevention. Circulation. 2003;107:363-9.
31. Gallos ID, Shemar M, Thangaratinam S, Papapstolou TK, Coomarasamy A, Gupta Jk. Oral progestogens vs levonorgestrel-releasing intrauterine system for endometrial hyperplasia: systematic review and metaanalysis. Am J Obstet Gynecol. 2010;203(6):547, el-10. [PubMed].
32. Garvey WT, Ryan DH, Look M, Gadde KM, Allison DB, Peterson CA, et al. Two year sustained weight loss and metabolic benefits with controlled-release phentermine/topiramate inobese and overweight adults (SEQUEL): a randomized, placebo-controlled, phase 3 extension study. Am J clin Nutr. 2012;95(2):297-308. (PMC free article) [PubMed].
33. Fauser BC, Tarlaztzis BC, Rebar RW, et al. Consensus on women's health aspects of polycystic ovary syndrome (PCOS): the Amsterdam ESHRE/ASRM-Sponsored 3rd PCOS Consensus Workshop Group. Fertil Steril. 2012;97(1):28-38. [PubMed].
34. Dokras A, Clifton S, Futterweit W, Wlid R. Increased prevalence of anxiety symptoms in women with polycystic ovary syndrome. Systematic review and meta-analysis fertile steril. 2010;97(1):225-30. [PubMed].
35. Fauser BC, Tarlaztzis BC, Rebar RW, et al. Consensus on women's health aspects of polycystic ovary syndrome (PCOS): the Amsterdam ESHRE/ASRM-Sponsored 3rd PCOS Consensus Workshop Group. Fertil Steril. 2012;97(1):28-38. [PubMed].

36. Hull MG. Epidemiology of infertility and polycystic ovarian disease: endocrinological and demographic studies. Gynecol Endocrinol. 1987;1:235-45. [PubMed].
37. Wild RA, Carmina E, Diamanti-kandarakis E, et al. Assessment of cardiovascular risk and prevention of cardiovascular disease in women with polycystic syndrome: a consensus statement by the Androgen Excess and Polycystic ovary Syndrome (AE-PCOS) Society. J Clin Endocrinol Metab. 2010;95(2):2038-49 [PubMed].
38. Rosenzweing JL, Ferrannini E, Grundy SM, et al. Primary prevention of cardiovascular disease and type 2 diabetes in patients at metabolic risk: an endocrine society clinical practice guideline. J Clin Endocrinol Metab. 2008;93(10):3671-89. [PubMed].
39. Conway G, Dewailly D, Diamanti-Kandarakis E, et al. The polycystic ovary syndrome a position statement from the European Society of Endocrinology. Eur J Endocrinol. 2014;171(4):1-29. [PubMed].
40. Legro RS, Arslanian SA, Ehrmann DA, et al. Diagnosis and treatment of polycystic ovary syndrome; an endocrine society clinical practice guideline. J Clin Endocrinol Metab. 2013;98(12):4565-92. [PubMed].
41. Wild RA, Carmina E, Diamanti-kandarakis E, et al. Assessment of cardiovascular risk and prevention of cardiovascular disease in women with polycystic syndrome: a consensus statement by the Androgen Excess and Polycystic ovary Syndrome (AE-PCOS) Society. J Clin Endocrinol Metab. 2010;95(2):2038-49. [PubMed].
42. Smith RA, von Eschenbach AC, Wender R, et al. ACs Prostate Cancer Advisory Committee. ACS Colorectal Cancer Advisory Committee. ACS Endomerial Cancer Advisorty Committee American. Cancer Society Guidelines for the early detection of cancer. Update of early detection guidelines for prostate, colorectal and endometrial cancer. Also: update 2001-testing for early lung cancer detection. CA Cancer J Clin. 2001;51(1):38-75. [PubMed].
43. Palomba S, Falbo A, Zullo F, Orio F Jr. Evidence-based and potential benefits of metformin in the polycystic ovary syndrome; a comprehensive review. Endocr Rev 2009;30(1):1-50. [PubMed].
44. Nieuwenhuis-Ruifrok Ae, Kuchenbecker WK, Hoek A, Middleton P, Norman RJ. Insulin Sensitizing drugs for weight loss in women of reproductive age who are overweight or obese: systematic review and meta-analysis. Hum Reprod Update. 2009;15(1):57-68. [PubMed].
45. Tang T, lard JM, Norman RJ Yasmin E, Balen AH. Insulin-sensitisng drugs metformin, rosiglitazone, pioglitazone, D-chiro-inositol for women with polycystic ovary syndrome, oligo amenorrhoea and subfertility. Cochrane Databasse Syst Rev. 2012(5); CD005552. [PubMed].

CHAPTER 15

Medicolegal Aspects of Polycystic Ovarian Disease

Hitesh J Bhatt

INTRODUCTION

After the inclusion of medical services under the ambit of consumer protection act, the awareness among patient about their rights has increased gradually and the rise of social media had added to it. Now doctor is accountable for all his professional conduct towards the patient not only under medical council act but under tort as well as criminal laws. Moreover, the trust in every relation is decreasing and more importance is being given to documentations. Even the sacred act of marriage needs compulsory registration! So doctors are no excuse and are expected to document everything they do in the best interest of the patient. As a doctor, we have habit of classifying every situation as per medical conditions, but the principals of law are not different for different medical conditions. The law remains same for each medical condition and each branch of medicine. Hence, the medicolegal aspect of polycystic ovarian disease (PCOD) can be the medicolegal aspect of any medical condition. What is more important is to understand the principal of law and the safeguards.

LEGAL IMPLICATIONS

First of all we must understand a few things as:
- What is negligence?
- What is civil negligence and what is criminal negligence?

What is Negligence?

The negligence is defined as "To do something what a prudent man in similar situation will not do (Act of commission) and not to do something what a prudent man in similar situation will do (Act of omission).

So, the conduct of the doctor in question shall be compared with the conduct of similar person, i.e. similarly qualified doctor dealing with similar case under similar circumstances. How such a colleague (Prudent person) would have treated the patient is the main question. This legal test or principal is called Bolam's test. How to find such a prudent person? This prudent person is a hypothetical situation. So, how such a prudent person would have acted is decided by various ways. Court shall consider textbook references, references from the journal and affidavit from a peer authenticating the treatment given by a doctor in question. Here comes the role of situation, court shall also consider that what was the situation at the time of mishap and that situation also becomes a deciding factor for negligence. For example, a case investigated and treatment given at primary health care by a gynecologist for menorrhagia cannot be compared with the similar case handled by similarly qualified gynecologist at tertiary care hospital. The expectation for specific investigations including Pap test, biopsy, blood investigations, CT scan, MRI, laparoscopy, hysteroscopy, etc. —whichever is necessary—are expected from a consultant sitting at higher center. Again a treatment given in emergency case cannot be compared with treatment given for planned case. The expectation of preparation to tackle the situation in later case is more than the previous case.

Civil Negligence and Criminal Negligence

We also must understand the basic difference between civil and criminal negligence.

Civil negligence is the breach of a duty to care or failure to fulfill one's duty, or a failure to follow the normal standards of conduct for a reasonable person. The negligent act must result in some injuries or loss or damage to the patient. Then patient claims for such damage in terms of some amount of rupees. The case is between two parties, the patient (plaintiff) and the service provider (the doctor).

Criminal negligence is different because the defendant is accused of intentionally acting in reckless fashion without regard to the safety of others, and as such, the offense falls under criminal codes. It needs high level of negligence then what is required to prove a civil negligence. The punishment here is fine or imprisonment or both. The case is filed by the State against the accused. There is role of police.

What are the Litigant Situations?

- When treatment is done without consent.
- When some complications have arisen.
- When charges are not communicated properly or charge more for the services and infrastructure.
- Rough behavior of the staff or doctor.

What Prevents Litigation or Saves a Doctor in Court?

- Proper communication.
- Proper documentation.

Communication

Communication includes general communication and consent. It says those who communicate well with patient shall never face the problems. Hiding things from patient or not explaining things for wont of time in busy outpatient department (OPD) can put you in trouble. If doctor himself is busy then he should appoint proper staff or counselors to communicate with the patients but avoiding communication is not the option. Any complication explained before surgery is well accepted by the patient then explaining it after it happens. Way of communication is the reflection of human nature. So if you communicate well, you shall be considered as one with good human nature.

Role of consent: Consent is an important aspect of communication while dealing with patient. After the landmark case of Sameera Kohli vs Dr Prabha Manchanda, where the Apex Court had discussed consent at length, the importance and necessity of consent came into limelight. Taking precedence of this case many other cases were decided where consents were not proper or treatment was done beyond the consent given.

In a case of Mrs Zeba Hamid vs Hajela Hospital and Ors. The patient was of primary infertility. She consented for diagnostic laparoscopy and hysteroscopy only. While the doctor did ovarian drilling and salpingectomy without consent. His intention must be good to save future expense and time but in the eyes of the law it was wrong. Apex court had said in case of Sameera Kohli vs Dr Prabha Manchanda that correctness of the treatment shall not make it legal treatment. So in present case the compensation was awarded in favor of the patient.

Documents

It is said that the things not documented has never happened. We Indians are very poor at documentation. In medical practice we must have various medical documents including case papers, consents, refer notes, reports, charts, X-rays, Forms, etc. Most doctors do not maintain OPD records. We must have copy of every document which our patient has. In court it is said that good documents means good defense, poor documents means poor defense and no documents means no defense. The documents have to be preserved for long time. Various guidelines by various bodies give different time frames as follows:
- Consumer Protection Act—2 years
- Civil Litigations—3 years
- Criminal Laws—No limit
- MTP Act (Section 5.1)—5 years
- PNDT Act (Section 9.6)—2 years
- Income Tax Act—8 years
- FOGSI Guidelines—5 years
- Medical Council Act—3 years
- ART Guidelines—10 years

We have to destroy documents after public notice.

CONCLUSION

- Most of the medicolegal problems are preventable.
- Communication and documentations are the keys to save you.
- Always keep in touch with current medical practice and update your knowledge regularly.
- In case of medicolegal problem always involve medicolegal expert to guide you.

- Never ignore nor reply to legal notice without consultation with medicolegal consultant.
- Medicolegal problems are part of practice, like bumps on a road so never get worried for any such problem. Have fearless practice.

KEY POINTS

- The law remains same for each medical condition and each branch of medicine.
- The negligence is defined as "To do something what a prudent man in similar situation will not do (Act of commission) and not to do something what a prudent man in similar situation will do (Act of omission).
- Civil negligence is the breach of a duty to care or failure to fulfill one's duty, or a failure to follow the normal standards of conduct for a reasonable person.
- Criminal negligence is different because the defendant is accused of intentionally acting in reckless fashion without regard to the safety of others, and as such, the offense falls under criminal codes.
- Way of communication is the reflection of human nature. So if you communicate well, you shall be considered as one with good human nature.
- It is said that the things not documented has never happened.
- The documents have to be preserved for long time. Various guidelines by various bodies give different time frames.
- Medicolegal problems are part of practice.

SECTION 5

MANAGEMENT

16. Lifestyle Modifications in Polycystic Ovarian Syndrome
17. Drilling the Ovaries: What is the Latest Evidence?
18. Hirsutism
19. Adjuvants in Polycystic Ovarian Syndrome
20. Recent Advances in Polycystic Ovarian Syndrome

CHAPTER 16

Lifestyle Modifications in Polycystic Ovarian Syndrome

T Ramani Devi

INTRODUCTION

Polycystic ovarian syndrome (PCOS) is a complex, common endocrine disorder affecting the women of reproductive age group. Incidence varies between 6 and 21% (Boyle et al, Yildiz et al).[1,2] PCOS is associated with reproductive, metabolic and psychological dysfunction. Most PCOS patients are obese and insulin resistant, which is the key factor for the syndrome.

Obese PCOS women have higher incidence of hyperinsulinemia when compared to their lean counterparts. Obesity particularly abdominal obesity is mediated by the development of insulin resistance, which is closely linked with the development of this condition and its clinical features, particularly menstrual irregularities and hyperandrogenemia. Hence, lifestyle modifications focusing predominately on diet, exercise and behavior are considered to be the preferred first-line treatment of PCOS management. Several studies have shown that weight loss of 5–10% in PCOS patients via caloric restriction can reduce hyper insulinemia and hyperandrogenism.

DIAGNOSIS OF POLYCYSTIC OVARIAN SYNDROME

Diagnosis is based on the internationally accepted Rotterdam criteria, NIH (National Institute of Health) criteria which include 2 out of 3 features must be present in order to make the diagnosis. More recently in 2009 the Androgen Excess and PCOS (AE-PCOS) society outlined its own criteria.

Criteria for Diagnosis of PCOS (2 Out of 3 Must be Present)

1. Oligo/anovulation.
2. Clinical (or) biochemical evidence of hyperandrogenism.
3. Polycystic appearing ovaries on imaging.
4. Other disorders like adrenal, thyroid dysfunction and hyperprolactinemia must be ruled out.

NIH criteria include, chronic anovulation, clinical (or) biochemical signs of hyperandrogenism. These two criteria should be present and other diagnosis must be excluded to allow the diagnosis of PCOS.

Definition of Lifestyle Modification

This consists of multifaceted approach of diet, exercise and behavioral therapy. According to NIH guidelines weight loss can be achieved within a short time by structured clinical setting. The weight loss should be at least 10% and should be maintained for more than 1 year (Wing RR, Phelan).[3] Those who succeed in long-term weight loss have the following behavior. They eat regular breakfast, low fat diet, weigh regularly and engage in high level of physical activity.

Many patients, who lose weight by dietary weight loss program, eventually regain weight (Anderson et al).[4] If initial weight loss is greater and when patients maintain regular healthier eating, control over eating, and self-monitor behavior, maintenance of weight loss is feasible (Elfhag and Rossner).[5]

Obesity and Insulin Resistance

Obesity is associated with insulin resistance and there is a parallel increase in the incidence of metabolic syndrome, Type II diabetes and cardiovascular disease (Reaven).[6]

Weight gain after adolescence is a predictor of hyperinsulinemia and menstrual disorders in PCOS. The prevalence of Type II diabetes is 10 times higher among young women with PCOS than healthy controls. Incidence of Type II diabetes is more common in obese PCOS than lean PCOS[7] (Legro et al).

Women with higher BMI were 13.7 times more likely to have insulin resistance than lower body mass index (BMI). Diet, exercise, behavioral modification and drug therapy can effectively reduce insulin resistance and reverse the menstrual abnormality, promote fertility, improve lipid profile and reduce the risk of diabetes and cardiovascular disease (Clark et al , Moran et al).[8,9] Lifestyle modification also improves the psychological disturbances like low self-esteem, anxiety and depression. 5–10% weight loss over a period of 4 weeks, improves the clinical presentation of PCOS, despite they remain clinically over weight. Weight loss essentially treats acute clinical dysfunction and long-term metabolic health.

DIET IN POLYCYSTIC OVARIAN SYNDROME

Diet should be low total calorie per day, low carbohydrate and fat, adequate proteins and vitamins. Traditional Indian food is high in carbohydrate and moderate in fat and protein. This type of food could have suited the people of previous generation, whereas current generation people have sedentary lifestyle which needs decreased caloric intake. Western dietary snacks and meals have been added to our dietary habit due to modernization. All these factors have led to increase in the prevalence of obesity and hence increased incidence of PCOS in Indian women.

Recommended caloric intake depends upon the weight of the patient, physical activity, age, gender and physiological status. Once should reduce 500 calorie per day to reduce weight. This can reduce ½ kg weight per week. Meal pattern and calorie need should be planned by nutritionist. Obese women tend to underestimate their calorie intake by 40–50%.

Carbohydrates

About 40–50% of the calorie intake must be from carbohydrate. Complex carbohydrate should be preferred over refined carbohydrate. Food with low glycemic index should be preferred to high glycemic index. Low glycemic diet will improve insulin sensitivity and possibly improve androgen profile of women with PCOS.[10,11] Simple carbohydrate like sugar, jiggery, etc. should be avoided. Individuals should be encouraged to consume four servings of vegetables and two servings of fruits every day. Long-term intake of fiber rich diet controls the blood sugar and improves the lipid profile.

Proteins

They have a vital role in the body and 20% of the total body weight is made-up of proteins. Proteins are needed for body building produce important enzymes, hormones neurotransmitters, tendon, ligament, antibodies and other body chemicals. PCOS women should select lean protein than high fat source of animal protein. Overall dietary carbohydrate can be substituted with lean protein which takes longer time to digest and gives a sense of satiety. Lean protein meals improve the overall insulin response in PCOS. About 25–30% of total calories should be in the form of protein, spread equally among all meals and snacks. This can stabilize blood sugars and prevent hypoglycemic and subsequent cravings.

Lipid Abnormalities in PCOS and Dietary Fat

2/3rds of women with PCOS have lipid abnormalities.[12] Dyslipidemia is due to hyperandrogenism, obesity, insulin resistance and hyperinsulinemia. Lipid abnormalities in PCOS are similar to diabetic patients like elevated total cholesterol and low-density lipoprotein (LDL) and decreased high-density lipoprotein (HDL).[13] Hyperinsulinemia and hyperandrogenism causes the adipocytes to undergo lipolysis and leads to increase in free fatty acids, which in turn stimulates the liver to produce triglycerides and very low density lipoprotein (VLDL).[14]

Dietary Fats and PCOS

Fat is essential for weight management and insulin resistance. Appropriate fat is needed for absorption of fat soluble vitamins, to decrease the overall risk of cardiovascular disease and gain reproductive benefit (As sex hormones are controlled by dietary fat). Fats also induce satiety.

Fats and oils are made-up of fatty acids. They are unsaturated fatty acids (Mono and Poly) and saturated fatty acids. Diet rich in monounsaturated fatty acids improves cholesterol levels, optimizes insulin levels and controls sugar.[15] Omega 3 and omega 6 fatty acids are types of poly unsaturated fatty acids and are essential fatty acids which humans cannot synthesize and are dependent on dietary sources. Omega 6: Omega 3 ratio in healthy diet should be 4: 1. Omega 3 fatty acids are essential for women with PCOS, as they have anti-inflammatory benefit. PCOS is a condition associated with low grade inflammation, as shown by elevation of proinflammatory markers.[16] It also supports healthy cardiovascular system, brain, mood, skin and immune function. It normalizes the lipid profile and improves insulin sensitivity.[17,18] Omega 3 fatty acids are found in fish, flax seed, nuts and leafy vegetables.

Saturated fatty acids increase the total and LDL cholesterol. Only 10% of the total calories should be saturated fatty acids. Consumption of transfats (hydrogenated fats like vanaspati) are proinflammatory and increase the risk of coronary artery disease. Hence, saturated fatty acids and trans-fat should be replaced by unsaturated fatty acids. Women with PCOS should have 25–30% of the calories from fat. Saturated fatty acids are found in meats, dairy products butter, cheese, cream, chicken skin, coconut, palm kernel and palm oil.

Diet should include lowest levels of saturated fat especially monosaturates. 3–7% of energy should be from polyunsaturated fats. Higher intake may relate to increased production of lipid peroxidase which is harmful.

Fruits and PCOS

Fruits are natural form of healthy diet should be encouraged in women with PCOS. They contain only carbohydrates and no proteins or fats. Fruits contain lot of fibers, vitamins, minerals and antioxidants. One serving of fruit will contain 60 calories and PCOS patients are recommended two servings per day. PCOS patients should avoid canned fruits and fruit juices. Fruits can be mixed with lean proteins and modest amount of fat like yogurt or nuts and low fat cheese. This will improve the satiety and stabilize blood sugars.

Vegetables and PCOS

Vegetables are high in fiber content vitamins, minerals and antioxidants. Non starchy vegetable should be preferred over starchy vegetables as they are low in calories and high in fiber content. This will not increase the weight or worsen the insulin resistance. They can be taken for three to four servings. The use of starchy vegetables should be limited as they increase the insulin levels.

Dietary Fibers

This is a complex carbohydrate present in vegetables, fruits and legumes.
They are not digested by gut and they form the unavailable carbohydrates in the food. Fenugreek is effective in controlling sugar and lipids.

Dietary Calcium

Dairy products contain calcium, proteins and other nutrients. Beyond bony health, calcium reduces the blood pressure and has relevance for calcium signaling. It is also suggested to have a role in fat metabolism. Calcium consumption should be 1200–1500 mg/day.[19,20]

Dietary Sodium and PCOS

PCOS women are prone for premature atherosclerosis and endothelial dysfunction. Sodium is found in various natural foods and additive food products. Processed food, pickles, *pappad*, dry fish contain preservatives like monosodium glutamate, sodium nitrate, sodium saccharin, sodium bicarbonate (baking soda) and sodium benzoate. Hence, sodium should be around 2300 mg/day (1 table spoon of salt). Adults with high blood pressure should not consume salt greater than 1500 mg/day.

Behavioral Modification in PCOS Management

Eating small, frequent, meals and snacks decreases the food cravings and prevents binges. It provides steady flux of energy and prevents hypoglycemia. Meal pattern should be 3 major meals and 3 snacks. Snacks should be around 60–100 calories. Breakfast should be 25–30% of total calories, lunch should be 35–40% of total calories and dinner should be 25–30% of total calories. Optimum meal plan is to consume breakfast within 1 hour of walking, snacks 2–3 hours later, eat lunch 2 hours later, snacks 2–3 hours later and 2 hours later dinner. Third snack may be substituted if needed after 2 hours of dinner.

Exercise and PCOS Management

Regular exercise is essential for weight management, physical and mental health. Physical activity reduces insulin levels, improves insulin sensitivity and optimizes lipid profile. It improves self-esteem, depression and anxiety in women with PCOS.

Exercise improves glucose homeostasis, relates to an upregulation of the expression activity of proteins involved in insulin signal transduction in the skeletal muscle.[21] Study by Vigorito et al, demonstrated, that programmed training-induced significant improvement of cardiopulmonary functional capacity, insulin sensitivity, reduced BMI and CRP levels.[22] Study by Brown et al also showed moderate intensity exercise also revealed the improvement lipid profile, without weight reduction, which will be useful in lean PCOS.[23] Hence, women with PCOS should be recommended to increase the physical activity, which can improve the overall metabolic picture and reduce the risk of cardiovascular morbidity.

EXERCISE RECOMMENDATIONS

Physical activity guidelines for Americans recommend that, physical activity should be 150 minutes per week of moderate intensity. Brisk walking, aerobics, dancing, gardening, playing baseball and volley ball, etc. are considered to by moderately intense exercise. Individuals can increase the intensity of exercise and reduce the timing to 75 minutes per week. Activities that strengthen muscles improve balance and preserve bone like weight training, resistant and weight-bearing aerobics are recommended for 2 days in a week.

KEY POINTS

- Majority of PCOS women are overweight.
- They benefit from weight reduction strategies.
- Successful weight loss is achieved through dietary modification and restrictions.
- Reduce simple carbohydrates, saturated fatty acids, omega 6 fatty acids, optimize dietary fiber and omega 3 fatty acids.
- Principle of no fasting or feasting should be followed. Frequent small meal pattern is ideal.
- Regular physical activity of moderate intensity along with dietary modification can enhance health benefit.
- Antiobesity drugs can also be tried.
- In morbidly obese individuals, bariatric surgery reverts the metabolic abnormalities.

REFERENCES

1. Boyle JA, Cunningham J, O'Dea K, Dunbar T, Norman RJ. Prevalence of polycystic ovary syndrome in a sample of Indigenous women in Darwin, Australia. Med J Aust. 2012;196:62-6.MedlineScience Google.
2. Yildiz BO, Bozdag G, Yapici Z, Esinler I, Yarali H. Prevalence, phenotype and cardiometabolic risk of polycystic ovary syndrome under different diagnostic criteria. Hum Reprod. 2012;27:3067-73. Abstract/FREE Full Text.
3. Wing RR, Phelan S. Long-term weight loss maintenance. American Journal of Clinical Nutrition. 2005;82:222S-225S.
4. Anderson JW, Konz EC, Frederich RC, et al. Long-term weight-loss maintenance: a meta-analysis of US studies. American Journal of Clinical Nutrition. 2001;74:579-84.
5. Elfhag K, Rossner S. Who succeeds in maintaining weight loss? A conceptual review of factors associated with weight loss maintenance and weight regain. Obesity Reviews. 2005;6:67-85.
6. Reaven GM. The insulin resistance syndrome: definition and dietary approaches to treatment. Annual Review of Nutrition. 2005;25:391-406.
7. Legro Rd, Kunelman AR, Dodson WC. Prevalence and predictors of risk for type 2 diabetes mellitus and impaired glucose tolerance in polycystic ovarian syndrome: a prospective, controlled study in 254 affected women. J ClinendocrinolMetab. 1999; 84:165-9.
8. Clark AM, Thornley B, Tomlinson L, et al. Weight loss in obese infertile women results in improvement in reproductive outcome for all forms of fertility treatment. Human Reproduction. 1998;13:1502-5.
9. Moran LJ, Noakes M, Clifton PM, et al. Short term energy restriction (using meal replacements) improves reproductive parameters in polycystic ovary syndrome. Asia Pacific Journal of Clinical Nutrition. 2004;13:S88.
10. Ehrmann DA, Barnes RB, Rosenfield RL, Cabaghn MK, Imperial J. Prevalence of impaired glucose tolerance and diabetes in women with polycystic ovarian syndrome. Diabetes Care. 1999;22:141-74.
11. Sathyapalan T. Atkin S. Mediators of inflammation in polycystic ovarian syndrome in relation to adiposity. Mediators Inflamm. 2010:758656.

12. Wild R. Dislipidemia in PCOS. Steroids. 2012;77:295-9.
13. Yildirim B, Sabir N, Kaleli B. Relation of intra abdominal fat distribution to metabolic disorders in non obese patients with polycystic ovary syndrome. Fertil Steril. 2003; 79:1358-64.
14. Potter van Loon BJ, Kluft C, Radder JK, Blankenstein MA, Medinders AE. The cardiovascular risk factor plasminogen activator inhibitor type is related to insulin resistance. Metabolism. 1993;42(8):945-9.
15. Lopex-Huetro E. The effect of EPA and DHA on metabolic syndrome patients: a systemic review of randomized controlled trials. Br J Nutr. 2012;107:S185-94.
16. Duleba AJ, Dokras A. Is PCOS an inflammatory process? Fertil Steril. 2012;97(1):7-12.
17. Bhathena S. Relationship between fatty acids and the endocrine system. Biofactors, 2000;13:35-9.
18. Parillo M, Rivellese AA, Ciardullo AV, Capaldo B, Giacco A, Genovese S. A high monounsaturated-fat/low-carbohydrate diet improves peripheral insulin sensitivity in non-insulin dependent diabetic patients. Metabolism. 1992;41(12):1373-8.
19. Dittas A. The role of vitamin D and calcium in type 2 diabetes. A systemic review and meta-analysis. J Clin Endocrional Metab. 2007;92(6):2017-29.
20. Shahar D. Does dietary calcium intake enhance weight loss among diabetic patients? Diabetes Care. 2007;30(3):485-9.
21. Hawley JA. Exercise as a therapeutic intervention for the prevention and treatment of insulin resistance. Diabetic Metab Res Rev. 2004;20:383-93.
22. Vigorito C, Gialluauria F, Palomba S, Cascella T, Manguso F, Lucci R. et al. Beneficial effects of a three-months structured exercise training program on cardiopulmonary functional capacity in young women with polycystic ovary syndrome. J Clin Endocrinol Metab. 2007;92(4):1379-84.
23. Brown AJ, Setji TL, Sanders LL. Lowry KP, Otvos JD, Kraus WE, Svetkey PL. Effects of exercise on lipoprotein particles in women with polycystic ovary syndrome. Med Sci Sports Exerc. 2009;41(3):497-504.

CHAPTER 17

Drilling the Ovaries: What is the Latest Evidence?

Vidhya V Bhat, Ritu Bijarnia

INTRODUCTION

Polycystic ovarian syndrome (PCOS) is a common endocrine disorder, characterized by menstrual irregularity and hyperandrogenism. This hyperandrogenemia leads to chronic anovulation, irregular periods, and infertility. It affects 5–10% women of reproductive age,[1] and is responsible for 75% cases of anovulatory infertility.[2]

American Society for Reproductive Medicine (ASRM) and the European Society of Human Reproduction and Embryology (ESHRE), define PCOS as presence of two out of the following three criteria: oligoovulation and/or anovulation, hyperandrogenism (clinical and/or biochemical), and ultrasound findings of polycystic ovaries [presence of ≥12 follicles in each ovary measuring 2–9 mm in diameter, and/or increased ovarian volume (>10 mL)] with the exclusion of other etiologies (Rotterdam ESHRE/ASRM Sponsored PCOS Consensus Workshop Group, 2004).[3]

A taskforce appointed by the Androgen Excess and PCOS (AE-PCOS) society in 2006, and published its criteria in 2009 emphasizing that in the society's opinion, PCOS should be considered as a disorder of androgen excess, as defined by the following: clinical and/or biochemical evidence of hyperandrogenism, evidence of ovarian dysfunction (oligoovulation and/or polycystic ovaries), exclusion of related disorders.[4,5]

The etiology of polycystic ovary syndrome remains unclear. Majority of investigators believe that PCOS is primarily an ovarian disorder,[6] while others believe it results from hypothalamic disturbance, hyperinsulinemia, a primary adrenal disorder, or a combination of these factors.[6,7]

MANAGEMENT

Treatment of PCOS includes a symptom-oriented approach to the presenting problem and a preventive strategy for the associated long-term morbidity. Weight reduction in obese patients improves symptoms and endocrine profile. Combined oral contraceptive pills are used for menstrual irregularities, while hyperandrogenic skin symptoms can be treated with oral contraceptive pills or with antiandrogenic therapy. Anovulatory infertility can be treated by insulin sensitizing measures (like lifestyle modification and metformin), clomiphene citrate (CC), and gonadotropins. Although most symptoms are managed medically, surgical intervention in the form of diathermic laparoscopic ovarian drilling (LOD) and laser plays a significant role in managing PCOS.

Clomiphene citrate is still the first-line medication for the induction of ovulation in PCOS women. Treatment with CC indicates a pregnancy rate of 36% and a miscarriage rate of 20%.[2] Resistance to CC is a challenging problem occurring in up to 40% of PCOS patients.[2,8,9] CC is commonly defined as failure to ovulate with a maximal dose of clomiphene citrate (150 mg/day for 5 days) and requires change of treatment mode.[2,10]

Gonadotropin therapy has classically been the next step for clomiphene citrate-resistant patients; treatment is associated with risk of ovarian hyper stimulation syndrome (OHSS), multiple gestation and recurrent abortions.[11,12]

Surgical management of PCOS includes bilateral ovarian wedge resection (BOWR, which was done in the past), transvaginal hydrolaparoscopy (THL), laparoscopic ovarian drilling (diathermy, laser).

Laparoscopic ovarian drilling is currently accepted as a successful second-line treatment for ovulation induction in clomiphene citrate-resistant women with PCOS[13] that can avoid or reduce the need for gonadotropins.

Ovarian drilling, or 'ovarian electrocautery', is the creation of multiple openings through the ovarian capsule using laparoscopy for surgical access. This can be accomplished electrosurgically using a pointed monopolar or bipolar electrode, or with laser energy (CO_2, argon, Nd: YAG, KTP).

Surgical treatment of polycystic ovaries to restore regular menstruation was described by Stein and Leventhal by in 1935. They did wedge resection of the ovaries in women with amenorrhea. Regular menstruation and spontaneous conception was achieved in them.[14,15]

This was called as bilateral ovarian wedge resection. This was not very popular because after a period of time, it was confirmed by Adashi et al (1981)[16] that women who underwent bilateral wedge resection had peritubal adhesions which in-turn caused infertility. With the advent of endoscopic surgeries different laparoscopic techniques were developed to induce ovulation in women with polycystic ovaries resistant to clomiphene citrate therapy. In 1984, Gjonnoess reported the laparoscopic ovarian drilling with a conception rate of 80%.[17]

Laparoscopic ovarian drilling should also be considered when the luteinizing hormone (LH), follicular-stimulating hormone (FSH) ratio is altered. Although gonadotropin treatment and laparoscopic ovarian drilling have demonstrated similar reproductive outcomes, Laparoscopic ovarian drilling has some advantages over gonadotropin treatment such as lower cost per pregnancy, improvement in menstrual regularity and better long-term reproductive performance and decreased rate of miscarriage due to PCO.

Criteria to consider an infertile patient for laparoscopic ovarian drilling:
- Diagnosed PCOS by Rotterdam criterion.
- Elevated androsternidione levels.
- Elevated Anti-Müllerian hormone (AMH)
- Ovarian volume—Calculated by the formula 0.523 × length × width × thickness of each ovary >10 cc
- LH: FSH >2.

Both gonadotropins and LOD have been considered equally effective as second-line management for CC resistant PCOS. The surgery may also be recommended for patients who need laparoscopic assessment of their pelvis, women who persistently hypersecrete LH, or who live too far away from the hospital for the intensive monitoring required during gonadotropin therapy. Extensive ovarian diathermy is not indicated to prevent hyper-responsiveness to exogenous gonadotropins.[18] Women with LH level >10 IU/L, normal BMI, and shorter duration of infertility have higher chances of achieving spontaneous ovulation post LOD.[19-21]

When Not to Perform LOD?

Laparoscopic ovarian drilling (LOD) is a surgical intervention and involves calculated irrevocable loss of ovarian reserve. Hence, the selection of patients should be done very meticulously.

LOD should not be considered for:
- Unmarried girls
- Reproductive age group patients who have completed family (noninfertility indications)
- Marked obesity (BMI>35 kg/m^2)
- Marked hyperandrogenism (testosterone >-4.5 nmol/L)
- Long duration of infertility (>3 years) seems resistant to LOD[20-23]

TECHNIQUES OF LAPAROSCOPIC OVARIAN SURGERY

Technique of Laparoscopic Ovarian Drilling

Patients are taken up in the immediate postmenstrual phase. All the cases are done under GA with Trendelenburg position. A diagnostic hysteroscopy is always done prior to laparoscopy. Pneumoperitoneum is created with veress needle, 10 mm umbilical port and two 5 mm lateral ports in the lower abdomen just above the anterosuperior iliac spine lateral to inferior epigastric vessels. Unilateral ports can also be put depending upon the surgeons comforts.

Inspection of the pelvis is done to rule out other factors of infertility or any pathology and ovaries are inspected for features of polycystic ovary. Chromopertubation is always done prior to performing a drilling. In case of blocked tubes, the decision for drilling should be reconsidered. The equipment for monopolar diathermy consists of electrosurgical unit and pointed needle electrode **(Fig. 17.1)**. This electrosurgical probe has a distil needle with conical tip measuring 8 mm in length and 2 mm in diameter and projecting from insulated solid cone, that prevents deep penetration and thermal damage of ovarian surface **(Fig. 17.2)**.

The ovary is lifted by suction cannula away from bowel and placed over the cervicouterine junction which forms a platform and easy to carry out the punctures. The monopolar needle is kept at right angles to the ovary. Antimesentric border of the ovary is chosen for drilling in view of less vascularity. Care should be taken to avoid injury to hilum, ovarian ligament and fallopian tube. The utero-ovarian ligament should not be grasped for fixation of the ovary

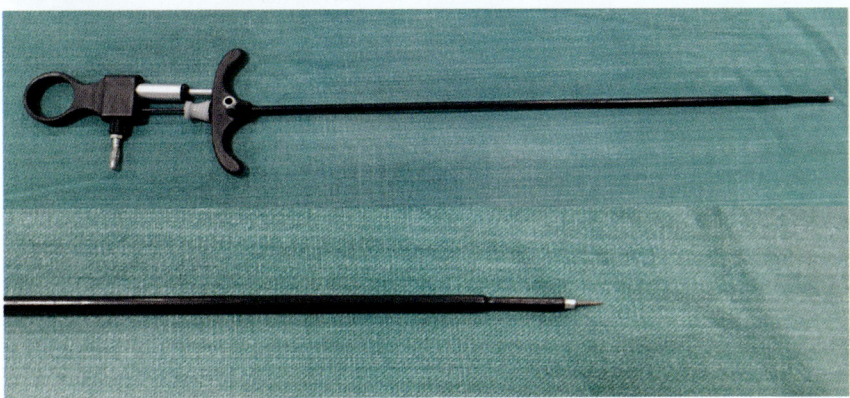

Fig. 17.1 Ovarian diathermy needle probe

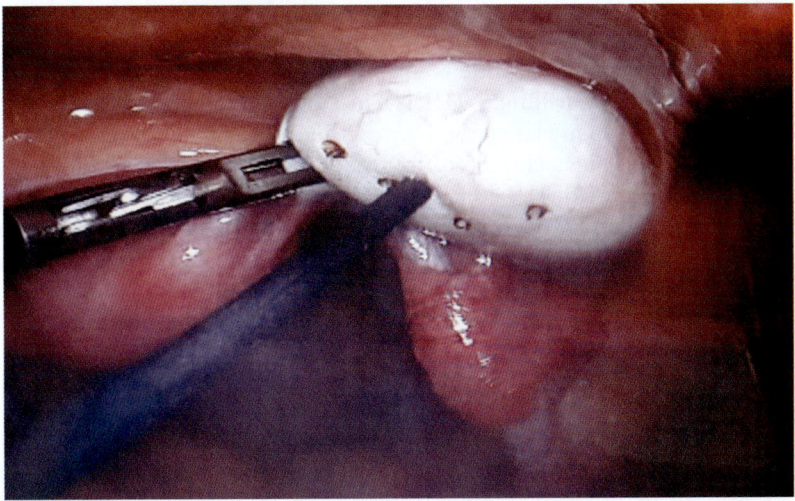

Fig. 17.2 Needle penetration. The full length of the needle is pushed into the ovarian capsule after stabilizing the ovary

in any case. Overly aggressive manipulation should avoid, since it can cause lacerations in the capsule, follicles and the utero-ovarian ligament, which can result in bleeding.

Power is set at 40 watts current in cutting mode, and full length of needle is inserted on each surface of the ovary at the depth of 4–6 mm on both the ovaries. Current is activated for 4 sec and 4 punctures done in each ovary. Take precaution not to injure the ovary by heat of prolonged coagulation current inside the ovarian tissue. A thorough suction irrigation is done with saline or ringer's lactate after the drilling. In our experience, we have noted that leaving 200 mL of Ringer's lactate in the pelvis avoids significant postoperative adhesions.

Ovaries of larger volume might need more punctures for optimum effects. We have conducted a study from 2003 to 2010, where in 829 diagnostic laparoscopies were carried out, of which 87 patients undergoing drilling were included in the study.

Laparoscopic ovarian drilling was carried out by doing multiple punctures using cutting current of 30–40 watts in 64 patients, while in 23 patients only 3–6 punctures were done. Better conception rates were observed over a period of two years in the group with multiple punctures. Laparoscopic ovarian drilling with short burst cutting current and multiple punctures has good outcome in terms of regularization of menstrual cycles, ovulation and conception.[24]

Amer et al. found that 4 punctures per ovary at 30 W for five seconds (150 J) per puncture, (600 J) energy per ovary to be the optimum number required to achieve the best results.[25]

Transvaginal Hydrolaparoscopy (THL)

A veress needle is used to enter the peritoneal cavity through the pouch of Douglas; approximately 300 mL of normal saline solution is instilled into the peritoneal cavity. Thereafter a special introducer with a 5-French caliber operative channel is inserted into the distended pouch of Douglas, which permits the introduction of a 2.9 mm scope with a 30-degree lens. After appropriate examination of the pelvic organs, a special bipolar electrode is introduced through the operating channel to carry out the ovarian drilling.[26] THL is a less traumatic and suitable outpatient procedure than diagnostic laparoscopy.[26,27] The risks of a general anesthetic are avoided, and there is less chance of trauma to major vessels. Fernandez et al. reported the usefulness of THL for the treatment of PCOS by ovarian drilling.[28,29] They performed ovarian drilling using bipolar electrosurgery by THL in 80 Clomiphene citrate resistant anovulatory women with PCOS. During a mean follow-up of 18 months, 73 (91%) patients recovered regular ovulatory cycles. The cumulative pregnancy rate was 60% for spontaneous and stimulated cycles, with 40% imputed to drilling alone.[29]

Laser Ovarian Surgery

Four lasers, including CO_2, Argon, Nd:YAG, KTP have been used to perform ovarian drilling in PCOS women. Electrosurgery is more effective than laser in achieving in ovulation and pregnancy, laser associated with higher risk of adhesion formation because of increased surface injury and expensive than electrosurgery. Effect of diathermy is long lasting and set-up is easier so electosurgery is preferred over laser for LOD.

Mechanism of Action: Laparoscopic Ovarian Drilling

The mechanism of action for the restoration of cyclical ovulation is not still understood. Different reasons are postulated by different surgeons:
1. *Stein and Leventhal (1935):* Postulated the bilateral ovarian-wedge resection decreased the mechanical crowding of the cortex by cysts, which again enabled the progress of normal gracifan follicle to the surface of the ovary.[14,15]
2. *Gjonnaess (1984):* Postulated that ovulation was either by ovarian stromal destruction or by extensive capsular damage with discharge of the contents of the follicle or by local capsular cautery of one specific but unidentified follicle.[17]

Flow chart 17.1 Mechanism of correction of hormonal milieu

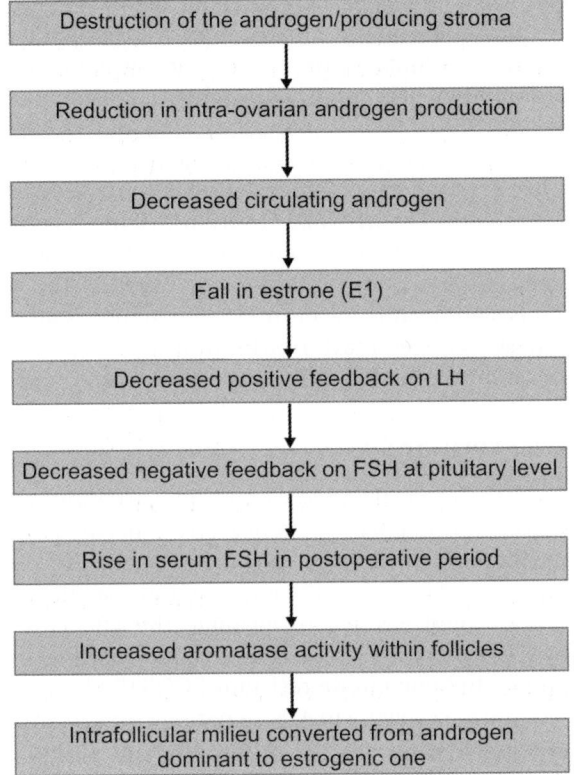

3. *Daniell and Miller (1989):* Suggested that physically opening the subcapsular cyst by laser, the follicular fluid which contains androgen is eliminated from the ovarian environment, in term lowering the androgen content of the ovaries thus triggering ovulation.[30]

Its beneficial effect is apparently due to destruction of the androgen producing stroma which leads to reduction in intra-ovarian androgen production and decreased circulating androgen,[31] it leads to fall in estrone (E1) which results in decreased positive feedback on LH and decreased negative feedback on FSH at pituitary level resulting rise in serum FSH in postoperative period leads to increased aromatase activity within follicles, so intrafollicular milieu converted from androgen dominant to estrogenic one. This leads to monofollicular maturation and ovulation **(Flow chart 17.1)**.

After laparoscopic ovarian drilling, the ovarian volume increases transiently, followed by a reduction. The serum LH concentration increases immediately after the procedure, and then decreases.[31,32] The LH pulse amplitudes are markedly reduced but the LH pulse frequencies do not change. Pituitary responsiveness to gonadotrophin-releasing hormone (GnRH) stimulation also decreases concomitantly with a decline in serum testosterone concentration, suggesting that the procedure has an indirect modulating effect on the pituitary-ovarian axis.[31] The FSH concentration generally increases rapidly, and thereafter demonstrates a cyclical rise in keeping with restoration of ovulation. Normal inhibin pulsatility is restored, in association with the onset of regular ovulatory cycles, reflecting the resumption of normal intra-ovarian paracrine signaling.[33] These endocrine changes which occur rapidly,[31] are sustained for several years[32] and result in recruitment of new cohort of follicles and restoration of ovulation in most of the subjects.

Ovary produces a number of growth factors such as insulin-like growth factor-1 (IGF-1), in response to tissue injury which sensitize the ovary to circulating FSH, leads to follicular growth. Laparoscopic ovarian drilling has been reported to decrease serum concentrations of vascular endothelial growth factor (VEGF) which are typically increased in patients with PCOS.[34] The ovarian stromal blood flow, which is significantly lower in PCOS patients, is also increased after the procedure. These changes may contribute to a decreased risk of ovarian hyperstimulation syndrome (OHSS) following laparoscopic ovarian drilling.

Ovulation and Pregnancy

Ovulation occurs after 2–4 weeks of LOD and menstruation occurs within 4–6 weeks in the responders. Regular ovulatory cycles occur in 70–80% of cases. Gjonaess with his multi-electrocauterization is PCOD achieved an ovulation rate 92 % and pregnancy rate of 69%. And the abortion rate was 15%.[17]

Farhi et al.[35] performed a study to evaluate the effect of ovarian electro cauterization and ovarian response to gonadotrophin stimulation and pregnancy rate in clomiphene citrate resistant PCOS. Reduced basal serum LH concentration and normal cyclicity in 41% of patients was recorded. When these patients were stimulated with gonadotrophin after the drilling, they required significantly less amount of gonadotrophin ampules and also higher ovulation and pregnancy rates. This shows increase in ovarian sensitivity to gonadotrophin after laparoscopic ovarian drilling.

Miscarriage

Increased LH levels are known to cause early pregnancy loss in women with PCOS. Ovarian drilling appears to decrease the spontaneous abortion rate associated with PCOS.[36,37] In a long-term follow-up study, Amer et al. reported a reduction in the miscarriage rate from 54% to 17% after laparoscopic ovarian drilling.[36] In a prospective randomized trial, the miscarriage rate following laparoscopic ovarian drilling was 21% less than that of control women with PCOS.[37]

Long-term Effects of LOD

Economic analyses of two RCTs suggest that LOD treatment of women with CC-resistant PCOS resulted in reduced direct and indirect costs.[38,39] The beneficial clinical and endocrinological effects and improvement in menstrual and reproductive performance of patients after LOD last for many years in significant number of PCOS women.[32,36]

Gjonnaess (1998) reported that over 50% of those who had the procedure continued to ovulate more than 10 years later.[40]

LOD and In Vitro Fertilization (IVF)

Gonadotropin treatment following laparoscopic ovarian drilling is associated with a lower duration of stimulation, lower total dose of gonadotropins and higher pregnancy rates. In women undergoing IVF, laparoscopic ovarian drilling improves reproductive outcome.[41] There is more orderly growth of follicles, serum estradiol concentrations are lower, and the rate of cycle cancellation is reduced, as is the incidence of ovarian hyperstimulation.[18,41-43] Laparoscopic ovarian drilling may therefore be useful in patients who have previously developed ovarian hyperstimulation syndrome (OHSS). Pretreatment with laparoscopic ovarian drilling was noted not to decrease the miscarriage rate after IVF.[18] A systematic review of published studies also failed to reveal a difference in the miscarriage rates between women undergoing laparoscopic ovarian drilling and those taking gonadotrophins.[44]

Repeat Laparoscopic Ovarian Drilling

Amer et al. assessed the effectiveness of a second laparoscopic ovarian drilling in 20 women with PCOS and infertility.[45] All 20 had drilling procedures 1-6 years before. About 12 of these responded positively to the first procedure, but their anovulatory status recurred; in the remaining eight women, the procedure did not yield any response. Following the second drilling procedure, 12 out of 20 (60%) started to ovulate and 10 out of 19 (53%) became pregnant. It is interesting to note that among the 12 women who had responded to the first procedure, 10 (83%) became ovulatory and eight became (67%) pregnant. However, of the eight who did not respond to the initial drilling, only two (25%) ovulated and were successful at achieving a pregnancy. Furthermore, statistically significant hormonal changes after repeat drilling, including reduction in serum LH, testosterone, and free androgen index, were only observed in the previous-responder group. The authors concluded that repeat laparoscopic ovarian drilling is highly effective in women who previously responded to the first procedure.

SAFETY AND COMPLICATIONS

Immediate Complications

Immediate complications are rare. Complications associated with ovarian drilling may be associated with anesthesia, establishment of the surgical access, and/or with the drilling procedure itself, which includes the use of energy, electrical or laser. Related to the drilling itself, the patient may experience bleeding from the drilling sites, laceration of the utero-ovarian ligament, which is frequently grasped to immobilize the ovary.

Late Complications

The use of excessive amounts of energy will destroy large numbers of follicles resulting in decreased ovarian reserve. The use of energy with an electrode introduced too deeply into the ovary may cause desiccation of the hilar vessels resulting in premature ovarian failure due to necrosis of the ovary.

Another important complication is the occurrence of postoperative adhesions. Adhesion formation seems to be more frequent with laser treatment than with electrocoagulation[46] and use of adhesion barriers does not reduce its incidence. Abdominal lavage and use of insulated needle electrocautery may help to reduce its occurrence.[46,47] Undoubtedly, the procedure must be carried out using a meticulous, atraumatic technique with proper respect to tissues.

ADVANTAGES

- Intensive monitoring of follicular development is not required after LOD, so the treatment is best suited to those for whom frequent ultrasound monitoring is impractical.
- Laparoscopic ovarian surgery can achieve unifollicular ovulation with very low risk of OHSS or multiple pregnancies.
- Laparoscopic ovarian surgery is an effective alternative to gonadotropin therapy for CC-resistant anovulatory PCOS with fewer side effects.
- Laparoscopic ovarian surgery is a single treatment using existing equipment.
- The risks of surgery are minimal and include the risks of laparoscopy, adhesion formation, and destruction of normal ovarian tissue.

In a recent Cochrane review, no evidence of a difference in the livebirth or miscarriage rates in women with clomiphene citrate-resistant PCOS undergoing LOD compared with gonadotropin treatment was reported.[48] Despite the fact that reduction in OHSS and multiple pregnancy rates in women undergoing LOD make this option attractive, unilateral LOD was found to be equally efficacious as bilateral drilling in inducing ovulation and achieving pregnancy in clomiphene citrate-resistant PCOS women, which makes it a more suitable option because of the reduced potential for adhesion formation.[49,50]

CONCLUSION

Laparoscopic ovarian drilling is a safe and cost-effective procedure in treating patients with clomiphene citrate resistant PCOS. We can be assured of a single treatment with unifollicular ovulation. The complications of clomiphene citrate and gonadotropin therapy like multiple pregnancy and ovarian hyperstimulation can be avoided. It is less costly and avoids intense, complex and inconvenient monitoring. It also increases the sensitivity to gonadotropin. Spontaneous correction of hormone levels prevents miscarriages. Main disadvantage of LOD is need for general anesthesia, adhesion formation and risk of ovarian failure. Since the procedure is easy and safe, it can be used as the first line of treatment in clomiphene resistant PCOS.

KEY POINTS

- LOD is a successful second-line treatment for ovulation induction in CC-resistant women with PCOS, can avoid or reduce the need for gonadotropins.
- Destruction of the androgen-producing stroma is its beneficial effect, which leads to reduction in intraovarian androgen production and decreased circulating androgen.
- LOD leads to increase in ovarian volume transiently, followed by a reduction.
- Ovulation occurs after 2-4 weeks of LOD and menstruation occurs within 4-6 weeks in the responders.
- Ovarian drilling appears to improves reproductive outcome, decrease the spontaneous abortion rate associated with PCOS
- Repeating LOD is highly effective in women who previously responded to the first procedure.
- The procedure must be carried out using a meticulous, atraumatic technique with proper respect to tissues.
- LOD is advantageous as it is a single treatment which will be followed by spontaneous unifollicular ovulation.

REFERENCES

1. Yavasoglu I, Kucuk M, Coskun A, et al. Polycystic ovary syndrome and prolactinoma association. Intern Med. 2009;48,611-3.
2. Homburg R. Polycystic ovary syndrome. Best Pract Res Clin Obstet Gynaecol. 2008;22, 261-74.
3. Rotterdam ESHRE/ASRM-Sponsored PCOS Consensus Workshop Group 2004 Revised 2003 consensus on diagnostic criteria and long-term health risks related to polycystic ovary syndrome. Fertility and Sterility. 2004;81:19-25.
4. Azziz R, Carmina E, Dewailly D, et al. Positions statement: criteria for defining polycystic ovary syndrome as a predominantly hyperandrogenic syndrome: an androgen excess society guideline. J Clin Endocrinol Metab. 2006;91(11):4237-45.
5. Azziz R, Carmina E, Dewailly D, et al. The androgen excess and PCOS society criteria for the polycystic ovary syndrome: the complete task force report. Fertil Sterile. 2009; 91(2):456-88.
6. Dunaif A. Insulin resistance and the polycystic ovary syndrome: mechanisms and implications for pathogenesis. Endocr Rev. 1997;18:774-800.
7. Gilling-Smith C, Willis DS, Beard RW, Franks S. Hypersecretion of androstenedione by isolated thecal cells from polycystic ovaries. J Clin Endocrinol Metab. 1994;79:1158-65.
8. Pritts EA. Treatment of the infertile patient with polycystic ovarian syndrome. Obstet Gynecol Survey. 2002;57:587-97.
9. Wolf LJ. Ovulation induction. Clin Obstet Gynecol. 2000;43:902-15.
10. Van Wely M, Bayram N, van der Veen F, et al. Predictors for treatment failure after laparoscopic electrocautery of the ovaries in women with clomiphene-citrate resistant polycystic ovary syndrome. Hum Reprod. 2005;20:900-5.

11. Beck JI. Boothroyd C, Proctor M, et al. Oral antioestrogens and medical adjuncts for subfertility associated with anovulation. Cochrane Database Syst Rev. 2005; 25,CD002249.
12. Farquhar C, Farquhar CM, Williamson K, et al. A randomized controlled trial of laparoscopic ovarian diathermy versus gonadotrophin therapy for women with clomiphene citrate-resistant polycystic ovary syndrome. Fertil Steril. 2002;78:404-11.
13. Sastre ME, Prat MO, Checa MA, et al. Current trends in the treatment of polycystic ovary syndrome with desire for children. Ther Clin Risk Manage. 2009;5:353-60.
14. Stein FI, Laventhol ML. Amenorrhoea associated with bilateral polycystic ovaries. American Journal of Obstetrics and Gynaeocology. 1935;29:181-91.
15. Stein FI, Duration of Fertility following ovarian wedge resection-stein-Leventhol syndrome. Western Journal of surgery obstetrics &Gynecology 1964,78:237.
16. Adashi EY, Rock JA, Guzick D, et al. Fertility following bilateral ovarian wedge resection: a critical analysis of 90 consecutive cases of the polycystic ovary syndrome. Fertility and sterility. 1981;36:320-25.
17. Gjonnaess H. Polycystic ovarian syndrome treated by ovarian electrocautery through the laparoscope. Fertility and Sterility 1984;49,956-60.
18. Rimington MR, Walker SM, Shaw RW. The use of laparoscopic ovarian electrocautery in preventing cancellation of in-vitro fertilization treatment cycles due to risk of ovarian hyperstimulation syndrome in women with polycystic ovaries. Hum Reprod. 1997;12:1443-7.
19. Gjonnaess H. Ovarian electrocautery in the treatment of women with polycystic ovary syndrome (PCOS): Factors affecting the results. Acta Obstetricia et Gynecologica Scandinavica. 1994;73:407-12.
20. Abdel GA, Khatim MS, Alnaser HM, Mowafi RS, Shaw RW. Ovarian electrocautery: responders versus non-responders. Gynecol Endocrinol. 1993;7:43-8.
21. Li TC, Saravelos H, Chow MS, Chisabingo R, Cooke ID. Factors affecting the outcome of laparoscopic ovarian drilling for polycystic ovarian syndrome in women with anovulatory infertility. Br J Obstet Gynaecol. 1998;105:338-44.
22. Duleba A, Banaszewska B, Spaczynski RZ, Pawelczyk L. Success of laparoscopic ovarian wedge resection is related to obesity, lipid profile and insulin levels. Fertility and Sterility. 2003;79:1008-14.
23. Stegmann BJ, Craig RH, Bay RC, et al. Characteristics predictive of response to ovarian diathermy in women with polycystic ovarian syndrome. American Journal of Obstetrics and Gynecology. 2003;79:1008-14.
24. Bhat V, Joshi P, Bhat BS, Manoj A, 2012 Outcome of laparoscopic ovarian drilling(LOD) with multiple versus fewer punctures.Indian Obstetrics and Gynecology Journal for Basic and Clinical Research 2013;3(1):32-34.
25. Amer S, Li T, Cooke ID. A prospective dose-finding study of the amount of thermal energy required for laparoscopic ovarian diathermy. Human Reproduction. 2003;18:1693-8.
26. Shibahara H, Fujiwara H, Hirano Y, Suzuki T, Obara H, Takamizawa S, et al. Usefulness of transvaginal hydrolaparoscopy in investigating infertile women with *Chlamydia trachomatis* infection. Hum Reprod. 2001;16:1690-3.
27. Fujiwara H, Shibahara H, Hirano Y, Suzuki T, Takamizawa S, Sato I. Usefulness and prognostic value of transvaginal hydrolaparoscopy in infertile women. Fertil Steril 2003;79:186-9.
28. Fernandez H, Alby JD, Gervaise A, et al. 2001 Operative transvaginal hydrolaparoscopy for treatment of polycystic ovary syndrome: a new minimally invasive surgery. Fertility and Sterility. 2001;75:607-11.
29. Fernandez H, Watrelot A, Alby JD, Kadoch J, Gervaise A, de Tayrac R, et al. Fertility after ovarian drilling by transvaginal fertiliscopy for treatment of polycystic ovary syndrome. J Am Assoc Gynecol Laparoscopy. 2004;11:374-8.

30. Daniell JF, Miller W. Polycystic ovaries treated by laparoscopic laser vaporization. Fertility and Sterility. 1989;51:232-6.
31. Rossmanith WG, Keckstein J, Spatzier K, Lauritzen C 1991 The impact of ovarian surgery on the gonadotrophin secretion in women with polycystic ovarian disease. Clinical Endocrinology (Oxford). 1991;34:23-30.
32. Amer SA, Gopalan V, Li TC, et al. Long-term follow-up of patients with polycystic ovarian syndrome after laparoscopic ovarian drilling: endocrine and ultrasonographic outcomes. Human Reproduction. 2002b;17:2851-57.
33. Lockwood GM, Muttukrishna S, Groome NP, et al. Midfollicular phase pulses of inhibin B are absent in polycystic ovarian syndrome and are initiated by successful laparoscopic ovarian diathermy: A possible mechanism regulating emergence of the dominant follicle. Journal of Clinical Endocrinology and Metabolism. 1998;83:1730-5.
34. Amin AF, Abd El-Aal D-EM, Darwish AM, Meki A-RMA. Evaluation of the impact of laparoscopic ovarian drilling on Doppler indices of ovarian stromal blood flow, serum vascular endothelial growth factor, and insulin-like growth factor-1 in women with polycystic ovary syndrome. Fertility and Sterility. 2003;79:938-41.
35. Farhi J, Soule S, Jacobs HS. Effect of laparoscopic ovarian electrocautery on ovarian response and outcome of treatment with gonadotropins in CC-resistant patients with polycystic syndrome. Fertility and Sterility. 1995;64:930-3.
36. Amer SA, Gopalan V, Li TC, et al. Long-term follow-up of patients with polycystic ovarian syndrome after laparoscopic ovarian drilling: clinical outcome. Human Reproduction. 2002a;17:2035-42.
37. Abdel Gadir A, Mowafi R, Alnaser H, et al. Ovarian electrocautery versus human menopausal gonadotrophins and pure follicle stimulating hormone therapy in the treatment of patients with polycystic ovarian disease. Clinical Endocrinology. 1990;33:585-92.
38. Farquhar CM, Williamson K, Brown PM, Garland J. An economic evaluation of laparoscopic ovarian diathermy versus gonadotrophin therapy for women with clomiphene citrate resistant polycystic ovary syndrome. Hum Reprod. 2004;19:1110-5.
39. Van Wely M, Bayram N, van der Veen F, Bossuyt PM. An economic comparison of a laparoscopic electrocautery strategy and ovulation induction with recombinant FSH in women with clomiphene citrate-resistant polycystic ovary syndrome. Hum Reprod. 2004;19:1741-5.
40. Gjonnaess H. Late endocrine effects of ovarian electrocautery in women with polycystic ovary syndrome. Fertility and Sterility. 1998;69:697-70.
41. Tozer AJ, Shawaf T, Zosmer A, et al. Does laparoscopic ovarian diathermy affect the outcome of IVF–embryo transfer in women with polycystic ovarian syndrome? A retrospective comparative study. Human Reproduction. 2001;16:91-5.
42. Farhi J, Soule S, Jacobs HS. Effect of laparoscopic ovarian electrocautery on ovarian response and outcome of treatment with gonadotropins in CC-resistant patients with polycystic syndrome. Fertility and Sterility. 1995;64:930-3.
43. Colacurci N, Zullo F, De Franciscis P, et al. In vitro fertilization following laparoscopic ovarian diathermy in patients with polycystic ovarian syndrome. Acta Obstetricia et Gynecologica Scandinavica. 1997;76:555-8.
44. Farquhar CM, Vandekerckhove P, Lilford R. Laparoscopic 'drilling' by diathermy or laser for ovulation induction in anovulatory polycystic ovary syndrome. The Cochrane Library, Issue 2, 2002a.
45. Amer SA, Li TC, Cooke ID. Repeated laparoscopic ovarian diathermy is effective in women with anovulatory infertility due to polycystic ovary syndrome. Fertility and Sterility. 2003;79:1211-5.

46. Naether OG, Fischer R, Weise HC, et al. Laparoscopic electrocoagulation of the ovarian surface in infertile patients with polycystic ovarian disease. Fertility and Sterility. 1993;60:88-94.
47. Felemban A, Tan SL, Tulandi T. Laparoscopic treatment of polycystic ovaries with insulated needle cautery: a reappraisal. Fertility and Sterility. 2000;73:266-9.
48. Farquhar C, Lilford, RJ, Marjoribanks J, et al. Laparoscopic 'drilling' by diathermy or laser for ovulation induction in anovulatory polycystic ovary syndrome. Cochrane Database Syst Rev. 2007;3:CD001122.
49. Roy KK, Baruah J, Moda N, et al. Evaluation of unilateral versus bilateral ovarian drilling in clomiphene citrate resistant cases of polycystic ovarian syndrome. Arch Gynecol Obstet. 2009;280:573-8.
50. Al-Mizyen E, Grudzinskas JG, Unilateral laparoscopic ovarian diathermy in infertile women with clomiphene citrate resistant polycystic ovary syndrome. Fertil Steril. 2007;88:1678-80.

CHAPTER 18

Hirsutism

Pooja Sharma Dimri, Chandana A

INTRODUCTION

Hirsutism is the excessive male pattern growth of facial or body hair affecting around 5–10%[1] of reproductive age women. Hirsutism can be seen as coarse, dark hair that may appear on the face, chest, abdomen, back, upper arms or upper legs. The etiology is androgen excess which reflects a state of hormonal imbalance. Polycystic ovary syndrome (PCOS), wherein the ovaries produce excess of androgens is the most common cause of hirsutism. Hirsutism negatively influences the psychological well-being, especially in the young females. Hence medical attention is important as delaying treatment makes the treatment more difficult and may have long-term health consequences.

In this chapter we shall review the pathophysiology, causes and treatment of hirsutism.

PATHOPHYSIOLOGY

Hair, especially on the scalp and face is important for social and sexual communication. Structurally, there are three types of hair:[2]
1. *Lanugo:* Soft hair, which cover the skin of the fetus and disappears within the first months of postpartum life.
2. *Vellus hair:* Soft but larger than lanugo hair and nonpigmented.
3. *Terminal hair:* Longer, pigmented and coarser in texture.

    Eyebrows, eyelashes, scalp hair, pubic, axillary hair in both sexes and much of the body and facial hair in men are composed of terminal hairs.[3]

    The hair cycle consists of rhythmic repetitive growth, regression and tissue remodeling events. The hair follicles have the ability to regenerate. Their number does not change but their size and type of hair changes with respect to several factors like androgens.

    Hair follicles pass through three major growth phases:
1. *Anagen (a stage of rapid growth):* It is about four months for facial hair. This is the reason it takes about six months to detect the effects of hormonal treatment for facial hirsutism. The duration of the anagen phase governs the hair cycle

length in different body regions. Scalp follicles have the longest anagen phase, and most normal scalp follicles are in the anagen phase[4].
- *Telogen (a stage of relative quiescence):* Lasts three to four months. Hair is released from the hair follicle and shed at the end of telogen and the next cycle is initiated.
- *Catagen (The involutional phase):* Lasts two to three weeks.

Hair growth disorders are due to the changes in the hair follicle cycle. Prolongation of the hair growth phase (anagen) is observed when vellus hairs evolve into terminal hairs (e.g. in hirsutism), whereas shortening of the anagen phase leads to hair loss.

Androgens and Hair Growth

Androgens are important for the normal growth of sexual hair. However, any excess or deficient androgen does lead to pathological hair growth. Androgens act differently in both the sexes and various parts of the body. The vellus hair is small, straight and fair in both the sexes before puberty. At the onset of puberty, due to increase in androgen levels, the vellus hair in pubic and axillary hair develop into terminal hair which become larger, curlier and darker.[5] The development of facial hair, male pattern pubic hair and trunk hair in men is due to androgen stimulation. In other body areas, such as the forehead and the cheeks, androgens increase the size of the sebaceous glands, but the hair in these areas remains vellus **(Box 18.1)**.

Synthesis of Androgens in Females[6]

- Testosterone—50% from peripheral conversion of other steroids, 25% each from ovaries and adrenal glands.
- Dihydrotestosterone (DHT) from conversion of testosterone by 5α-reductase in the hair follicle.
- Androstenedione from ovaries and adrenals.
- Dehydroepitestosterone (DHEA) from adrenals.

The major androgens in the serum of normal cycling women are DHEAS, dehydroepiandrosterone, androstenedione, testosterone and DHT in descending order of serum concentrations.[7]

Hirsutism is the result of interaction between circulating androgen concentrations, local factors and the variability in end organ sensitivity of the hair follicle to androgens.[8] Hence all women do not respond the same to circulating androgen levels and have variable response. Serum free or

BOX 18.1 Androgen-sensitive sites of hair growth

More common	Less common
• Upper lip • Beard area • Breasts • Lower abdomen • Inner thighs • Lower back	Chest and sternum Upper abdomen Upper back

bioavailable testosterone concentrations correlate positively with hirsutism scores, while sex hormone-binding globulin (SHBG) concentrations correlate negatively with hirsutism scores.[9,10] When androgen production in increased, SHBG is suppressed, hence there is an increase in free testosterone levels, which have an increased metabolism, thereby reducing the serum concentrations of testosterone.

CAUSES OF HIRSUTISM

- Increased androgen production
    - PCOS
    - *Adrenal disorders:* Cushing's syndrome and congenital adrenal hyperplasia
    - Androgen producing ovarian and adrenal tumors
    - XY females
- Increased free androgens
    - Insulin resistance
    - Obesity
    - PCOS
- Increased local activity of 5α reductase
- Medications
    - Androgen therapy—Testosterone injections, creams, patches
    - Danazol
    - Sodium valproate, phenytoin
    - Anabolic steroids
    - Cyclosporine
    - Progestins
    - Diazoxide
    - Minoxidil
    - Glucocorticoids.

EVALUATION AND DIAGNOSIS

History and Physical Examination

- Age of onset (puberty, middle age, menopause)
- Rate of onset of symptoms (gradual or sudden).
- Loss of breast tissue or loss of normal female body contour, clitoromegaly, increased libido, increased muscle mass as in shoulder girdle, malodorous perspiration, etc.
- Any signs or symptoms of virilization (acne, deepening of voice, infrequent menstruation)
- History of weight gain
- History of diabetes
- Drug history
- Functional causes are peripubertal and slow in onset with a family history of hyperandrogenism mostly and signs of virilization or defeminization are rare.
- Androgen secreting tumors are sudden and rapid in onset with severe virilization and defeminization.

- Oligo or amenorrhea, infertility point towards ovarian dysfunction associated with PCOS, nonclassic congenital adrenal hyperplasia (NCCAH) or even androgen-secreting tumors. Since PCOS is frequently associated with insulin resistance, abdominal obesity or acanthosis nigricans are frequent physical findings.
- Pelvic examination to exclude pelvic masses such as in cases of androgen producing ovarian tumors.
- Abdominal palpation to rule out ovarian mass
- Grading
  - Modified Ferriman-Gallwey scoring system (mFG) is currently considered the 'gold' standard for the clinical evaluation of hirsutism.[11]
  - It scores 9 of the 11 body areas (upper lip, chin, chest, upper and lower back, upper and lower abdomen, arm, forearm, thigh and lower leg) originally proposed by Ferriman and Gallwey (1961). But excludes the lower legs and forearms cause these areas are sensitive to very low androgen concentrations even in healthy women.
  - It is scored as zero when no terminal hair growth is seen. If minimally visible—a score of 1, if hair growth is more than minimal—a score of 2, a score of 3 is that of a not very hairy male while a score of 4 is that typically observed in well-virilized healthy adult males.
  - Total scores range from 0–36. Hirsutism has been usually graded as mild up to a score of 15, moderate from 16–25, and severe above 25. However, because terminal body hair growth has substantial racial and ethnic variability, the cut-off value of the mFG score should be ideally established for the population to which it is applied.[2]
  - To improve the quality of assessment, patients should be advised to avoid use of electrolysis or lasers for at least 3 months, depilation or waxing for 4 weeks, and cautioned not to shave at least 5 days prior to evaluation.[11,12]

Laboratory Evaluation

Measuring serum androgens and other steroid concentrations is essential for establishing the etiology of hirsutism. The magnitude of the increase in serum androgen levels may correlate with the metabolic and cardiovascular associations of functional causes of hyperandrogenism, including PCOS.[13]

- *Testosterone:* Free testosterone levels are much more sensitive than the measurement of total testosterone for the diagnosis of hyperandrogenic disorders. Serum testosterone may be normal or high in case of benign pathology as PCOS and congenital adrenal hyperplasia (CAH) but would be definitely raised (>200 ng/mL) in case of malignant tumor of the adrenal or ovary.[14]
- *Dehydroepiandrosterone sulfate (DHEAS):* Raised DHEAS (>700 µg/dL) indicates an adrenal cause, benign or malignant.[14]
- *17-hydroxy-progesterone:* For suspected congenital adrenal hyperplasia. It is done in early morning between 07.00 and 09.00 hours in the early follicular phase of the menstrual cycle. Levels less than 200 ng/dL exclude the disease. Levels between 300 and 1,000 ng/dL require an ACTH stimulation test. In this cosyntropin (synthetic ACTH), 250 µg, is administered intravenously and

levels of 17-hydroxyprogesterone are measured before and one hour after the injection. Poststimulation values (>1,000 ng/dL) constitute a positive test.[14]
- *Twenty-four-hour urine free cortisol:* It is required if Cushing's syndrome is suspected.
- Luteinizing hormone (LH)/follicle-stimulating hormone (FSH) ratio greater than 3 is indicative of PCOS.[14]
- Prolactin would be raised in hyperprolactinemia due to hypothalamic disease or a pituitary tumor.
- *Serum TSH:* Hypophyseal hypothyroidism can act as a cofactor in hirsutism causing raised thyroid-stimulating hormone (TSH).[14]

Imaging

- Pelvic ultrasonography can be done to detect an ovarian neoplasm or a polycystic ovary.
- Magnetic resonance imaging (MRI) or computed tomography (CT) of the adrenal region is useful for diagnosis.

MANAGEMENT OF HIRSUTISM

The goals of the correct management of hirsutism are to ameliorate the hirsutism and reproductive complaints, to prevent and treat the possible associated metabolic derangements and to treat the underlying cause.

Principles of management to be discussed with affected women at the onset of therapy.[15]
- Treatment will never be curative; therefore chronic treatment will likely be necessary.
- The effects of drugs are not evident before several months of administration.
- Treatment should take into account the characteristics and expectations of the individual patient.
- Treatment must be monitored by an expert.

Lifestyle Modification

Changes in the existing lifestyle, which involves physical exercise, dietary advice, behavioral changes or combined treatment is important for the management of androgen excess and for the cardiovascular protection in women with PCOS.[13]

However lifestyle modifications alone do not cure hirsutism but the rate of attenuation may be slower. Patients with PCOS as the etiology should be counseled for lifestyle modifications after having explained the need for additional approach.[2] Patients should be advised against smoking as it could interfere with the treatment of hirsutism, when oral contraceptive pills (OCPs) are being considered.[16]

Cosmetic Procedures

Hair removal complements medical treatment. In mild or localized cases, cosmetic methods may be sufficient as a single therapy when terminal hair localizes in the most exposed areas such as the face. It is important for the patient to be aware that any treatment for hirsutism will not treat existing hair.

Topical Treatment

Eflornithine hydrochloride 13.9% is a topical preparation for mild facial hirsutism. It inhibits hair growth by irreversibly inhibiting ornithine decarboxylase. It does not remove hair, but rather slows hair growth. It can be used alone or in combination with other therapies.[17] The Endocrine Society guidelines suggest the addition of eflornithine to photoepilation therapy in women who desire a more rapid initial response.[18]

Temporary Methods

Include bleaching, plucking, shaving and waxing. They are safe and change the rate of hair growth. Results are better when used in combination with pharmacological intervention. Local discomfort is the most common disadvantage.

Permanent Methods

Include electrolysis, laser therapy and intensed pulsed light.

Electrolysis destroys the dermal papilla resulting in permanent amelioration of hirsutism in the treated area. If competently performed, it does not cause scarring. Disadvantages are discomfort, postinflammatory erythema, whealing and small crusts. Since follicles are treated one at a time, it is impractical to use electrolysis to treat very large areas of the body.

Laser therapy and intense pulsed light: The available lasers operate in the red or near-infrared wavelengths and depend on selective photothermolysis. The melanin pigment in the follicle absorbs the selected wavelength leading to hair follicle destruction. Hence laser hair removal is most successful in patients with lighter skin colors and dark colored hairs.[19] Laser treatments may be used on large areas of the body. Without concurrent medical treatment, new hair does grow. It is best to delay laser or electrolysis treatment for at least 6 months after beginning medical treatment so that the growth of new terminal hairs will be reduced.

PHARMACOLOGIC INTERVENTION

It is necessary when hirsutism is moderate to severe or is widespread in androgen-sensitive areas.

Oral Contraceptive Pills

Combined oral contraceptive pills containing estrogen and progestin have been the mainstay for hirsutism therapy for decades.

Mechanism of Action[20,21]

- Inhibition of luteinizing hormone secretion and therefore LH dependent ovarian androgen production.

- Increased hepatic synthesis of sex hormone-binding globulin by estrogen, resulting indecreased concentrations of serum free testosterone and other SHBG-bound androgens.
- Inhibition of adrenal androgen secretion.

The decrease in circulating free androgens results in an improvement in the hirsutism, provided that OCPs are administered chronically.

Choice of OCPs

Must balance, the greater efficacy of third generation pills against the safer coagulation profile of second generation OCP, especially in adolescents, smokers and hypertensive women.
- A neutral (low androgenicity) progestin, such as desogestrel or gestodene.
- An antiandrogen such as cyproterone acetate, chlormadinone acetate
- Spironolactone derivative drospirenone

All of these drugs provide adequate normalization of testosterone levels.[22] Besides, OCPs provide the contraception recommended for the concomitant use of antiandrogens, to regularize menstrual cycles in women with PCOS, which in turn reduces the risk of endometrial hyperplasia. Hence the recommendations of OCPs as first line therapy are:[15]
- As a single drug in women with mild hirsutism.
- As an adjuvant to antiandrogen administration in women with moderate or severe hirsutism and to provide adequate contraception to these patients.
- To guarantee regular menstrual bleeding in hirsute patients with PCOS presenting with oligo- or amenorrhea.

Approximately 60–100% of women with hirsutism demonstrate improvement on oral contraceptives.[23] Oral contraceptive pills reduced the amount of hairs, but the reduction was not consistent across the studies, although two OCPs (ethinyl estradiol 35 µg + cyproterone acetate 2 mg compared to ethinyl estradiol 30 µg + desogestrel 0.15 mg) appeared to be effective in a way that can be considered important for women with hirsutism.[24]

Antiandrogens

Antiandrogens (androgen receptor blockers and 5α-reductase inhibitors) are possibly the most effective drugs for hirsutism. According to Cochrane database, of the antiandrogen drugs, flutamide wasconsidered to be more effective. Spironolactone was also effective but data were only available for the physicians' assessments. Finasteride did not show convincing effectiveness based on the evaluations of the hirsute women. The addition of cyproterone acetate (an antiandrogen) to OCP seemed to enhance the beneficial effect of OCPs on hair reduction:[24]

Recommendations for prescribing an antiandrogen:[15]
- Combined with OCPs in women presenting with moderate or severe hirsutism or in those with a milder hirsutism who do not reach a satisfactory control of hair growth using OCPs alone after 1 year of treatment.
- As single drugs in women in whom OCPs are contraindicated, warranted that areliable contraceptive method is used.

Considering their similar efficacy and potential for side-effects, it is suggested to prescribe finasteride (5 mg/day), cyproterone acetate or spironolactone (100 mg/day) instead of flutamide (250–750 mg/day) when an antiandrogen is needed, as flutamide is known to cause hepatotoxicity although safe at doses below 250 mg/day.[25]

Insulin-sensitizing Drugs

Insulin sensitizers are mainly used for PCOS because insulin resistance contributes to the pathogenesis of this disorder. Insulin sensitizers improve insulin resistance and menstrual dysfunction and may decrease serum androgen concentrations. The best available evidence for their possible efficacy for hirsutism comes from a systematic review and meta-analysis. Meta-analysis of eight metformin trials found no significant reduction in Ferriman-Gallwey scores with metformin when compared with placebo.[26] 2008 Endocrine Society guidelines suggests against their routine use for hirsutism[27] as metformin has minimal or no benefit and rosiglitazone though modestly effective for hirsutism is associated with weight gain and possible adverse cardiovascular effects.[26] According to Cochrane database insulin sensitizers and lifestyle modification did not have any demonstrable benefit in terms of the severity of hirsutism.[24]

Gonadotropin-releasing Hormone Agents

Gonadotropin-releasing hormone agents (GnRH) analogs act by inhibiting ovarian steroidogenesis. The studies of these drugs in the management of hirsutism are quite limited.[28] These drugs induce a reversible menopause requiring combined use with OCPs and its very high economic cost, this class of drugs should be restricted, if used at all, to the very selected patients with severe hyperandrogenism of ovarian origin that do not respond to other drugs.[2]

Glucocorticoids

They are used for the treatment when hirsutism is due to congenital adrenal hyperplasia. Consistent reports regarding its role and safety is not available and it is less effective on hirsutism compared with OCPs or antiandrogens.[2]

KEY POINTS

- Hirsutism is excessive growth of male pattern hair, due to androgen excess which reflects hormonal imbalance.
- PCOS is the most common cause of hirsutism.
- Androgen excess is the main underlying pathology which has various effects on the growth of type of hair at different androgen sensitive areas.
- Thorough history and physical examination directs to the underlying cause.

- Modified Ferriman Gallwey scoring system (mFG) is currently considered the 'gold' standard for the clinical evaluation of hirsutism.
- Various laboratory parameters help in differentiating the causes of hirsutism.
- Treatment of hirsutism should be a combination therapy.
- In cases of mild hirsutism, cosmetic therapy with or without combination of pharmacological therapy is recommended. For women undergoing direct hair removal methods, pharmacologic therapy to be added or continued to minimize hair regrowth.
- For any pharmacologic therapy, waiting for a minimum of six months before making changes in dose or type of medication or adding a medication is advised.
- Oral contraceptive pills (OCPs) is recommended as the first line therapy.
- If suboptimal cosmetic result after six months of OC monotherapy, suggest adding an antiandrogen.
- Use of flutamide for hirsutism is restricted because of its potential hepatotoxicity
- Insulin-lowering drugs, GnRh analogs and glucocorticoids are not recommended for the treatment of hirsutism.

REFERENCES

1. Sachdeva S. Hirsutism: Evaluation and treatment. Indian J Dermatol. 2010; 55:3-7
2. Escobar-Morreal HF, Carmina E, Dewailly D, Gambineri A, Kelestimur F, Moghetti P, Pugeat M, Qiao J, Wijeyaratne CN, Witchel SF, Norman RJ. Epidemiology, diagnosis and management of hirsutism: a consensus statement by the Androgen Excess and Polycystic Ovary Syndrome Society. Human Reproduction Update. 2012;18(2):146-70.
3. Uno H. Biology of hair growth. Semin Reprod Endocrinol. 1986;4:131-41.
4. Randall VA. Androgens and hair growth. Dermatol Ther. 2008;21:314-28.
5. Marshall WA, Tanner JM. Variations in pattern of pubertal changes in girls. Arch Dis Child. 1969; 44:291–303.
6. Metwally M. Hirsutism–review. Obstetrics, Gynaecology and Reproductive Medicine. 2012;22(8):211-4.
7. Burger HG. Androgen production in women. Fertil Steril. 2002; 77 Suppl 4:S3–S5.
8. Deplewski D, Rosenfield RL. Role of hormones in pilosebaceous unit development. Endocr Rev. 2000; 21:363
9. Karrer-Voegeli S, Rey F, Reymond MJ, et al. Androgen dependence of hirsutism, acne, and alopecia in women: retrospective analysis of 228 patients investigated for hyperandrogenism. Medicine (Baltimore). 2009;88:32.
10. McManus SS, Levitsky LL, Misra M. Polycystic ovary syndrome: clinical presentation in normal-weight compared with overweight adolescents. Endocr Pract. 2013; 19:471.
11. Yildiz BO, Bolour S, Woods K, Moore A, Azziz R. Visually scoring hirsutism. Hum Reprod Update. 2010;16(1):51-64.
12. Lizneva D, Gavrilova-Jordan L, Walker W, Azziz R, Androgen excess: investigations and management, Best Practice and Research Clinical Obstetrics and Gynaecology (2016) (accepted manuscript).
13. Wild RA, Carmina E, Diamanti-Kandarakis E, Dokras A, Escobar-Morreale HF, Futterweit W, Lobo R, Norman RJ, Talbott E, Dumesic DA. Assessment of cardiovascular

risk and prevention of cardiovascular disease in women with the polycystic ovary syndrome: a consensus statement by the Androgen Excess and Polycystic Ovary Syndrome (AE-PCOS) Society. J Clin Endocrinol Metab. 2010; 95:2038-49.
14. Lin-Su K, Nimkarn S, New MI. Congenital adrenal hyperplasia in adolescents: Diagnosis and management. Ann NY Acad Sci. 2008;1135:95-8.
15. Escobar-Morreale HF. Diagnosis and management of hirsutism. Ann NY Acad Sci. 2010;1205:166-74.
16. Somani N, Turvy D. Hirsutism: an evidence-based treatment update. Am J Clin Dermatol. 2014;15:247-66.
17. Mihailidis J, Dermesropian R, Taxel P, Luthra P, Jane M, Grant-Kels. Endocrine evaluation of hirsutism. International Journal of Women's Dermatology. 2015. pp. 90-4.
18. Martin KA, Chang RJ, Ehrmann DA, Ibanez L, Lobo RA, Rosenfield RL. Evaluation and treatment of hirsutism in premenopausal women: an Endocrine Society Clinical Practice guideline. J Clin Endocrinol Metab. 2008;93:1105-20.
19. Sanchez LA, Perez M, Azziz R. Laser hair reduction in the hirsute patient: a critical assessment. Hum Reprod Update. 2002;8:169-81.
20. Granger LR, Roy S, Mishell DR Jr. Changes in unbound sex steroids and sex hormone binding globulin—binding capacity during oral and vaginal progestogen administration. Am J Obstet Gynecol. 1982;144:578?
21. Madden JD, Milewich L, Parker CR Jr, et al. The effect of oral contraceptive treatment on the serum concentration of dehydroisoandrosterone sulfate. Am J Obstet Gynecol. 1978;132:380.
22. Sobbrio GA, Granata A, D'Arrigo F, Arena D, Panacea A, Trimarchi F, Granese D, Pulle C. Treatment of hirsutism related to micropolycystic ovary syndrome (MPCO) with two low-dose oestrogen oral contraceptives: a comparative randomized evaluation. Acta EurFertil. 1990;21:139-141.
23. Burkman RT, Jr. The role of oral contraceptives in the treatment of hyperandrogenic disorders. Am J Med. 1995;98(1A):130S-6S.
24. van Zuuren EJ, Fedorowicz Z, Carter B, Pandis N. Interventions for hirsutism (excluding laser and photoepilation therapy alone). Cochrane Database of Systematic Reviews 2015, Issue 4. Art. No.: CD010334.
25. Ibanez L, Jaramillo A, Ferrer A, de Zegher F. Absence of hepatotoxicity after long-term, low-dose flutamide in hyperandrogenic girls and young women. Hum Reprod. 2005;20:1833-36.
26. Cosma M, Swiglo BA, Flynn DN, et al. Clinical review: Insulin sensitizers for the treatment of hirsutism: a systematic review and metaanalyses of randomized controlled trials. J Clin Endocrinol Metab. 2008;93:1135.
27. Martin KA, Chang RJ, Ehrmann DA, et al. Evaluation and treatment of hirsutism in premenopausal women: an endocrine society clinical practice guideline. J Clin Endocrinol Metab. 2008;93:1105.
28. van der Spuy ZM, Tregoning S. Gonadotrophin-releasing hormone analogues for hirsutism (Protocol). Cochrane Database Syst Rev. 2008;CD001126

CHAPTER 19

Adjuvants in Polycystic Ovarian Syndrome

Apoorva Pallam Reddy, Yasodhara Pallam Reddy

INTRODUCTION

Polycystic ovarian syndrome (PCOS) is the most common endocrinopathy, affecting 6–10% of women of reproductive age.[1] Even though the incidence varies based on the diagnostic criterion used, PCOS is undisputedly the most prevalent cause of female anovulatory infertility affecting women across their lifespan. Establishing ovulation in PCOS women is the first step towards conception and often considered the most challenging part. Various modalities have been used over decades individually and in combination to achieve this.

Clomiphene citrate (CC) is the traditional first-line treatment for chronic anovulation in PCOS. However, 20–25% of PCOS women fail to ovulate with incremental doses of clomiphene citrate. In addition, clinical data revealed a discrepancy between ovulation rates (75–80%) and conception rates (30–40%) during CC treatment.[2]

In cases that failed to ovulate despite using maximum dose of ovulogens, the proposed second-line intervention includes either exogenous gonadotropins or laparoscopic ovarian surgery (LOS).[3] Use of gonadotropins is expensive and is associated with significant risk of hyperstimulation, whereas LOS is invasive and has its own pit falls in the long run.

It is at this crossroads, that a wide variety of adjuvants have been tried to increase the incidence of ovulation and eventually pregnancy rates. Although there is not enough literature to seal the deal for a single drug or a combination of drugs, this chapter aims at presenting to you the best available evidence for most commonly used adjuvants.

RATIONALE FOR USE OF ADJUVANTS

Even though insulin resistance (IR) is not considered a diagnostic criterion in PCOS (ESHRE/ASRM, 2004), it plays a central role in the pathogenesis of PCOS.

An estimated prevalence of IR among PCOS patients of 60–70% has been reported (Deugarte et al. 2005). Of all the abnormalities in insulin metabolism identified in women with PCOS, defective insulin receptor signalling that adversely affect the insulin-mediated glucose transport into the muscles, is the

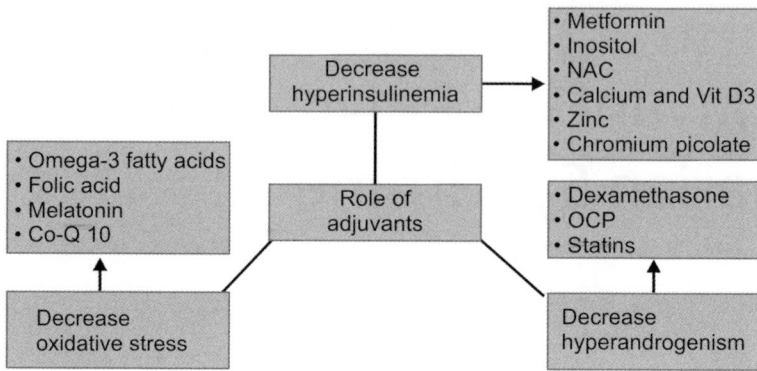

Flow chart 19.1 Role of adjuvants

Abbreviations: NAC, N-acetyl-l-cysteine; OCP, oral contraceptive pill; CoQ10, coenzyme Q10

most significant. The insulin-mediated glucose uptake is reduced by 35–40% in PCOS women independent of obesity. This combined with impaired suppression of hepatic gluconeogenesis causes prolonged elevation in blood glucose levels which further stimulates pancreatic beta cells for insulin production leading to hyperinsulinemia.[4]

This compensatory hyperinsulinemia of PCOS directly stimulates testosterone production by ovarian thecal cells, promoting the hyperandrogenic state that is responsible for hirsutism, acne, alopecia, higher waist to hip ratio, alters the follicular milieu from a pro-ovulatory (estrogenic) environment to an anovulatory or atretic milieu (androgenic) with menstrual disturbances and the microcystic appearance of the ovaries that characterize this syndrome. It noteworthy that insulin receptors on the ovary, ironically, remain sensitive to insulin, or perhaps hypersensitive to it, even when classic target tissues such as muscle and fat manifest resistance to insulin action.[5]

In addition, hyperinsulinemia inhibits the hepatic production of sex hormone binding globulin, further increasing circulating free testosterone levels.[6]

Hence, insulin impedes ovulation, either by directly affecting follicular development, or by indirectly increasing intraovarian androgen levels or altering gonadotropin secretion.

Further, decreased production of adiponectin and decreased activity of the enzyme lipoprotein that is commonly seen in PCOS women, cause aberrant fat metabolism increasing the oxidative levels.[7]

The adjuvants used in PCOS aim at decreasing the insulin resistance, balancing the oxidative stress and thus subsequently reduce the hyperandrogenic environment finally achieving ovulation. **Flow chart 19.1** depicting the various adjuvants and their role in PCOS.

ADJUVANTS USED

Metformin

Metformin, a biguanide, is the most widely used adjuvant in PCOS worldwide. Its primary action is to inhibit hepatic glucose production, but it also increases the sensitivity of peripheral tissues to insulin. It lowers circulating total and free androgen levels through its effect on both the ovaries and adrenal gland suppressing their androgen production, reducing pituitary luteinizing hormone and increases the production of sex hormone binding globulin by the liver [Bailey and Turner, 1996], resulting in improvement of the clinical sequelae of hyperandrogenism.

Metformin versus Placebo

Lord and colleagues (Lord et al. 2003) compiled many early studies on metformin and concluded that metformin was an effective first-line treatment to induce ovulation in PCOS patients and emphasized that it should be used in conjunction with a change in lifestyle. After analysing 7 studies, 46% of women on metformin ovulated whereas only 24% of women on placebo ovulated. The authors concluded that metformin is superior to placebo in inducing ovulation in PCOS women.

A Cochrane review of seven RCTs involving 702 women found that the clinical pregnancy rate for metformin versus placebo was significantly increased [Peto odds ratio (OR) 2.31, 95% confidence interval (CI), 1.52 to 3.51]. However, there was no evidence that metformin improved live birth rates, compared with placebo (pooled OR 1.80, 95% CI 0.52 to 6.16, 3 trials, 115 women).[8]

> Metformin is superior to placebo in inducing ovulation when used unaided by other ovulogens.

Metformin versus Clomiphene Citrate in Nonobese PCOS

Many researchers have opined that there is no difference in the ovulation induction rates between clomiphene citrate and metformin when used in nonobese individuals (Tang et al. 2010, Karimzadeh and Javedani, 2010, Johnson et al. 2010; Johnson, 2011). A systematic review and meta-analysis of RCTs found that there was insufficient evidence to establish a difference between metformin and clomiphene citrate in terms of ovulation, pregnancy, live birth, miscarriage and multiple pregnancy rates in women with PCOS who are nonobese with a BMI <32 kg/m^2.[9]

Tang et al. reported in their Cochrane review that addition of metformin might be beneficial in improving clinical pregnancy and ovulation rates. However, there is no evidence that it improves live-birth rates whether it is used alone or in combination with clomiphene citrate (CC), or when compared with CC. Therefore, the use of metformin as a first-line treatment in improving reproductive outcomes in women with PCOS appears to be limited.[10]

For obese women, on the other hand, the pregnancy and live-birth rates appeared to be overwhelmingly higher for clomiphene versus metformin (Tang et al.), further supported by a Malaysian RCT in which most of the women were obese and again, clomiphene was found to be superior to metformin for obese women with anovulatory PCOS.[11]

Nonobese PCOS women fail to show any advantage of a combination treatment.

In the review of current literature, Johnson opined that, contrary to the international consensus recommendation, research shows that metformin is a very suitable alternative to clomiphene as a first line ovulation induction treatment for nonobese women with anovulatory PCOS. In fact, metformin carries some potential advantages over clomiphene, including no known adverse endometrial effect, no known increase in multiple pregnancy rate (unlike that associated with CC) and thus no requirement for inconvenient and costly monitoring of ovulation induction cycles, and no concern over long-term adverse effects on the ovaries.

> - Metformin achieves similar ovulation rates as that of clomiphene citrate when used in nonobese individuals. However, the minimum duration to achieve the effect is much higher (3 months) and the compliance is poorer for metformin.
> - Obese individuals have significantly higher ovulation rates with CC than Metformin. Hence, use of metformin alone is not recommended in obese women.

Role of Metformin in CC-Resistant Cases

Clomiphene resistance, defined as failure to ovulate after receiving 150 mg of CC daily for 5 days per cycle, for at least three cycles, is common and occurs in approximately 15–40% in women with PCOS. Many investigators have demonstrated an improvement in insulin sensitivity and a significant decrease in serum insulin and free testosterone levels after long-term treatment with metformin for 5–8 weeks.[12]

In a placebo-controlled RCT by Neena et al. amongst 36 CC resistant cases, metformin-clomiphene citrate therapy in significantly increases ovulation and pregnancy rates (p <0.001).[13]

Creanga et al. 2008 in a meta-analysis, confirmed that metformin in combination with CC increased the likelihood of ovulation [OR 4.39, 95% CI 1.94–9.96, number-needed- to-treat (NNT) 3.7] and pregnancy (OR 2.67, 95% CI 1.45– 4.94, NNT 4.6) in comparison with CC alone, especially in CC-resistant and obese PCOS patients.[14]

In a systemic review of the available literature, Gill et al. found a significant improvement not only in the ovulation rates, but also in the pregnancy rates when metformin was added to CC-resistant PCOS women for ovulation induction. However, the optimal treatment regime remains ambiguous.[15]

> - Use of metformin as an adjuvant has a definite role in CC-resistant women.
> - It should be considered before moving on to second line of ovulogens (Gonadotrophins/LOD).

Metformin versus Laparoscopic Ovarian Drilling

Two RCTs compared the combination of metformin and CC with LOD, showing that both are effective approaches to treat CC-resistant infertile PCOS patients. In 50 primary infertile patients with CC-resistant PCOS, Palombo et al. 2010 found no significant difference between the 2 groups in pregnancy and live-birth rates per cycle (13.1% versus 16.3% and 11.2% versus 14.1%, respectively). However, the ovulation rate per cycle was significantly lower in LOD group than in metformin/CC group (56.5% versus 72.0%).[16]

On the other hand, in a well-designed adequately powered RCT by Hashim et al. comprised of 282 anovulatory women with CC-resistant PCOS, reported no significant difference between the 2 groups in ovulation and pregnancy rates per cycle (67% versus 68.2% and 15.4% versus 17%, respectively).

However, a significant difference with respect to midcycle endometrial thickness was found (9.2 ± 1.2 mm versus 7.6 ± 1.1 mm), in metformin/CC and LOD groups, respectively.[17]

LOD is an invasive procedure involving short terms risks due to anesthesia and surgery as well as long-term squeal. Use of metformin is as effective as LOD in achieving ovulation and positive reproductive outcomes. If compliance is achieved, then metformin is a good alternative to LOD.

> Metformin with CC is as effective as LOD for ovulation induction and has the advantage of being noninvasive.

Metformin with Gonadotropins for Ovulation Induction

The use of gonadotropins for ovulation induction in conjunction with metformin was the subject of interest since the introduction of gonadotropins for ovulation induction.

A meta-analysis of 7 RCTs involving 1023 cycles showed that metformin improved live-birth [odds ratio (OR) = 1.94, 95% confidence interval (CI) 1.10 to 3.44; P = 0.020] and pregnancy (OR = 2.25, 95% CI 1.50 to 3.38; p <0.0001) rates, in patients with PCOS who receive gonadotropins for ovulation induction. Further, a significant reduction of cancellation rate and total dose of gonadotropin was observed after metformin administration (OR = 0.41, 95% CI 0.24 to 0.72, P = 0.002). There was no significant effect of metformin on the miscarriage rate.

The authors concluded that an add on of metformin for all PCOS women requiring gonadotrophins for ovulation induction has a positive impact on the live-birth rate.[18]

> Addition of metformin with gonadotropins during ovulation induction for PCOS women might improve the live-birth rate.

Metformin in IVF

A recent Cochrane review of 9 RCTs involving 816 PCOS women undergoing IVF/ICSI concluded that adding metformin to the ovarian stimulation treatment improves clinical pregnancy rates and decreased incidence of OHSS. However, it had no impact on live-birth rate or miscarriage rate. The analysis was done on all PCOS women and no subgroup evaluation was done.[19]

Qublan et al. 2009 have reported that the addition of metformin to their regular stimulation protocol had a positive effect on the quality of the oocytes and embryos.

In a retrospective analysis of 101 centers performing a total of 50,800 annual IVF cycles, 10.4%(n = 5,260) reported metformin use during IVF cycles. However, specific indications for use of metformin like PCOS with habitual abortions (67%), had prior poor egg quality (61%), had high serum insulin levels (56%). Less reported was PCOS with obesity/anovulation (29%), PCOS with multiple manifestations (23%) and glucose intolerance and insulin resistance (23%) were used. When used for a duration of 3 months at a dose of 1500–2000 mg/day, 70% of IVF cycles reported increased pregnancy rates and decreased miscarriage rates with the use of metformin.[20]

It might be logical to suggest that certain subgroups of PCOS might benefit from supplementation of metformin during ART cycles.

> - A subgroup of PCOS patients with habitual abortions, poor oocyte quality and elevated serum insulin levels might benefit from supplementation of metformin at 1500–2000 mg/day 3 months prior to cycle and continue throughout pregnancy.
> - Metformin significantly reduces the risk of OHSS in all PCOS women.

Metformin Effect on Body Mass Index

A meta-analysis by Nieuwen Huis-Ruifrok et al. in 2009, it was reported that metformin treatment was associated with a significant reduction in BMI compared with placebo. They also reported an effect related to both the dose and duration of treatment.

Two other groups, evaluating this effect, reported independently, that the combination of low-calorie diet and metformin led to a significant reduction in visceral fat [Gambineriet al. 2006, 2004; Pasquali et al. 2000].

In a randomized double-blind placebo-controlled trial consisting of 100 severely obese (mean BMI 34.6 kg/m^2) insulin-resistant children aged 6–12 years, randomized to 1,000 mg metformin (n = 53) or placebo (n = 47) twice daily for 6 months, children prescribed metformin had significantly greater decreases in BMI (difference 21.09 kg/m^2, CI 21.87 to 20.31, p = 0.006), body weight (difference 23.38 kg, CI 25.2 to 2 1.57, p, 0.001), BMI Z score (difference between metformin and placebo groups 20.07, CI 20.12 to 20.01, p = 0.02), and fat mass (difference 21.40 kg, CI 22.74 to 20.06, p = 0.04). Fasting plasma glucose (p = 0.007) and homeostasis model assessment (HOMA) insulin-resistance index (p = 0.006) also improved more in metformin-treated children than in placebo-treated children.[21]

> Metformin seems to be of definite benefit in reducing BMI, especially in obese women when used in along with lifestyle changes. The higher the BMI, the greater the benefit.

Metformin and Miscarriage

Polycystic ovarian syndrome women have a much higher risk of miscarriage compared with non-PCOS women at an estimated 30–50%. However, this risk has been attributed to obesity more than the oocyte quality. Metformin was thought to improve the ovarian artery impedance and perifollicular vascularization which theoretically can bring ovarian follicular development in line with normal women [Palomba et al. 2006].

Further, improvements in uterine artery blood flow along with several other implantation markers and positive effect on trophoblastic invasion during the first phases of nidation have also been reported in PCOS patients receiving metformin [Palomba et al. 2006]. Miscarriage occurred in 62–73% of pregnancies without metformin and 9–36% of pregnancies in the same women when metformin was taken.

Several observational studies have also shown that metformin decreases the incidence of miscarriage in PCOS patients.

A prospective clinical-controlled trial concluded that metformin use in pregnant patients with an abnormal glucose tolerance test and history of recurrent spontaneous abortions effectively reduced the chances of first trimester abortion with improved chances of a successful pregnancy.[22]

A metanalysis of 17 RCTs reported that preconception use of metformin had no beneficial effect on the miscarriage rate [Palombaet al. 2009]. However, the major pitfall of this review has been that, in all the RCTs metformin was discontinued after the confirmation of pregnancy.[23] Hence, the results of this trial should be interpreted with caution.

> The benefits of metformin use to decrease miscarriage rate can only be achieved when it is used in PCOS women with abnormal OGTT, history of recurrent miscarriage and when continued throughout the pregnancy.

Metformin and Gestational Diabetes Mellitus

Women with PCOS are more likely than healthy women to suffer from pregnancy-related problems like gestational diabetes mellitus and hypertensive states in pregnancy. The use of metformin therapy in these patients throughout pregnancy may have beneficial effects (Boomsma et al. 2006).

Glueck and colleagues reported a prevalence of GDM of 7% among pregnant PCOS women who continued taking metformin throughout pregnancy compared with 30% among those who did not. Both groups were instructed on healthy dietary practices.

A prospective study done on 98 pregnant women with PCOS who received metformin (1700–3000 mg/day) before conception and up to 37 weeks of pregnancy versus 110 normal pregnant controls, showed a significant reduction of pregnancy complications, such as gestational diabetes and gestational hypertension but an insignificant decrease in pre-eclampsia incidence with comparable mean neonatal Apgar scores, weight and length between the two groups. Continued metformin use throughout the entire pregnancy, had diminished incidences of fetal growth restriction, preterm labor, and increased live-birth rates. There were also no congenital anomalies, intrauterine deaths or stillbirths reported in the test subjects, suggesting metformin use is not related to teratogenicity.[24]

On the contrary, in a double-blinded randomized, placebo-controlled study, done on 257 pregnant women with PCOS, aged 18–42 years, who either received metformin or placebo from first trimester to delivery, failed to demonstrate any reduction of pregnancy-related complications, such as gestational diabetes, pre-eclampsia and preterm delivery in the metformin group.[25]

A systemic review of literature by Zhou et al. suggested that only non-RCT studies have shown a positive impact on pregnancy complications and none of the RCTs showed any benefit of routine use of metformin in pregnancy.[26]

> There is no role of universal prophylactic use of metformin in pregnant PCOS women to prevent pregnancy-related complications.

Effective Dose and Duration

Optimal dose and duration of metformin is probably the single most important factor determining the efficacy of the drug and a substantial area of conflict. The lack of uniformity amongst the dose used in the studies, makes it highly difficult to compare and infer from.

Harborne et al. compared the doses of 1,500 and 2,550 mg/day in obese patients (BMI >30) and in patients with morbid obesity (BMI >40). Those investigators reported a greater weight reduction in patients receiving 2,550 mg/day and concluded that the long-term effect of metformin is better with greater doses.[27]

In an RCT where 1500 mg of metformin was used in anovulatory PCOS, the subgroup with IR showed significant improvement in ovulation and improved insulin sensitivity assessed by fasting glucose to insulin ratio (FGIR) progressively beginning from 4 weeks of therapy.[28]

Although there is no universal consensus on the minimum effective dose, most authors opine on using 1500 mg/day as the least effective dose.

> 1500–2000 mg/day of metformin for a minimum of 3 months should be administered to achieve optimal benefits of the drug.

Side Effects

The main side effects associated with metformin treatment are the gastrointestinal symptoms of nausea, diarrhea, flatulence, bloating, anorexia, metallic taste and abdominal pain. These symptoms occur with variable degrees in patients and in most cases resolve spontaneously. The severity of side effects can be reduced by gradual administration of metformin and titrating the dose increase guided by the severity of symptoms.

A start dose of 500 mg daily during the main meal of the day for 12 weeks can lessen the side effects. A weekly or biweekly increase by 500 mg a day can then be pursued as required until a maximum dose of 2500–2550 mg/day is reached depending on the clinical benefit and side effects.

If the dose increase results in worsening of the side effects, the current dose can be maintained for 2–4 weeks until tolerance is developed Nestler, 2008]. Slow release metformin can be associated with fewer side effects.[29]

> Gastrointestinal side-effects may be minimized by titrating the dose and consuming with food.

Caution with Metformin

Metformin can also lead to vitamin B12 malabsorption in the distal ileum in approximately 10–30% of patients which is an effect dependent on age, dose and duration of treatment (Ting et al. 2006). Rarely, lactic acidosis can occur, mainly in diabetic patients, which is a serious condition that can potentially be fatal. However, unless there is a contraindication to taking metformin such as renal disease the risk of lactic acidosis is negligible (Salpeter et al. 2003a, 2003b).[29]

> Long-term usage and higher doses of metformin may cause vit B12 deficiency. Hence supplementation is recommended.

Inositol

Inositol is a polyalchol existing in nine different stereoisomers, two of which have been shown to be insulin mediators: myo-inositol (MI) and D-chiro-inositol (DCI).

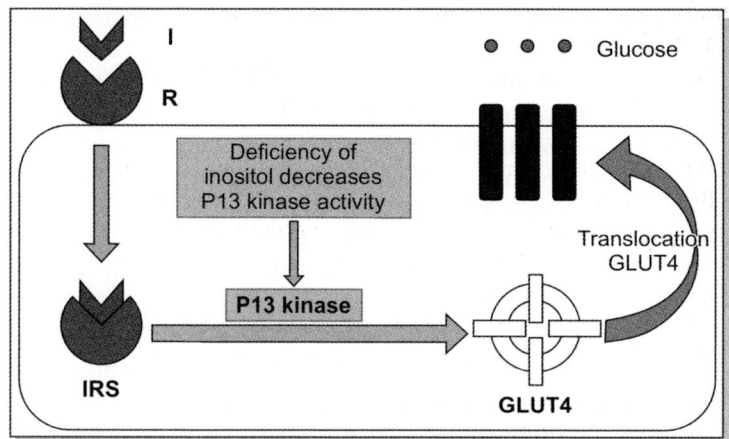

Fig. 19.1 Deficiency of inositol decreases PI3 kinase activity
Abbreviations: I, Insulin; R, Insulin receptor; IRS, Insulin receptor substrate; PI3, Phosphotidylinositol 3 kinase; GLUT4, Glucose transporter type 4

There have been numerous studies demonstrating significant low serum levels of inositol in PCOS women. In the ovary, DCI is involved in insulin-mediated androgen synthesis, whereas MI mediates glucose uptake and follicle-stimulating hormone (FSH) signaling.

In human ovaries, 99% of the intracellular pool of inositol consists of MI and the remaining part consists of DCI; imbalance of ovarian MI and DCI concentrations, like a putative Myo-Ins deficiency, might impair the FSH signaling, as observed in PCOS patients.

In vivo DCI is synthesized by an epimerase that converts MI into DCI and, depending on the specific needs of the two different molecules, each tissue has a typical conversion rate.[30,31]

Role of DCI in the treatment of PCOS was first realized in 1999 by Nestler et al. In their study, 19 out of 22 obese hyperinsulinemic PCOS patients treated with 1.2 g/day DCI showed restored ovulation and an improvement of the hormonal profile compared with the placebo group. Recent studies showed that 4 g/day MI, besides improving hormonal profile and restoring ovulation, can induce regular menses in both lean and obese PCOS patients.[32]

Furthermore, a direct correlation of MI concentration in the follicular fluid and high oocyte quality has been found. Additional studies also showed that MI supplementation rather than DCI, is able to improve oocyte quality.[33]

Interestingly, in both studies, a drop in the amount of recombinant FSH (rFSH) administered and the number of canceled cycles were observed.

The explanation for this can be correlated to the interesting D-chiro-inositol paradox proposed by Gianfranco Carlomagno et al. Ovaries, unlike other tissues such as muscle and liver, never become insulin resistant. Therefore, it could be speculated that PCOS patients with hyperinsulinemia likely present an enhanced MI to DCI epimerization in the ovary; this would result in an increased DCI/MI ratio (i.e., overproduction of DCI), which, in turn, would lead to an MI deficiency in the ovary. This MI depletion could eventually be responsible for the poor oocyte quality observed in these patients.[34]

In a double blinded RCT done by Carlomagno et al. patients in study group undergoing IVF were treated with 4g of MI and 400 mg of folic acid for 3 months before starting ovarian stimulation and throughout pregnancy. Patients assigned to placebo group were treated with 400 mg of folic.

Total rFSH units ($p < 0.05$) and number of stimulation days ($p < 0.05$) were significantly reduced in the MI group. Fertilization and cleavage rates were higher in the MI group (73.1% vs 67%, $p < 0.01$ and 72.4% vs 87.8%, $p < 0.01$). Furthermore, grade I embryos were higher in the MI group (72.4% vs 87.8%, $p < 0.01$); this will likely reflect the increase in biochemical pregnancy rate observed (33.5% vs 23.5%, $p < 0.01$). Clinical pregnancy showed a positive trend in the MI group (20.5% vs 18.4%, $p < 0.06$).

Based on the findings, the authors recommending supplementing MI routinely in ART cycles might be of added benefit.[35]

A systemic review of 12 RCT till 2016 by Unfer et al. suggested that myo-ins supplementation improves several of the hormonal and reproductive disturbances of PCOS; furthermore, the analysis lends prominence to the pivotal role of inositol(s), mainly myo-ins and D-chiro-ins, as a safe and effective therapy for PCOS, including an enhanced oocyte follicular development and oocyte maturation and in stimulation and pregnancy outcomes in IVF procedures.[36]

> The available literature suggests that inositiol supplements at a minimum of 2 g/day add benefit to reproductive outcome in PCOS patients.

N-Acetyl Cysteine (NAC)

N-acetyl-cysteine (NAC) is an antioxidant derivative from the amino acid L-cysteine. NAC has been shown to influence both the insulin secretion in pancreatic β-cells, as well as the regulation of insulin receptors in human erythrocytes. Moreover, NAC has antioxidant effects via increasing the cellular levels of reduced glutathione.[37]

In recent years, a limited number of studies have shown the possible benefits of NAC administration in improving induction of ovulation outcomes in patients with PCOS. The possible beneficial effects of NAC on ovulation in CC-resistant PCOS patients has been proposed and studied extensively.

In 2007, Badawy et al. noted that the addition of NAC to a CC regimen in patients with PCOS would increase ovulation rates significantly.[38]

Gayatri et al. showed significant effects of NAC on the clinical features, biochemical markers of insulin resistance, hormonal levels, anovulation, and oxidative stress inhibition in PCOS women. Considering their positive effect on insulin resistance and limited adverse effects, they recommended using NAC as adjuvants for ovulation induction.[39]

A prospective double-blind clinical trial, by Salehpour et al. on 46 PCOS women showed 6 weeks use of NAC can increase ovulation rate and HDL levels and decrease weight, body mass index (BMI), and waist/hip ratio, fast blood sugar (FBS), serum insulin, total cholesterol, LDL levels, and HOMA-IR index while luteinizing hormone (LH), Follicle-stimulating hormone (FSH), prolactin, LH/FSH levels and glucose/insulin ratio were the same with no significant changes.[40]

Another study of Salehpour et al. showed that using of NAC as an adjuvant in Clomiphene citrate cause an increase in number of follicles >18 mm, mean endometrial thickness on the day of hCG administration, ovulation and pregnancy rates with no adverse side-effects and no cases of ovarian hyperstimulation syndrome. Similar results were achieved by EL-Gharib et al. 2014. Improved conception rate was noted when NAC was supplemented to CC, probably owing to mucolytic action of N-acetyl cysteine recuperating cervical mucus quality (conception rate 12.5% vs. 2.5%).[41]

The study by Rizk et al. was the only trial to have shown benefit of combination of CC and NAC by increasing ovulation and pregnancy rates in CC-resistant PCOS patients.[42]

However RCT by Abu Hashim et al. (2010) showed that the efficacy of metformin-CC combination therapy is higher than that of NAC-CC for inducing ovulation and achieving pregnancy among CC-resistant PCOS patients.

Dosages and duration of NAC varied between all the studies ranging from 1.2 to 1.8 g/day for 5 days to 5–6 weeks.

> The current available evidence endorses against the use of NAC in CC resistant PCOS and proposes a possible benefit for using it only as a supplement to PCOS women responding to CC.

Calcium and Vitamin D

Some studies back the effect of vitamin D deficiency on pathophysiology of PCOS and even insulin resistance. Pal et al. found that 3 months supplementation with vitamin D and calcium (Ca) can reduce androgen sowing to their direct effect on the ovarian and/or adrenal steroid genesis pathway. Firouzabadi et al. also found calcium and vitamin D supplementation can make a positive effect on weight loss, follicle maturation, menstrual regularity, and improvement of hyperandrogenism, in infertile women with PCOS.

In a clinical trial of 80, PCOS women supplemented with calcium and Vitamin D (1000 mg/day calcium plus 50,000 IU/2 weeks for 4 weeks) in addition to metformin therapy resulted in a better outcome in a variety of PCOS symptoms including menstrual regularity, and ovulation.[43]

> Calcium and vit D3 supplementation is beneficial in PCOS women.

Zinc

Zinc (Zn), one of the most important trace elements, is essential for more than 300 different cellular processes. Zn also is a basic element for many vital functions including homeostasis, immune responses, oxidative stress, and apoptosis and in other words, for health, either physically or mentally and also is involved in fertility and reproduction.

Besides, zinc is important for insulin synthesis and action in both, normal and diabetes mellitus condition.[44]

Although some studies did not find any significant differences between women with and without PCOS regarding to serum Zn levels, Tabrizi et al. in a randomized, double-blind, placebo-controlled parallel groups trial on 65

PCOS women showed that 8 wk supplementation with 50 mg of zinc in the zinc sulphate form can arise serum zinc significantly and also reduce homeostasis model of assessment-insulin resistance score, fasting serum total cholesterol, LDL-C, triglyceride, testosterone, and TG/HDL-C ratio in comparison with placebo.[45]

They further added that zinc supplementation for PCOS women may have some beneficial effects on cardio metabolic risk factors.

Folic Acid

Polycystic ovary syndrome is one of the conditions that are associated with elevated homocysteine levels. Homocysteine is a product of methionine metabolism and can cause cytotoxic effects on vascular endothelium.[46]

Folic acid is one of the supplements which have a well-known physiological effect on Hcy reduction. According to Palomba et al. 6 months treatment with metformin and folic acid, could cause a significant improvement in all the markers of structure and function of the vascular endothelium and this improvement was significantly different between folic acid supplementation and placebo groups.[47]

Regarding this matter, Kazerooni et al. in a prospective clinical trial on 70 Iranian hyperhomocysteinemic PCOS women reported that 3 months folic acid supplementation could significantly decreased Hcy levels in these women regardless of insulin resistance status although this reduction was higher in women without IR. These researchers believe that IR can have effect on Hcy responses to folic acid.[48] 3 months of folic acid supplementation as a part of the preconception care would be beneficial in ways more than one.

Omega-3 Fatty Acids

Omega-3 fatty acids, at first were found in fatty fish. Fish oil that is the main source of dietary omega-3 fatty acids have several healthy effects including anti-inflammatory, antithrombotic, antiarrhythmic and antiatherogenic effects. While insulin resistance is an important component in the pathogenesis of PCOS, this syndrome is associated with inflammatory factors, so polyunsaturated fatty acids (PUFA) may treat PCOS with the help to decrease insulin resistance and androgen excess.[49]

Rafraf et al. in their study found omega-3 fatty acids for 8 weeks can decrease total cholesterol (TC), triglyceride, low density lipoprotein (LDL), malonodialdehyde (MDA), and increase high density lipoprotein (HDL), but make no changes in total antioxidant capacity (TAC). These researchers concluded that omega-3 fatty acids are useful for PCOS women in order to reduce lipids and lipid peroxidation levels and improves metabolic disturbances.[50]

> Folic acid, zinc and omega-3 fatty acids play a role in reducing the oxidative stress and improving metabolic profile.

Chromium Picolate

Chromium picolinate is a chemical compound sold as a nutritional supplement to prevent or treat chromium deficiency. This compound is derived from chromium and picolinic acid. Small quantities of chromium are needed for glucose utilization by insulin in normal health, but deficiency is extremely rare.

In a RCT by et al. women with CC resistant PCOS were given either 1500 mg of metformin/day or 200 mcg of chromium picolate daily for 3 months. Chromium picolinate significantly decreased fasting blood sugar (FBS), serum levels of fasting insulin after 3 months of treatment (p = 0.042). In comparison to the patients who received chromium picolinate, those who received metformin had significantly lower levels of testosterone (p = 0.001) and free testosterone (p = 0.001) after 3 months of treatment. There was no significant difference between the two study groups regarding ovulation (p = 0.417) and pregnancy rates (p = 0.500). The authors emphasized on the positive role of chromium picolate in CC resistant cases and proposed that it maybe better tolerated than metformin.[51]

Melatonin

The role of melatonin (N-acetyl-5-methoxytryptamine), a small lipophilic indoleamine, in human reproduction is still unknown.

Melatonin, as well as its metabolites, are claimed to be broad-spectrum antioxidants and free radical scavengers, and their role is to quench reactive oxygen species (ROS) as well as reactive nitrogen species. Elevated melatonin in preovulatory follicles, as seen in normal women, is likely to protect granulosa cells and oocyte from free radicals that are induced during ovulation.[52]

Although the circulating levels of melatonin are elevated in PCOS women, the ovarian follicular fluid levels are significantly reduced and this fall is responsible for follicular atresia because of increased oxidative stress and consequent follicular damage.[53]

Rosanna et al. from Italy are currently investigating the role of melatonin in PCOS women through a RCT. Till the results of the study are published the role of supplementing melatonin for PCOS women is questionable.

> There is no role of supplementing melatonin alone in PCOS women.

Dexamethasone

In some CC-resistant PCOS women, addition of glucocorticoids (e.g. dexamethasone 0.5 mg or prednisone 5 mg hs) to the CC treatment regimen will achieve ovulation when CC alone has failed. Adjunctive glucocorticoid treatment is perhaps most useful in those having serum DHEA-S levels greater than 200 µg/dL, but can also be empirical, continued if successful and promptly discontinued when it is not.[54]

In a study of 230 women with PCOS who failed to ovulate with 200 mg of CC for 5 days, addition of 2 mg of dexamethasone from 5 to 14 days is associated with a higher ovulation rate and cumulative pregnancy rate.[55]

Compared with the placebo, dexamethasone reduced testosterone by 27%, androstenedione by 21%, dehydroepiandrosterone sulphate by 46% and free testosterone index by 50% in women with PCOS treated with diet and lifestyle advice, and metformin. Given the potential side effects and risks of chronic glucocorticoid administration, continued treatment should be limited to those who respond and extended durations of treatment avoided.[56]

In a single-blinded RCT, supplementation of 0.5 mg of dexona 4 times a day in PCOS women undergoing ART cycles, pregnancy rate in the group receiving dexamethasone was 17.5% significantly higher versus 4.3% in the placebo group ($p<0.05$). The mean number of embryos in the patients received dexamethasone was 6.7 ± 4.3, significantly greater than placebo which was 4.9 ± 4.9 ($p<0.05$). The mean number of gonadotropin ampoules used in the group received dexamethasone was 3.5 ± 1.6, significantly lower versus the placebo which was 5.3 ± 2.5 ($p<0.05$). The mean number of oocytes in the group received dexamethasone was 11.8 ± 8 and in the placebo group was 9.6 ± 5.8 that was not significant.[57]

Dexamethasone at 2 mg/day dose is effective in reducing androgen levels and achieving ovulation chiefly in those women with severe hyperandrogenism and hirsutism (DHEA-S >200 µg/dL).

Oral Contraceptive Pills (OCPs)

For many decades oral contraceptive pills (OCPs) have been standard therapy for women with PCOS not seeking pregnancy. There have been several advantages of treatment with OCPs, including immediate regularization of menses, amelioration of hirsutism and acne and foremost protection from the development of endometrial carcinoma. The importance of these benefits is undisputed. However, off late there has been a concern whether OCPs might also exert adverse metabolic effects with long-term consequences, especially in a group of women with known insulin resistance and predisposition to type 2 diabetes. Long-term RCTs are required to assess the effect of prolonged supplementation of OCP over the frequency of metabolic syndrome.

Administration of OCP to women seeking pregnancy in order to achieve a favorable hormonal milieu is not acceptable and there is no added benefit of using it as a precursor to ovulation induction cycles.

Statins

Statins are inhibitors of mevalonate pathway and possess antioxidant and anti-inflammatory pathway. Inhibition of HMG-CoA reductase results in both a reduction in cholesterol synthesis and with decreased production of other biologically important products of the mevalonate pathway. As cholesterol is the substrate for androgen synthesis, decrease in the LDL levels is projected to improve the ovarian steroidogenesis.

Both *in-vitro* and clinical studies provide consistent and encouraging data supporting the concept that statins may be useful in the treatment of many aspects of PCOS, including reduction of hyperandrogenemia, and various metabolic aspects. However, the role of statins is limited in women of reproductive age group seeking pregnancy as statins are teratogenic. Their use should be restricted to women who are either not sexually active or using reliable contraception.[58]

Routine use of statins is not advised for PCOS women seeking pregnancy.

Coenzyme Q10 (CoQ10)

Coenzyme Q10 (CoQ10) is a fat-soluble coenzyme, found in the inner mitochondrial membrane that plays a crucial role in the production of cellular energy and acts as an antioxidant. Of late, there has been much buzz around the use of CoQ10 in making the oocytes, especially in poor responders. Animal studies have reported that CoQ10 increases the reproductive lifetime of female mice by about 30% and that animals that receive more CoQ10 produce more and healthier eggs and show improved ovarian response and various consistent hormonal changes (Bentov et al. 2010). Researchers found that mitochondrial dysfunction may contribute to the onset of metabolic syndrome including obesity, insulin resistance, abnormal lipid profile and an increased risk of coronary heart diseases later in life (Luce et al. 2010).

A prospective randomized controlled trial by Refaeey et al. evaluated the effect of combined oral coenzyme Q10 (CoQ10) and clomiphene citrate for ovulation induction in 101 clomiphene-citrate-resistant PCOS patients.

Numbers of follicles >14 mm and 18 mm, endometrial thickness on the day of human chorionic gonadotropin (8.82 ± 0.27 mm versus 7.03 ± 0.74 mm) and ovulation rates [54/82 cycles (65.9%) in the CoQ10 group and 11/71 cycles (15.5%) in the control group] were significantly higher in the CoQ10 group. Even clinical pregnancy rate was significantly higher in the CoQ10 group (19/51, 37.3%) versus the control group (3/50, 6.0%). The authors opined that CoQ10 is a safe, well-tolerated cheap adjuvant that can improve ovulation rates chiefly in CC resistance.[59]

The use of CoQ10 in *in-vitro* culture of bovine embryos results in superior rate of early embryo cleavage and blastocyst formation, higher percentage of expanding blastocysts and a larger inner cell mass (Gosden, 2002; Perez et al. 2000). Also, the potential for embryo implantation is correlated with the ATP content of the embryo (Lerkom et al. 1995; Van Blerkom et al. 2000)

> Coenzyme Q 10 has shown positive impact on improving oocyte quality in PCOS women.

CONCLUSION

Currently, there is an extensive list of adjuvants available that claim to improve the fertility outcome in PCOS women. It is safe to say that there will be many more new additions to this list in the times to come. Despite having identified the syndrome decades back, no clear-cut consensus over the treatment regimens has been possible. This can principally be attributed to the disparity in the research methodology and the constant evolution of new drugs claiming to be superior. Metformin is the oldest and most effect adjuvant available so far. It definitely has a role in improving fertility outcomes when the right subjects are chosen. Inositol is a promising new addition supplementing fertility in PCOS. Judicious selection of adjuvants based on the expected outcome, for a hand-picked group of patients will not only give an ideal response but also save the patient from being given a cocktail of medicines.

KEY POINTS

- The concept of using adjuvants in PCOS is to improve insulin resistance, hyperandrogenemia and oxidative stress.
- Metformin:
  - Metformin is superior to placebo in inducing ovulation when used unaided by other ovulogens
  - Metformin achieves similar ovulation rates as that of clomiphene citrate when used in non-obese individuals. However, the minimum duration to achieve the effect is much higher (3 months) and the compliance is poorer for metformin
  - Obese individuals have significantly higher ovulation rates with CC than metformin. Hence, use of metformin alone is not recommended in obese women
  - Use of metformin as an adjuvant has a definite role in CC-resistant women.
  - It should be considered before moving onto second line of ovulogens (Gonadotropins/LOD)
  - Metformin with CC is as effective as LOD for ovulation induction and has the advantage of being noninvasive
  - Addition of metformin with gonadotropins during ovulation induction for PCOS women significantly reduces OHSS risk and might improve the live-birth rate.
  - A subgroup of PCOS patients with habitual abortions, poor oocyte quality and elevated serum insulin levels might benefit from supplementation of metformin at 1500–2000 mg/day for 3 months prior to cycle and continue throughout pregnancy
  - There is no role of universal prophylactic use of metformin in pregnant PCOS women to prevent pregnancy-related complications
  - 1500–2000 mg/day of metformin for a minimum of 3 months should be administered to achieve optimal benefits of the drug
- Inositiol supplements at a minimum of 2 g/day add benefit to reproductive outcome in PCOS patients
- The current available evidence endorses against the use of NAC in CC resistant PCOS and proposes a possible benefit for using it only as a supplement to PCOS women responding to CC
- Dexamethasone at 2 mg/day dose is effective in reducing androgen levels and achieving ovulation chiefly in those women with severe hyperandrogenism and hirsutism (DHEA-S >200 µg/dL)
- Administration of OCP to women seeking pregnancy in order to achieve a favorable hormonal milieu is not acceptable and there is no added benefit of using it as a precursor to ovulation induction cycles
- Coenzyme Q 10 has shown positive impact on improving oocyte quality in PCOS women.

REFERENCES

1. Knochenhauer ES, Key TJ, Kahsar-Miller M, Waggoner W, Boots LR, Azziz R. Prevalence of the polycystic ovary syndrome in unselected black and white women of the south eastern United States: a prospective study. J Clin Endocrinol Metab. 1998; 83:3078-82.
2. Yen SS. Chronic anovulation caused by peripheral endocrine disorders. In: Yen SS, Jaffe RB, eds. Reproductive endocrinology; physiology, pathophysiology, and clinical management, 3rd ed. Philadelphia: Saunders; 1991. pp. 576-630.
3. Best practices of ASRM and ESHRE: a journey through reproductive medicine Fertility and Sterility®. 2012;98(6):0015-0282.
4. Ciaraldi TP, el-Roeiy A, Madar Z, Reichart D, Olefsky JM, Yen SS. Cellular mechanisms of insulin resistance in polycystic ovarian syndrome. J Clin Endocrinol Metab. 1992;75(2):577-83.
5. Nestler JE, Jakubowicz DJ, de Vargas AF, Brik C, Quintero N, Medina F. Insulin stimulates testosterone biosynthesis by human thecal cells from women with polycystic ovary syndrome by activating its own receptor and using inositolglycan mediators as the signal transduction system. J Clin Endocrinol Metab. 1998;83:2001-5.
6. Nestler JE. Role of hyperinsulinemia in the pathogenesis of the polycystic ovary syndrome, and its clinical implications. Semin Reprod Endocrinol. 1997;15:111-22.
7. Manneras-Holm L, Leonhardt H, Kullberg J. Adipose tissue has aberrant morphology and function in PCOS: enlarged adipocytes and low serum adiponectin, but not circulating sex steroids, are strongly associated with insulin resistance. J Clin Endocrinol Metab. 2011;96(2):E304-11.
8. Tang T, Lord JM, Norman RJ, et al. Insulin-sensitising drugs (metformin, rosiglitazone, pioglitazone, D-chiroinositol) for women with polycystic ovary syndrome, oligo amenorrhoea and subfertility. Cochrane Database Syst Rev. 2012;5:CD003053.
9. Michael F. Metformin versus clomiphene citrate for infertility in non-obese women with polycystic ovary syndrome: a systematic review and meta-analysis Marie L. Misso1,2, Costello Human Reproduction Update. 2013;19(1): 2–11.
10. Tang, T et al. (2010). Insulin-sensitising drugs (metformin, rosiglitazone, pioglitazone, D-chiro-inositol) for women with polycystic ovary syndrome, oligo amenorrhoea and subfertility. Cochrane Database of Systematic Reviews, Issue 1. Art. No. CD003053
11. Zain MM, Jamaluddin R, Ibrahim A, et al. Comparison of clomiphene citrate, metformin, or the combination of both for first-line ovulation induction, achievement of pregnancy, and live birth in Asian women with polycystic ovary syndrome: a randomized controlled trial. Fertil Steril 2009;91:514-21.
12. Kocak M, Caliskan E, Simsir C, Haberal A. Metformin therapy improves ovulatory rates, cervical scores, and pregnancy rates in clomiphene citrate–resistant women with polycystic ovary syndrome. Fertility and Sterility. 2002;77(1)10-6.
13. Chuni N; Efficacy of sequential treatment of metformin and clomiphene citrate in clomiphene resistant women with polycystic ovary syndrome. J Obstet Gynecol India. 2007;57(1):69-72.
14. Creanga AA, Bradley HM, McCormick C, Witkop CT. Use of metformin in polycystic ovary syndrome: a meta-analysis. Obstetrics & Gyne, 2008.
15. Sabraj Gill A, Ailsa Gemmell A, Rebecca Colleran. Does Metformin combined with Clomiphene Citrate improve fertility-related outcomes in Clomiphene resistant women with PCOS? A systematic review. Middle East Fertility Society Journal. 2014;19:81-88.
16. Palomba S, et al. Laparoscopic ovarian diathermy vs. clomiphene citrate plus metformin as second-line strategy for infertile anovulatory patients with polycystic ovary syndrome: a randomized controlled trial. American Journal of Obstetrics and Gynecology. 2010;202(6):577.e1-8.

17. Abu HH, El Lakany N, Sherief L. Combined metformin and clomiphene citrate versus laparoscopic ovarian diathermy for ovulation induction in clomiphene-resistant women with polycystic ovary syndrome: A randomized controlled trial. The Journal of Obstetrics and Gynaecology Research. 2011;37(3):169-77.
18. Palomba, et al. Reproductive Biology and Endocrinology. Metformin and gonadotropins for ovulation induction in patients with polycystic ovary syndrome: a systematic review with meta-analysis of randomized controlled trials. 2014,12:3.
19. Tso LO, Costello MF, Albuquerque LE, Andriolo RB, Macedo CR. Cochrane Database Syst Rev. Metformin treatment before and during IVF or ICSI in women with polycystic ovary syndrome. 2014;18;(11):CD006105
20. Wu H, Zhao Y, Yemini M. Metformin use in patients undergoing in vitro fertilization treatment: results of a worldwide web-based survey Mindy S. Christianson, corresponding. J Assist Reprod Genet. Published online 2015 Jan 30. 2015;32(3): 401-6.
21. Yanovski A, Krakoff J, Salaita CG. Effects of Metformin on Body Weight and Body Composition in Obese Insulin-Resistant Children A Randomized Clinical Trial Jack. Diabetes. 2011.60:477-85.
22. Zolghadri J, Tavana Z, Kazerooni T, Soveid M, Taghieh M. Relationship between abnormal glucose tolerance test and history of previous recurrent miscarriages, and beneficial effect of metformin in these patients: a prospective clinical study. Fertil Steril. 2008;90(3):727-30.
23. Palomba S, Falbo A, Orio F Jr, Zullo F. Effect of preconceptional metformin on abortion risk in polycystic ovary syndrome: a systematic review and meta-analysis of randomized controlled trials. Fertil Steril. 2009 Nov; 92(5):1646-58.
24. De Leo V, Musacchio MC, Piomboni P, Di Sabatino A, Morgante G. The administration of metformin during pregnancy reduces polycystic ovary syndrome related gestational complications. Eur J Obstet Gynecol Reprod Biol. 2011;157(1):63-6.
25. Vanky E, Stridsklev S, Heimstad R, Romundstad P, Skogøy K, Kleggetveit O, Hjelle S, von Brandis P, Eikeland T, Flo K, Berg KF, Bunford G, Lund A, Bjerke C, Almås I, Berg AH, Danielson A, Lahmami G, Carlsen SM. Metformin versus placebo from first trimester to delivery in polycystic ovary syndrome: a randomized, controlled multicenter study. J Clin Endocrinol Metab. 2010 Dec; 95(12):E448-55.
26. Zhuo Z, Wang A, Huimin Yu. Effect of Metformin Intervention during Pregnancy on the Gestational Diabetes Mellitus in Women with Polycystic Ovary Syndrome: A Systematic Review and Meta-Analysis. Journal of Diabetes Research Volume 2014 (2014), Article ID 381231.
27. Harbone LR, et al. Metformin and weight loss in obese women with polycystic vary syndrome (PCOS): comparison of doses. J Clin Endocrinol Metab. 2005;90:1-24.
28. Eisenhardt S, Schwarzmann N. Early Effects of Metformin in Women with Polycystic Ovary Syndrome: A Prospective Randomized, Double- Blind, Placebo-Controlled Trial. The Journal of Clinical Endocrinology & Metabolism 91(3):946–952 Printed in U.S.A. Copyright © 2006 by The Endocrine Society doi: 10.1210/jc.2005-1994.
29. Lashen H. Role of metformin in the management of polycystic ovary syndrome. Ther Adv Endocrinol Metab. 2010;1(3):117-28 DOI: 10.1177/ 2042018810380215.
30. Sun TH, Heimark DB, Nguygen T, Nadler JL,Larner J. D-chiro-Inositol—its functional role in insulin action and its deficit in insulin resistance. Int J Exp Diabetes Res. 2002;3:47-60.
31. Both myo-inositol to chiro-inositol epimerase activities and chiro-inositol to myoinositol ratios are decreased in tissues of GK type 2 diabetic rats compared to Wistar controls. Biochem Biophys Res Commun. 2002;293:1092-8.
32. Costantino D, Minozzi G, Minozzi E, Guaraldi C. Metabolic and hormonal effects of myo-inositol in women with polycystic ovary syndrome: a double blind trial. Eur Rev Med Pharmacol Sci. 2009;13: 105–10.

33. Papaleo E, Unfer V, Baillargeon JP, Fusi F, Occhi F, de Santis L. Myo-Inositol may improve oocyte quality in intracytoplasmic sperm injection cycles. A prospective, controlled, randomized trial. Fertil Steril. 2009;91:1750-4.
34. Carlomagno G, et al. The D-chiro-inositol paradox in the ovary. Fertility and Sterility. 2011;95(8).
35. Carlomagno G, Montanino Oliva M, Roseff SJ, Myo-Inositol: Ovarian stimulation and ivf outcomes. Fertility and Sterility. 2012;98(3):S74-S75.
36. Unfer V, John E. Effects of Inositol(s) in Women with PCOS: A Systematic Review of Randomized Controlled Trials. Nestler, International Journal of Endocrinology Volume 2016, Article ID 1849162, 12 pages
37. Thakker D, Raval A, Patel I, Walia R. N-acetylcysteine for polycystic ovary syndrome. A systemic review and meta-analysis of randomized controlled clinical trials. Obstet Gynecol Int. 2015.
38. Badawy A, State O, Abdelgawad S. N-Acetyl cysteine and clomiphene citrate for induction of ovulation in polycystic ovary syndrome: A cross-over trial. Acta Obstet Gynecol Scand. 2007;86:218-22.
39. Gayatri K, Saubhagya Kumar J, Basanta Kumar B. Metformin and N-acetyl Cysteine in Polycystic Ovarian Syndrome-A comparative study. Indian J Clin Med. 2010;1:7-13.
40. Salehpour S, Tohidi A, Akhound MR, Amirzargar N. N Acetyl Cysteine, A novel Remedy for Poly Cystic Ovarian Syndrome. Int J Fertil Steril. 2009;3:66-73.
41. Salehpour S, Akbari Sene A, Saharkhiz N, Sohrabi MR, Moghimian F. N-acetylcysteine as an adjuvant to clomiphene citrate for successful induction of ovulation in infertile patients with polycystic ovary syndrome. J Obstet Gynaecol Res 2012;38:1182-86.
42. Rizk AY, Bedaiwy MA, Al-Inany HG. N-acetylcysteine is a novel adjuvant to clomiphene citrate in clomiphene citrate-resistant patients with polycystic ovary syndrome. Fertil Steril. 2005;83:367-70
43. Tehrani HG, Mostajeran F. The effect of calcium and vitamin D supplementation on menstrual cycle, body mass index and hyperandrogenism state of women with poly cystic ovarian syndrome. J Res Med Sci. 2014;19(9):875-80.
44. Dosa MD, Adumitresi CR, Hangan LT, Nechifor M. Copper, Zinc and Magnesium in Non-Insulin-Dependent Diabetes Mellitus Treated with Metformin. http://dx.doi.org/10.5772/ 48230.
45. Sohrabvand F, Shirazi M, Shariat M. Fatemeh Mahdiyin. Serum zinc level in infertile women with and without polycystic ovary syndrome: a comparative study. Tehran Univ Med J. 2013;71:157-63.
46. Grodnitskaya EE, Kurtser MA. Homocysteine metabolism in polycystic ovary syndrome. Gynecol Endocrinol. 2012;28:186-9.
47. Palomba S, Falbo A, Giallauria F, Russo T, Tolino A, Zullo F, et al. Effects of Metformin With or Without Supplementation With Folate on Homocysteine Levels and Vascular Endothelium of Women With Polycystic Ovary Syndrome. Diabetes Care. 2010;33: 246-51.
48. Kazerooni T, Asadi N, Dehbashi S, Zolghadri J. Effect of folic acid in women with and without insulin resistance who have hyperhomocysteinemic polycystic ovary syndrome. Int J Gynecol Obstet. 2008;101:156-60.
49. Kasim-Karakas SE, Almario RE, Gregory L, Wong R, Todd H, Lasley BL. Metabolic and endocrine effects of a polyunsaturated fatty acid-rich diet in Polycystic Ovary Syndrome. J Clin Endocrinol Metab. 2004;89:615-20.
50. Rafraf M, Mohammadi E, Farzadi L, Asghari-Jafarabadi, Sabour S. [Effects of ω-3 Fatty Acid Supplementation on Glycemic Status and High Sensitive C-Reactive Protein in Women with Polycystic Ovary Syndrome]. J Ardabil Univ Med Sci. 2012; 12: 373-83. (In Persian).
51. Amooee MD, Mohammad Ebrahim Parsanezhad MD. Original article Metformin versus chromium picolinate in clomiphene citrate-resistant patients with PCOs:

A double-blind randomized clinical trial Sedigheh. Iran J Reprod Med. 2013;11(8): 611-618.
52. Reiter RJ, Tan DX, Maldonado MD. Melatonin as an antioxidant: Physiology versus pharmacology. J Pineal Res. 2005;39:215-6.
53. Jain P, Jain M, Haldar C, Singh TB, Jain S. Melatonin and its correlation with testosterone in polycystic ovarian syndrome. J Hum Reprod Sci. 2013;6:253-8.
54. Isaacs JD Jr, Lincoln SR, Cowan BD. Extended clomiphene citrate (CC) and prednisone for the treatment of chronic anovulation resistant to CC alone. Fertil Steril. 67:641, 1997.
55. Parsanezhad ME, Alborzi S, Motazedian S, Omrani G. Use of dexamethasone and clomiphene citrate in the treatment of clomiphene citrate-resistant patients with polycystic ovary syndrome and normal dehydroepiandrosterone sulfate levels: a prospective, double-blind, placebo-controlled trial. Fertil Steril. 2002;78(5):1001-4.
56. Vanky E, KÅ. Six-month treatment with low-dose dexamethasone further reduces androgen levels in PCOS women treated with diet and lifestyle advice, and metformin Salvesen Human Reproduction. Volume 19, Issue 3Pp. 529-33.
57. Impact of dexamethasone on pregnancy outcome in PCOs women candidate for IVF/ICSI, a single-blind randomized clinical trial studies Zahra Basirat, Mahtab Zeinalzadeh. Middle East Fertility Society Journal (2016) 21,184-8.
58. Athyapalan T, Stephen LA. Evidence for statin therapy in polycystic ovary syndrome. Ther Adv Endocrinol Metab. 2010 Feb; 1(1): 15–22. doi: 10.1177/2042018810367984 PMCID: PMC3474609.
59. Abdelaziz El Refaeey, Amal Selem, Ahmed Badawy. Combined coenzyme Q10 and clomiphene citrate for ovulation induction in clomiphene-citrate-resistant polycystic ovary syndrome. Reproductive BioMedicine Online. 2014;29:119-24.

Recent Advances in Polycystic Ovarian Syndrome

Parul Kotdawala, Shalini Gainder

INTRODUCTION

Polycystic ovarian syndrome (PCOS) is a heterogeneous syndrome, which manifests variably from adolescence as oligomenorrhea, hirsutism or obesity, goes on to affect the reproductive performance of the female by causing anovulation. Some may even be severely affected by metabolic syndrome, diabetes mellitus or endometrial carcinoma.

Tremendous research efforts are dedicated to unravel PCOS's underlying pathophysiological and genetic basis, while medical innovation constantly tackles the specific hurdles in formulating the best treatment protocols for its various aspects.

In the basic research arena, the main two fronts that has been explored in the last few years are the genomic origins as well as the subcellular, organ-specific (liver, muscle, adipose tissue) and metabolic derivations. The main tools that are used in the genomic approach are whole-genome analysis studies and association studies of specific candidate genes in defined groups of PCOS patients versus normal ovulatory women. Altogether, it appears that PCOS is the result of a primary ovarian defect, modified by body mass and its direct correlate, serum insulin.[1]

CLASSIFICATION OF PCOS: IS THERE A NEED FOR A NEW CONSENSUS?

The classification of Rotterdam which is the most used is not fully reliable. Firstly, it lacks sensitivity and/or specificity of each item taken one by one. Secondly, this can fail in challenging clinical situations, particularly, in women with hypothalamic anovulation and associated polycystic ovarian morphology (PCOM). Conversely, this classification excludes asymptomatic women with PCOM.

Oligomenorrhea

Women with oligomenorrhea or amenorrhea have about a 90% chance of being diagnosed with PCOS, and up to 95% of affected adults have oligomenorrhea or amenorrhea. Menstrual cycles in women with PCOS may become more regular later in life. Irregular menses are associated with increased metabolic risk. It remains unclear whether PCOS patients have a longer reproductive life span.

Hyperandrogenemia

Hirsutism is present in approximately 70% of women with PCOS, but hyperandrogenemia should be evaluated biochemically in all women suspected of having PCOS. By comparison, acne and alopecia are not commonly associated with hyperandrogenemia and therefore should not be regarded as evidence of hyperandrogenemia. For women with PCOS in whom hirsutism is a major concern, treatment is focused on reduction of androgen production, decreasing the fraction of circulating free testosterone (T), and limiting androgen bioactivity to hair follicles. In those women with PCOS who have acne vulgaris, clinical benefit may be derived from many systemic therapeutic modalities. Because terminal hair turnover occurs slowly, at least 6 months of treatment is generally considered the minimal interval to see a response.[2]

Often oral contraceptives pills (OCPs) are prescribed which cause augmentation of serum hormone binding globulin in combination with an antiandrogen to block androgen action at the hair follicles. Antiandrogens include spironolactone (an aldosterone-antagonist diuretic), flutamide (an androgen receptor antagonist), and finasteride (a 5a-reductase type 2 inhibitor). In general, the addition of an antiandrogen to OCPs has not appeared to increase the overall treatment benefit. Each of these agents have been shown to reduce hirsutism, and all appear (without head-to-head comparisons) to have equivalent efficacy.

Antiandrogens should be combined with OCP. Prolonged (>6 months) medical therapy for hirsutism is necessary to document effectiveness.

Ultrasonography in PCOS

Currently, the sonographic assessment of ovaries is one of the obligatory criteria for the diagnosis of PCOS according to the Rotterdam consensus (2003) and Androgen Excess & PCOS Society (2006). This criterion is determined by the presence of ≥12 follicles within the ovary with a diameter of 2–9 mm and/or ovarian volume ≥10 cm.[2] Such an ultrasound image in one gonad only is sufficient to define polycystic ovaries. The coexistence of polycystic ovaries with polycystic ovary syndrome is confirmed in over 90% of cases irrespective of ethnic factors or race. However, because of the commonness of ultrasound features of polycystic ovaries in healthy women, the inclusion of this sign to the diagnostic criteria of polycystic ovary syndrome is still questioned. The assessment of anti-Müllerian hormone levels as an equivalent of ultrasound features of polycystic ovaries is a promising method.[3]

Using newer ultrasound technology and a reliable grid system approach to count follicles, recently it has been concluded that a substantially higher threshold of follicle counts throughout the entire ovary (FNPO)-26 versus 12 follicles-is required to distinguish among women with PCOS and healthy women from the general population.[4]

PCOS Phenotypes

Recently a newer type of categorization has been used to describe which presents a better understanding of the syndrome.[5]

The presentation of PCOS can be categorized into discrete phenotypes, depending on the features used in the diagnostic criteria and recently the use of this categorization has found increasing use in literature.
1. Phenotype A, clinical and/or biochemical hyperandrogenism (HA) and oligo-/anovulation (OA) and polycystic ovarian morphology at ultrasound (PCOM).
2. Phenotype B, HA with OA only.
3. Phenotype C, HA with PCOM only; and phenotype D, OA with PCOM only. Phenotype A and B are addressed as classical PCOS.

The PCOS phenotypes at metabolic risk should be better identified. In one study, the classic phenotype and, to a lesser extent, the ovulatory phenotype were independently associated with insulin resistance, whereas the normoandrogenic phenotype was not.[3]

Some authors proposed that the name PCOS be retained for the reproductive phenotypes and that a new name be created for the phenotypes at high metabolic risk.[5] It is not clear, however, that every patient would fit such a clear-cut classification. The scientific use of the Rotterdam classification is also a major issue, particularly for genetic studies. The phenotypic variability of PCOS, as defined by the Rotterdam classification, may be partly genetically determined, as indicated by the study where independent associations were found between some SNPs and each of the Rotterdam criteria separately. However, as seen in daily practice, some patients with PCOS may "mutate" from one phenotype to another, depending on the extrinsic factors of the disease such as age, weight, or environment. Thus, OA and to a lesser degree HA regress with age,[6] and conversely overweight women with PCOS are more prone to ovulation disorder and HA than lean women.[7]

Polycystic Ovarian Morphology

Should these women be excluded from the definition? They are not subfertile,[8] but at baseline, the serum AMH and FSH level is increased or decreased, respectively.[9] When stimulated, they have PCO-like features in terms of androgen secretion[10] or follicle response to controlled ovarian hyperstimulation (COH).[11] In a recent genetic study, a specific single-nucleotide polymorphism (SNP) in the *C9ORF3* gene was associated with isolated PCOM.[12]

Adolescent PCOS

The PCOS might be over diagnosed in adolescents or conversely unrecognized because it is difficult to assess the U/S criteria. There is no overall agreement as to how to diagnose PCOS in adolescence. Acne is common during the adolescent years, whether or not PCOS is present, whereas hirsutism—associated with PCOS—typically develops over time. Hyperandrogenemia may be a more consistent marker for PCOS during the teenage years. In all young women, irregular menses are common in the years immediately after menarche. As many as 85% of menstrual cycles are anovulatory during the first year after menarche, and up to 59% are still anovulatory during the third year after menarche.

Based on few available data, guidelines for diagnosing PCOS during adolescence have recently been proposed.[13] During adolescence, a positive diagnosis of PCOS should require all elements of the Rotterdam consensus (and not just two out of three). In addition, it may be better to define hyperandrogenism as hyperandrogenemia (elevated blood androgens found using sensitive assays) and discount clinical findings such as acne and alopecia, with the exception of documented progressive hirsutism. Oligomenorrhea should be present for at least 2 years, and the diagnosis of polycystic ovaries by abdominal ultrasound should also include increased ovarian volume (>10 cm^3).

Thus, the diagnosis of PCOS should be considered only in girls who had menarche at least 2 years before diagnosis. By use of these parameters, clinicians may confirm the diagnosis PCOS only in adolescents who have hyperandrogenism, oligomenorrhea, and polycystic ovaries on ultrasound. When the diagnosis cannot be confirmed, the patients should be observed closely until adulthood, and the diagnosis should be reconsidered if the symptoms persist.

PCOM also changes with age, while the influence of the weight seems minimal or negligible. It is the same for the plasma level of anti-Müllerian hormone (AMH). It, nevertheless, remains that some women with PCOS appear to be "protected" from OA or HA, for reasons that remain unresolved to date and that genetics may help elucidate. When assessing women for PCOS, it is important to consider the following points, which are addressed further in the guideline.[14] In young women, menstrual cycles may take up to 2 years to regulate after menarche. Irregular cycles persisting into the third year postmenarche should be investigated for PCOS. If commencing a young woman on hormonal contraception after 12 months of irregular cycles, consideration should also be given to assessment of PCOS before commencement of the hormonal contraception.[15]

Ultrasound is not reliable in the diagnosis of polycystic ovaries in adolescent and young women. Up to 70% of young women may have polycystic ovaries on ultrasound initial investigations must exclude other causes of the presentation. These include thyroid function tests and prolactin and follicle stimulating hormone (FSH) levels.

TREATMENT OF PCOS

Lifestyle modification should be the first-line of treatment of obese infertile women.[16] However, it has been observed that these women lack motivation and probably a stringent follow-up is needed because if there is no improvement then delaying ovulation induction makes no sense.

Ovulation Induction in PCOS

It is ideal to treat these anovulatory women with clomiphene citrate starting with a dose of 50 mgs given for 5 days and if they fail to ovulate then escalating the dose to 100 mgs, subsequently to 150 mgs and establish the dose at which ovulation occurs. The ovulation rates are very high (75–80%), and the reported conception rates are disappointing (30–40%). At the dose of 150 mgs some women who failed to ovulate with lower dose would show ovulation but the conception still remains low because a higher dose of clomiphene results in negative effect on endometrium which remains thin.[17]

The other protocol which has recently been published is the *Stair Step Protocol*, where clomiphene citrate is used in the same cycle in the escalating dose if ovulation fails to occur and at that very time a dose hike of 50 mg is given and ultrasound performed after 5 days to confirm ovulation. The benefit is that in a single cycle the dose at which ovulation occurs is established and time is saved.

If women fail to ovulate with clomiphene citrate the other drug used was aromatase inhibitor, letrozole which was proven beneficial and in some cases had a better effect. The doses tried were 2.5 mg, 5 mg and 7.5 mg. However, due to lack of approval and literature to suggest its adverse affect in causing malformation has led to a ban in sale for treating anovulation, still this is a drug of choice in women where endometrial hyperplasia or endometrial carcinoma occurs.

Gonadotropins are needed in women who do not ovulate with oral drugs, low dose step-up protocol is ideal where the starting dose of FSH is used in as low dose as 37.5 IU and slowly increasing to the level where monofollicular ovulation occurs. There is a high chance of ovarian hyperstimulation and this may lead to cycle cancellation

Laparoscopic ovarian drilling was initially done more judiciously to treat resistant PCOS who failed to ovulate but now with the recent literature that it may have an impact on the ovarian reserve and lead to adhesions formation. This has led to restricted use.

Metformin—the Rise and Fall

The use of metformin as first-line pharmacological treatment option for ovulation induction in PCOS has sparked a heated discussion.[18] Clomiphene citrate (CC) remains the first-line therapy and therefore metformin as per the literature available be considered in a selective group of women with insulin resistance where it benefits. With regard to the use of metformin for induction of ovulation, two randomized controlled trials (RCTs) have indicated that metformin does not increase live-birth rates above those observed with CC alone in either obese or normal weight women with PCOS. There seems to be no advantage to adding metformin to CC in women with PCOS.[19-21]

The Cochrane review found no conclusive evidence that metformin treatment before or during ART cycles improved live birth rates in women with PCOS. However, the use of this insulin-sensitizing agent increased clinical pregnancy rates and decreased the risk of ovarian hyperstimulation syndrome (OHSS).[17] It has little proven benefit in adolescent group with hyperinsulinemia.

Inositols and PCOS

Insulin resistance is the main factor in the pathogenesis of PCOS. It causes theca cell stimulation resulting in increase synthesis of androgens. Hyperglycemia also results in decrease synthesis of sex hormone binding globulin thereby causing increase in the free androgen levels. Insulin sensitizing agents like metformin are successfully being used in the treatment of insulin resistant PCOS. Recently the role of second messengers to insulin, inositols is being evaluated in the treatment of PCOS. The two major sterio-isomers of inositols are myoinositol (myolns) and d-chiroinositol (chirolns). The normal physiological plasma concentration of these is 40:1 with myolns in abundance. This physiological ratio is disturbed in PCOS. Chirolns at its low physiological level is known to increase insulin sensitivity, decrease androgen levels and increases frequency of ovulation. However, high levels of chirolns are detrimental for ovarian function. An insulin dependent enzyme NAD/NADH epimerase is activated in the ovaries which converts myolns in to chirolns. The increased release of high levels of chirolns under insulin stimulation results in increase androgen synthesis by theca cells. In addition, it hinders the uptake of myolns in the ovarian cells resulting in disruption of their physiological ratio. This is known as chiroln ovarian paradox. The supplementation of myolns in PCOS females has shown to counteract the symptoms of metabolic syndrome, improve the quality of oocytes and the frequency of ovulation. It also decreases the duration and dose of FSH treatment required for triggering ovulation. Thus, besides improving ovarian function in PCOS females it also improves the systemic features of PCOS like glucose and lipid metabolism and hyperandrogenism. Some clinicians use the combination of chirolns and myolns in physiological plasma ratio (40:1).[20,21]

Estrogen–Progesterone Pills in PCOS

Overall, the benefits of oral contraception pills (OCPs) outweigh the risks in most patients with PCOS. Women with PCOS are more likely to have contraindications for OCP use than normal women. There is no evidence for differences in effectiveness and risk among the various progestogens and when used in combination with a 20 versus a 30 mg daily dose of estrogen. Subsequent fertility is not negatively affected by OCPs. There is no definitive evidence that the type of OCP determines efficacy of hirsutism control. These pills can be used for management of PCOS and also for long-term management in women not desiring fertility.

IMPACT ON QUALITY OF LIFE

Patients with PCOS are an at-risk group for psychological and behavioral disorders and reduced quality-of-life (QOL).[22-24] Studies have been hampered by the existence of only one validated disease-specific questionnaire, The QOL Questionnaire for Women with PCOS (PCOSQ).[25]

The PCOSQ cannot be used to evaluate the prevalence of emotional and other disorders (e.g., sexual or eating disorders). However, from other validated measures, it appears that patients with PCOS are at higher risk for developing significant psychological difficulties (i.e., depression, anxiety) compared with healthy and other controls and may also be at risk for eating disorders and sexual and relational dysfunction, though this evidence is inconsistent.[22] It has been suggested that women with PCOS should undergo psychological screening to improve their long-term prognosis.

OBESITY AND ITS IMPACT: ROLE OF BARIATRIC SURGERY IN PCOS

Excess adiposity was also associated with poorer metabolic health in PCOS. Women with PCOS who had a greater body mass index (BMI) had higher fasting insulin levels and greater insulin resistance. Similarly, the effect of fat distribution on ovarian function is unclear. Some studies found that a higher trunk/leg fat ratio or upper/lower region fat ratio is associated with higher levels of testosterone.[27,28] Central obesity was associated with greater fasting insulin levels, greater insulin area under the curve, and greater insulin resistance (HOMA). Treatment with antiobesity drugs can be used in morbid obesity consensus.

It has been suggested that women with a BMI > 35 kg/m^2 after failed attempts at weight loss for more than 1 year may consider bariatric surgery.[28] Bariatric surgery has been shown in randomized controlled trials to be beneficial for patients with a BMI above 30 kg/m^2 with type 2 DM.[29]

Bariatric surgery is known to improve markers of PCOS influencing fertility, including anovulation, hirsutism, hormonal changes, insulin resistance, sexual activity and libido.[30] However, small for gestational age (SGA) and preterm birth have emerged as potential complications associated with births after bariatric surgery.

Therefore, bariatric surgery could be considered to improve fertility outcomes in women with PCOS who are anovulatory, have a BMI ≥ 35 kg/m^2, and who remain infertile despite undertaking an intensive structured lifestyle management program involving reducing dietary energy intake, exercise and behavioral interventions preferably for a minimum of 6 months.

CARDIOVASCULAR HEALTH FACTORS

Life-long metabolic dysfunction in women with PCOS exaggerates the risk for cardiovascular diseases (CVDs) with aging, particularly after menopause. This metabolic dysfunction is based upon insulin resistance, which occurs in most women with PCOS and is independent of and additive with obesity. The severity of carotid-intima media thickening, coronary artery calcification, and to a lesser extent aortic calcification is greater in women with PCOS.

Postmenopausal women with existent hyperandrogenemia and premenopausal menstrual irregularity have a larger number of cardiovascular events than controls. All surrogate markers of cardiovascular risk are higher in PCOS (adjusted for age and BMI), but the association of these markers with cardiovascular events in PCOS remains unclear. Endothelial dysfunction in PCOS is related to abdominal obesity and insulin resistance.

GENETICS AND PCOS

There is ample evidence for a genetic basis of PCOS.

It is clear that abnormalities of glucose/insulin homeostasis are more common in first-degree relatives of women with PCOS than in a reference population. These women do have an additional risk for gestational diabetes. Genes that have been recently identified as contributing to the genotype and phenotype of Type

2 diabetes are being extrapolated as candidate genes in the etiology of PCOS. The evidence that such genes play a part in the genetic etiology of PCOS is somewhat conflicting.[31,32] Interestingly enough despite the recognition that genetic basis for this syndrome, going through recent literature it seems that much investigative effort has been channeled into the study of possible role for genes that do not have a significant presence or function in the ovary, namely those functional in carbohydrate and energy-substrate metabolism.

Multiple inherited genes are responsible for the occurrence. In India, the prevalence of PCOS was 22.5% by Rotterdam and 10.7% by Androgen Excess Society criteria. Mild PCOS is one of the most common phenotype occurring in about 52.6% of women. In the presentation of the syndrome some genes are up regulated and some genes are down regulated. Although the genetics and mechanism of PCOS are not yet understood, computational tools may be helpful in finding the cause of this syndrome using various structural aspects.

Accumulation of reports on the two arms of genetic studies on PCOS, the first regarding genes related to the general metabolic pathways and the second related to genes within the ovary. Various genetic studies have been carried out to see the connection in general. The effort to define genes that may play a role in any pathology involves the comparison of DNA from a group of affected individuals (in this case those with PCOS) and a group of control subjects (normal ovulatory women). The more modest approach would target a gene of possible relevance to the pathology and compare either the full sequences or a known associated single-nucleotide polymorphism (SNP), whereas the more robust approach involves what is called whole-genome analysis study or genome-wide association study (GWAS), which documents only a set of SNP. The former, if it finds a difference, may indicate a more straightforward direction for functional study, whereas the latter necessitates a longer stride to define the genes that are in the vicinity of the differing SNP and their possible relevance to the pathology. GWAS are relatively scarce, compared with single-gene comparisons, and we will start with the studies on single genes. Interestingly, probably because of the inclusion of populations such as Han Chinese, in whom PCOS is diagnosed in many normal BMI women, GWAS results have pointed to few genes (as will be discussed in greater detail) that are involved in carbohydrate metabolism, but the majority have not been found to be associated. This might be a further support to the notion that there is an exaggerated effect of the association of PCOS with obesity in Caucasians on the direction of research. Taken together, despite several correlations found between genotypes and clinical responses, no comprehensive view on the role of any of the gene products involved in carbohydrate metabolism was reached, which would better explain the clinical picture of PCOS. Genes associated with cardiovascular risk have also been identified. The path that this research has taken is 2-fold. At one end are the gene expression studies, which do not provide direct data to explain deranged function, whereas at the other end one finds detailed in vitro studies of cell functions, which get closer to the explanation of the pathophysiology of PCOS. A true focus point for all interest in PCOS, as a pathology of deranged ovarian function, is the genes that were documented as expressed in the ovary. These include those involved in gonadotropin signaling, insulin signaling, steroidogenic machinery and growth factors as well as their receptors.

Other studies[33] have been targeted to study the steroid regulating genes. The androgen receptor (AR) was studied by several Groups although some correlations of genotypes with the clinical picture have been found, no functional data connects all these in a cascade of steroidogenic steps to a comprehensive view, which consistently captures the basics of the deranged steroid hormone milieu in PCOS. One could view either of two situations. At one end stands the overt derangement, associated with a known genetic variant, which explains a clinical syndrome such as PCOS. At the other end it is possible to contemplate that a combination of partial defects in a cascade of steps towards the production of steroids can accumulate to provide the full-scale derangement. It would be prudent to test in vitro the steroidogenic capacity of granulosa and theca cells which harbor some or all of the aforementioned genotypes.

Insulin signaling genes have also been identified. It is widely accepted that insulin signal transduction might be disturbed in PCOS, but no study has gone beyond association to try to test a functional effect of the specific variant.[34,35] Future studies should be targeted to elucidate the local ovarian expression and function of these genes, singularly or in a concerted way, to verify to what extent various polymorphic, minimally different, proteins affect ovarian cell function. Some recent studies have examined PCOS from other perspectives evaluating mutations in different other locations such as the FSH receptor (FSHR), interleukin receptor, MTHFR mutation, oxidative phosphorylation (OXPHOS) complex and mitochondrial enzymes as well as GDF9, BMP15, AMH and AMHR2. Taken together, the data on gene expression and DNA methylation do not converge yet to suggest a specific metabolic or signaling cascade that is consistently and significantly affected in PCOS.

Some in vitro studies to understand the cell function of theca cells have been carried out.

ANIMAL MODELS OF PCOS

Humans are mono-ovulatory mammals, while essentially small laboratory animals and the pig are polyovulatory. Hence, it is doubtful if any model from the latter can truly reflect pathological processes in the former. Nevertheless, the inability to probe the human scenario has led the extensive efforts to develop such models. Of the large, mono-ovulatory animal models, primates are difficult and expensive to use, thus sheep are reasonable subjects. In humans, it is difficult to separate the maternal genetic contribution from the respective prenatal intrauterine hormonal exposure. Thus, the foundations of the deranged insulin ovarian response in women with PCOS, which cannot be directly approached, cannot be reliably attributed to either of the two. It is desirable, that, if in the future human granulosa and theca cells could be derived from pluripotent stem cells, this issue will become approachable in vitro.

There are certain obvious obstacles, as there is no true animal model, and obtaining human tissue is very limited. Yet transcriptomic and proteomic analyses have gone a remarkable distance, which should allow detailed workup of small cellular samples. This in turn can enable the harvest of theca cells and granulosa cells, from either 'stuck' antral follicles or true leading follicles, as well as corpora lutea from women with PCOS. Preliminary evidence from either blastocysts from

PCOS patients or follicular fluid and cumulus cells at oocyte retrieval during IVF support the potential productivity of this path.

PREGNANCY IN PCOS WOMEN

Women with PCOS who desire a pregnancy may be at increased risk for adverse pregnancy outcomes, and this may be exacerbated by obesity and/or insulin resistance. Health should be optimized before conception, with advice about smoking cessation, lifestyle, diet, and appropriate vitamin supplementation (e.g., folic acid). Miscarriage rates are not increased in natural conceptions in women with PCOS, independent of obesity. Miscarriage rates after induction of ovulation mirror those found in other infertile populations. Women with PCOS should be observed closely during pregnancy as they may be at increased risk for the development of GDM, gestational hypertension, and associated complications. Pregnancy-associated risks are greater in women diagnosed by more classic (NIH) criteria as opposed to nonhyperandrogenic women. Babies born from women with PCOS may have increased morbidity and mortality. There is no evidence for improved live-birth rates or decreased pregnancy complications with the use of metformin either before conception or during pregnancy. However, metformin can be continued in pregnancy if there is blood sugar derangement. The impact on pregnancy and outcome of in vitro fertilization (IVF) cycle may be explained by the effects of obesity and/or metabolic, inflammatory, and endocrine abnormalities on ovulatory function, oocyte quality, and endometrial receptivity.

Ovarian hyperandrogenism and hyperinsulinemia may promote premature granulose cell luteinization, and paracrine dysregulation of growth factors may disrupt the intrafollicular environment and impair cytoplasmic and/or nuclear maturation of oocytes.[36] These features are not universal, and oocyte quality, fertilization, and implantation rates in an individual woman with PCOS can be normal.[37] During early pregnancy, the embryo may be exposed to androgen excess in utero. This may have long-term effects, particularly on female offspring. Fetal hyperandrogenism may disturb epigenetic programming, in particular those genes regulating reproduction and metabolism. Data in relation to the risk of miscarriage in women with PCOS are conflicting, although miscarriage rates are generally thought to be comparable with other subfertile populations.[38,39] When pregnancy occurs in women with PCOS, there is a higher incidence of gestational diabetes (GDM) (40% to 50%) and associated fetal macrosomia, gestational hypertensive disorders (such as preeclampsia and pregnancy-induced hypertension) (5%), and birth of small-for-gestational-age (SGA) babies (10% to 15%).[40]

PCOS AND CANCER

There are moderate quality data to support those women with PCOS have a 2.7-fold (95% confidence interval [CI], 1.0–7.3) increased risk for endometrial cancer. Most endometrial cancers are well differentiated and have a good prognosis. Limited data exist that do not support the conclusion that women with PCOS are at increased risk for ovarian cancer and breast cancer.

PERIMENOPAUSE AND MENOPAUSE

Age may improve many manifestations of PCOS, including normalizing ovarian size and morphology, T levels, and oligo-ovulation before menopause. The long-term risk for morbidity and mortality among postmenopausal women with a history of PCOS is uncertain.[41,42] There is no established phenotype for PCOS after menopause. Women with PCOS who have transitioned through menopause will have increased rates of obesity, diabetes, and cardiovascular events. Most reports tend to show normal or increased bone mineral density in women with PCOS. Alternative data suggest they have higher rates of stroke and CVD.[43-46]

KEY POINTS

- PCOS may "mutate" from one phenotype to another, depending on the extrinsic factors of the diseases.
- Overweight women with PCOS are more prone to ovulation disorder and HA than lean women.
- In young women, menstrual cycles may take up to 2 years after menarche to become regularized.
- Irregular cycles persisting into the third year postmenarche should be investigated for PCOS.
- Ultrasound is not reliable in the diagnosis of polycystic ovaries in adolescent and young women.
- Lifestyle modification should be the first-line of treatment of obese infertile women.
- The benefits of administering OCP outweigh the risks in most patients with PCOS.
- PCOS women should undergo psychological screening to improve their long-term prognosis.
- Central obesity was associated with greater fasting insulin levels, greater insulin area under the curve, and greater insulin resistance (HOMA).
- Women with BMI >35 kg/m^2 after failed attempts at weight loss for more than 1 year may consider bariatric surgery.

REFERENCES

1. Shlomo IB, Johnny S, Younis JS. Basic research in PCOS: are we reaching new frontiers? Reprod Biomed Online. 2014;28(6):669-83.
2. Fauser JM, Tarlatzis BC, Rebar RW, Legro RS, Adam H, Balen AH, Lobo R, et al. Consensus on women's health aspects of polycystic ovary syndrome (PCOS): the Amsterdam ESHRE/ ASRM-Sponsored 3rd PCOS Consensus Workshop Group. Fertil Steril. 2012;97(1):28-38.
3. Broekmans FJ, Knauff EA, Valkenburg O, et al. PCOS according to the Rotterdam consensus criteria: change in prevalence among WHO-II anovulation and association with metabolic factors. BJOG. 2006;113(10):1210-7.

4. Bachanek M, Abdalla N, Cendrowski K, Sawicki W. Value of ultrasonography in the diagnosis of polycystic ovary syndrome-literature review. J Ultrason. 2015;15(63):410-22.
5. Lujan ME, Jarrett BY, Brooks ED, Reines JK, Peppin AK, Muhn N, Haider E, Pierson RA, et al. Updated ultrasound criteria for polycystic ovary syndrome: reliable thresholds for elevated follicle population and ovarian volume. Hum Reprod. 2013;28(5):1361-8.
6. Azziz R. Introduction: Determinants of polycystic ovary syndrome. Fertil Steril. 2016;106(1):4-5.
7. Dunaif A, Fauser BC. Renaming PCOS two-state solution. J Clin Endocrinol Metab. 2013;98(11):4325-8.
8. Elting MW, Korsen TJ, Rekers-Mombarg LT, et al. Women with polycystic ovary syndrome gain regular menstrual cycles when ageing. Hum Reprod. 2000;15(1):24-8.
9. Kiddy DS, Hamilton-Fairley D, Bush A, et al. Improvement in endocrine and ovarian function during dietary treatment of obese women with polycystic ovary syndrome. Clin Endocrinol (Oxf). 1992;36(1):105-11.
10. Hassan MA, Killick SR. Ultrasound diagnosis of polycystic ovaries in women who have no symptoms of polycystic ovary syndrome is not associated with sub fecundity or subfertility. Fertil Steril. 2003;80(4):966-75.
11. Catteau-Jonard S, Bancquart J, Poncelet E, et al. Polycystic ovaries at ultrasound: normal variant or sillent polycystic ovary syndrome? Ultrasound Obstet Gynecol. 2012;40(2):223-9.
12. Chang PL, Lindheim SR, Lowre C, et al. Normal ovulatory women with polycystic ovaries have hyperandrogenic pituitary ovarian responses to gonadotropin-releasing hormone-agonist testing. J Clin Endocrinol Metab. 2000;85(3):995-1000.
13. Sigala J, Sifer C, Dewailly D, et al. Is polycystic ovarian morphology related to a poor oocyte quality after controlled ovarian hyperstimulation for intracytoplasmic sperm injection? Results from a prospective, comparative study. Fertil Steril. 2015; 103(1):112-8.
14. Cui L, Li G, Zhong W, et al. Polycystic ovary syndrome susceptibility single nucleotide polymorphisms in women with a single PCOS clinical feature. Hum Reprod. 2015; 30(3):732-6.
15. Carmina E, Oberfield SE, Lobo RA. The diagnosis of polycystic ovary syndrome in adolescents. Am J Obstet Gynecol. 2010;203:201-5.
16. Teede HJ, Misso ML, Deeks AA, et al. Assessment and management of polycystic ovary syndrome: summary of an evidence-based guideline. Med J Aust. 2011;195:S65-112.
17. Cochrane Database of Systematic Reviews. The effect of a healthy lifestyle for women with polycystic ovary syndrome. Cochrane Database of Systematic Reviews. 2011.
18. Tso LO, Costello MF, Albuquerque LT, Andriolo RB, Macedo CR. Metformin in women with polycystic ovary syndrome for improving fertility. Cochrane Database of Systematic Reviews, 2014. Issue 11. Art No. CD0061 05.DOI
19. Johnson NP. Metformin use in women with polycystic ovary syndrome. Ann Transl Med. 2014;2(6):56.
20. The Thessaloniki ESHRE/ASRM-Sponsored PCOS Consensus Workshop Group. Consensus on infertility treatment related to polycystic ovary syndrome. Fertil Steril. 2008;89:505-22.
21. Glocker MH, Davidson K, Kochman L, Guzick D, Hoeger K. Improvement in quality-of-life questionnaire measures in obese adolescent females with polycystic ovary syndrome treated with lifestyle changes and oral contraceptives, with or without metformin. Fertil Steril. 2010;93:1016-9.
22. Legro RS, Barnhart HX, Schlaff WD, Carr BR, Diamond MP, Carson SA, et al. Clomiphene, metformin, or both for infertility in the polycystic ovary syndrome. N Engl J Med. 2007;356:551-66.
23. Lowenstein EJ. Diagnosis and management of the dermatologic manifestations of the polycystic ovary syndrome. Dermatol Ther. 2006;19:210-23.

24. Futterweit W, Dunaif A, Yeh HC, Kingsley P. The prevalence of hyperandrogenism in 109 consecutive female patients with diffuse alopecia. J Am Acad Dermatol. 1988;19:831-6.
25. Cela E, Robertson C, Rush K, Kousta E, White DM, Wilson H, et al. Prevalence of polycystic ovaries in women with androgenic alopecia. Eur J Endocrinol. 2003;149:439-42.
26. Kaufman KD. Androgen metabolism as it affects hair growth in androgenetic alopecia. Dermatol Clin. 1996;14:697-711.
27. Douchi T, Ijuin H, Nakamura S, Oki T, Yamamoto S, Nagata Y. Body fat distribution in women with polycystic ovary syndrome. Obstet Gynecol. 1995;86:516-9.
28. Douchi T, Yoshimitsu N, Nagata Y. Relationships among serum testosterone levels, body fat and muscle mass distribution in women with polycystic ovary syndrome. Endocr J. 2001;48:685-9.
29. Scholtz S, Le Roux, C, Balen, AH. The role of bariatric surgery in the management of female fertility. Scientific Advisory Committee Opinion Paper 2015. Royal College of Obstetricians and Gynaecologists.
30. Busetto L, Dixon J, De Luca M, Shikora S, Pories W, Angrisani L. Bariatric surgery in class I obesity: a Position Statement from the International Federation for the Surgery of Obesity and Metabolic Disorders (IFSO). Obes Surg. 2014;24:487-519.
31. Malik SM, Traub ML. Defining the role of bariatric surgery in polycystic ovarian syndrome patients. World J Diabetes. 2012;3:71-9.
32. Biyasheva A, Legro RS, Dunaif A, Urbanek M. Evidence for association between. Polycystic ovary syndrome (PCOS) and TCF7L2 and glucose intolerance in women with PCOS and TCF7L2. J Clin Endocrinol Metab. 2009;94:2617-25.
33. Barber TM, Golding SJ, Alvey C, Wass JA, Karpe F, Franks S, et al. Global adiposity rather than abnormal regional fat distribution characterizes women with polycystic ovary syndrome. J Clin Endocrinol Metab. 2008;93:999-1004.
34. Jones MR, Mathur R, Cui J, Guo X, Azziz R, Goodarzi. Independent confirmation of association between metabolic phenotypes of polycystic ovary syndrome and variation in the type 6 17beta-hydroxysteroid dehydrogenase gene. J Clin Endocrinol. Metab. 2009;94:5034-8.
35. Mukherjee S, Shaikh N, Khavale S, Shinde G, Meherji P, Shah N, Maitra A. Genetic variation in exon 17 of INSR is associated with insulin resistance and hyperandrogenemia among lean Indian women with polycystic ovary syndrome. Eur J Endocrinol. 2009;160,855-62.
36. Mutharasan P, Galdones E, Penalver Bernabe B., Garcia OA, Jafari N, Shea LD, Woodruff TK, Legro RS, Dunaif A, Urbanek M. Evidence for chromosome 2p16.3 polycystic ovary syndrome susceptibility locus in affected women of European ancestry. J Clin Endocrinol Metab. 2013;98:E185-E190.
37. Dumesic DA, Padmanabhan V, Abbott DH. Polycystic ovary syndrome and oocyte developmental competence. Obstet Gynecol Surv. 2008;63:39-48.
38. Weghofer A, Munne S, Chen S, Barad D, Gleicher N. Lack of association between polycystic ovary syndrome and embryonic aneuploidy. Fertil Steril. 2007;88:900-5.
39. Tang T, Lord JM, Norman RJ, Yasmin E, Balen AH. Insulin-sensitising drugs (metformin, rosiglitazone, pioglitazone, D-chiro-inositol) for women with polycystic ovary syndrome, oligo amenorrhoea and subfertility. Cochrane Database Syst Rev. 2010;1:CD003053.
40. Vanky E, Stridsklev S, Heimstad R, Romundstad P, Skogoy K, Kleggetveit O, et al. Metformin versus placebo from first trimester to delivery in polycystic ovary syndrome: a randomized, controlled multicenter study. J Clin Endocrinol Metab. 2010; 95:E448-55.
41. Boomsma CM, Eijkemans MJ, Hughes EG, Visser GH, Fauser BC, Macklon NS. A meta-analysis of pregnancy outcomes in women with polycystic ovary syndrome. Hum Reprod Update. 2006;12:673-83.

42. Mulders AG, Laven JS, Eijkemans MJ, de Jong FH, Themmen AP, Fauser BC. Changes in anti-Müllerian hormone serum concentrations over time suggest delayed ovarian ageing in normogonadotrophic anovulatory infertility. Hum Reprod. 2004;19:2036-42.
43. Davison SL, Bell R, Donath S, Montalto JG, Davis SR. Androgen levels in adult females: changes with age, menopause, and oophorectomy. J Clin Endocrinol Metab. 2005;90:3847-53.
44. Alsamarai S, Adams JM, Murphy MK, Post MD, Hayden DL, Hall JE, et al. Criteria for polycystic ovarian morphology in polycystic ovary syndrome as a function of age. J Clin Endocrinol Metab. 2009;94:4961-70.
45. Hudecova M, Holte J, Olovsson M, Sundstrom Poromea I. Long-term follow- up of patients with polycystic ovary syndrome: reproductive outcome and ovarian reserve. Hum Reprod. 2009;24:1176-83.
46. Tehrani FR, Solaymani-Dodaran M, Hedayati M, Azizi F. Is polycystic ovary syndrome an exception for reproductive aging? Hum Reprod. 2010;25:1775-81.

Index

Page numbers followed by *f* refer to figure and *t* refer to table

A

Abortions, spontaneous 159
Acne 44
Adrenal 218
   disorders 219
   glands 56
   hyperplasia, congenital 219
   insufficiency 148
   region, computed tomography of 221
   steroidogenesis, abnormalities of 55
   tumors 219
Aldosterone antagonists 148
Alopecia 144
Amenorrhea 3
American Cancer Society Guideline 186
American Society for Reproductive
      Medicine 22, 34, 119, 141, 184, 204
Anabolic steroids 219
Androgen 218
   excess 18, 20, 31
   secreting tumor 29
   synthesis of 218
   therapy 219
Androstenedione 218
Anesthesia 92
   local 92
Anovulation 21
Antiandrogens 148, 150, 223
Anti-Müllerian hormone 54, 79, 110, 111
Antral follicle count 40
Anxiety 172
   disorder 171
Aromatase inhibitors 67
Assisted reproductive technology 78, 79,
      92, 130, 156

B

Bariatric surgery 65
Barker hypothesis 156
Berberine 72
Binge-eating disorder 172
Bipolar disorder 171
Bleeding 93
   laparoscopic cauterization of 94*f*

Blood pressure
   diastolic 180
   systolic 180
Body mass index 18, 55, 184, 198, 232, 236
Bone morphogenetic protein 111
Bowel injury 93

C

Calcium 237
Cancer 256
Carcinoma, endometrial 47*f*
Cardiovascular diseases 164, 253
Catagen 218
Chromium picolate 238
Chronic ovulatory dysfunction 18, 21
Clomiphene citrate 65, 65, 205, 227, 229, 251
Cognitive behavioral therapy 175
Color Doppler pulse repetition frequency 36
Combined oral contraceptive 73
   therapy 73
Consumer Protection Act 193
Cushing's syndrome 29, 53, 219, 221
Cyclic progesterone 150
Cyclosporine 219
Cyproterone acetate 149
Cyst formation 81

D

Danazol 219
Deep venous thrombosis 148
Dehydroepiandrosterone sulfate 220
Dehydroepitestosterone 218
Depressive disorder 171
Desogestrel 147
Dexamethasone 73, 239
Diabetes mellitus 3, 57, 93, 132, 164, 182, 183
   gestational 155, 159, 160, 233
Diazoxide 219
Dietary
   calcium 200
   fats 199
   fibers 200
   sodium 201
Dihydrotestosterone 146, 218

Drospirenone 147, 148
Dyslipidemia 182, 199

E

Eating disorders 172
Embryo transfer 79, 83
Endometriosis 93
Endometrium 46, 134
Endoplasmic reticulum 66
Epidermal growth factor 111
Estrogen 150
    progesterone pills 252
    replacement therapy 174
Ethynodiol diacetate 147
European Society for Human Reproduction
    and Embryology 22, 34, 53
Excessive follicular growth 54

F

Fasting
    blood sugar 239
    glycemia 184
Fears 172
Fertility 51, 102
Fibroblast growth factor 111
Finasteride 149
Fistula 93
Flow index 37
Flutamide 64, 149
Folic acid 238
Follicle
    arrangement of 44
    number per ovary 19
    stimulating hormone 10, 11, 65, 78,
        108, 174, 221, 235, 236
Follicular
    arrest 54
    fluid 114
    number per ovary 40
    stimulating hormone, hypofunction of
        54
Free androgen index 173
Frozen pelvis 93

G

Global vascular indices vascularity index 36
Glucocorticoids 219, 224
Glucose intolerance 57
Gonadotropin 56, 67, 68
    releasing hormone 54, 80, 146
    agents 224
    stimulation 209
    therapy 68
    principles of 67
Granulosa cells 79, 107

H

Hair growth 218
    androgen sensitive sites of 218
Hemoperitoneum 95
    management of 96
Hemorrhage 93
Heparin 148
Hepatic dysfunctions 148
High density lipoprotein 180, 238
Higher total cholesterol, low-density
    lipoprotein 171
Hirsutism 107, 144
    causes of 219
    management of 221
Human
    chorionic gonadotropin 11, 135
        agonist 80
    menopausal gonadotropin 69, 132
    reproductive medicine 112
Hyperandrogenemia 18, 21, 22, 26, 107-
    109, 131, 136, 197, 199, 158, 248
Hyperinsulinemia 34, 43, 54, 55, 107-109,
    144, 199
Hyperplasia, endometrial 47f
Hyperprolactinemia 197, 221
Hyperstimulated large fragile ovaries 93
Hypertension 93, 134
    gestational 159
Hypophyseal hypothyroidism 221
Hypothalamic disease 221
Hypothalamic pituitary-gonadal axis 57
    disruption of 55

I

In vitro
    fertilization 78, 79, 107, 117, 211
    maturation 86, 108, 118
Infection 93
Infertility 53, 93, 107
Inositol 234, 251
Insulin 56
    like growth factor 80, 111
    resistance 55, 57, 182, 198, 219
    sensitizing
        agents 145
        drugs 224

Intracytoplasmic sperm injection 117
Intraovarian resistance index 35
Intrauterine
   growth retardation 10
   insemination 69
Intravenous sedation 92

K

Klinefelter's syndrome 10

L

Lactation issues 159, 161
Lanugo 217
Laparoscopic ovarian
   drilling 73, 85, 135, 205, 208, 210, 211, 230
      role of 83, 85
      technique of 206
   surgery 227
      technique of 206
Laser ovarian surgery 208
Levonorgestrel 147
Low density lipoprotein 199, 238
Luteinizing hormone 11, 174, 205, 221, 236
   hypersecretion of 54, 107, 108

M

Melatonin 72, 239
Menopause 257
Menstrual dysfunction 3, 107, 180
Mental disorders 170
Metabolic syndrome 132, 180
Metformin 64, 70, 148, 149, 228-234, 251
   role of 83, 84, 230
Minoxidil 219
Miscarriage 210, 232
Modified Ferriman Gallwey scoring system 220, 225
Multifetal gestation 159

N

N-acetylcysteine 71, 236
National Cholesterol Education Program Guidelines 182
National Institute of Health 21, 22, 53, 170, 197
Needle penetration 207f
Neonatal intensive care unit 155, 159
Nonclassical congenital adrenal hyperplasia 28, 222
Norethindrone acetate 147
Norgestrel 147

O

Obesity 57, 93, 158f, 183, 186, 198, 199, 219
   abdominal 180
Obstructive sleep apnea 184, 187
Oligoanovulation 22
Oligomenorrhea 21, 26, 247
Omega-3 fatty acids 238
Oocyte 10
Oogenesis 109
Oral contraceptive pills (OCPs) 85, 135, 139, 147, 148, 150, 222, 225, 228, 240, 248, 252
   choice of 223
Oral glucose tolerance test 184
Ovarian
   diathermy needle probe 207f
   hyperstimulation syndrome 81, 205, 210, 211 251
   steroidogenesis, dysregulation of 55
   stimulation 61, 70, 93
   stromal flows 35f
   surface 94f
      bleeding 93
   torsion 95, 96f
   volume 38, 44
      calculation of 19
Ovaries 56, 218
   3D power Doppler, volume of 36f
   baseline scan of 34
   longitudinal and transverse sections of 35f
   normal 41f
Overhyperstimulation syndrome 74
Ovulation 65, 210
   induction 61, 65, 67, 73, 79, 231, 250
      management of 62
      principles of 65
      pathophysiology of 62
Ovulatory dysfunction 18, 20, 22, 24, 31

P

Peak systolic velocity 35
Pelvic
   abscess 93
   infection 97
   injury 98
Peripheral polycystic pattern 45f
Phenytoin 219
Pituitary tumor 221

Polycystic ovarian
　disease 138
　　medicolegal aspects of 191
　morphology 20, 24, 31, 39, 247, 249
　syndrome (PCOS) 3, 9, 10, 17, 22t, 27t,
　　34, 39, 43, 46, 51, 53, 61, 62, 68, 74,
　　78, 79, 82, 107, 108, 109, 129-131,
　　133, 133t, 134t, 138, 141, 142, 144,
　　155-157, 168, 180, 186, 197, 198, 204,
　　227, 247
　　classification of 247
　　long-term sequel of 180
　　management of 150t
　　nonhyperandrogenic 23
　　ovulatory 23
　　pathogenesis of 139f, 140
　　pathophysiology of 157
　　phenotypes 249
　　prevalence of 5t
　　treatment of 250
Polycystic ovaries 3, 34, 41, 41f, 45f, 110,
　　116, 157f, 158
　dense hyperechoic stroma of 42f
　ultrasound criteria of 37
Polyfollicular syndrome 34
Polyunsaturated fatty acids 238
Potassium supplementation 148
Premature adrenarche 142
Progestin 219
　intrauterine device 185

R

Randomized controlled trials 251
Renal insufficiency 148
Retroperitoneal hematoma 93
Rotterdam criteria, 2003 21
Royal College of Obstetricians and
　　Gynaecologists 18

S

Schizophrenia 171
Sclerocystic ovaries 34
Serotonin norepinephrine reuptake
　　inhibitors 175
Serum anti-Müllerian hormone 30
Sex hormone-binding globulin 11, 56, 61,
　　130, 140, 142, 146, 158, 160, 219
Single-nucleotide polymorphism 254
Small for gestational age 10, 256
Spironolactone 149

Stein-Leventhal syndrome 4
Stroke 148
Stromal
　abundance 40, 43
　ovarian cells 110
　vascularity 45

T

Telogen 218
Testosterone 218, 220
　injections 219
Theca cell 110
　function 110f
Thiazolidinediones 64
Thrombosis 148
Thyroid
　disease 28
　dysfunction 197
　stimulating hormone 221
Total intravenous anesthesia 92
Transvaginal
　hydrolaparoscopy 208
　oocyte retrieval 92
Tricyclic antidepressants 175
Triglycerides 180
Tumor necrosis factor 56

U

Urinary tract injury 93

V

Vaginal vault bleeding 93
Valproic acid 171
Vascular endothelial growth factor 82
Vascularity index 37
Very low density lipoprotein 199
Visceral adiposity index 132
Vitamin D 237

W

Waist circumference 180
Weight loss 64

Z

Zinc 237
Zona pellucida 117